Clinical Cancer Genetics

Clinical Cancer Genetics

Risk Counseling and Management

Kenneth Offit, M.D., M.P.H.

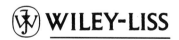

A John Wiley & Sons, Inc. Publication

NEW YORK • CHICHESTER • WEINHEIM • BRISBANE • SINGAPORE • TORONTO

Address All Inquiries to the Publisher
Wiley-Liss, Inc., 605 Third Avenue, New York, NY 10158-0012

Printed in the United States of America

While the author and publisher believe that the medical recommendations, drug selection and dosage, and the specification and usage of equipment, devices, and tests as set forth in this book, are in accord with current recommendation and practice at the time of publication, they accept no legal responsibility for any errors or omissions, and make no warranty, express or implied, with respect to material contained herein. In view of ongoing research, equipment modifications, changes in governmental regulations, and the constant flow of information relating to medical practice, drug therapy, drug reactions, cancer screening recommendations and the use of equipment and devices, the reader is urged to review the current medical practice standards and evaluate the information provided in the package insert or instructions for each drug, piece of equipment, test result or device for, among other things, any changes in the instructions or indication of dosage or usage and for added warnings and precautions. The clinical examples included in this text have been modified to protect confidentiality; any resemblance to specific families is coincidental.

Cover illustration: Spectral karyotype (courtesy of Dr. R. S. K. Chaganti)

Library of Congress Cataloging-in-Publication Data

Offit, Kenneth.
 Clinical cancer genetics : risk counseling and management /
Kenneth Offit.
  p. cm.
 "A Wiley-Liss publication."
 Includes index.
 ISBN 0-471-14655-2 (cloth : alk. paper)
 1. Cancer—Genetic aspects. 2. Genetic counseling. 3. Cancer—
Risk factors. I. Title.
 [DNLM: 1. Neoplasms—genetics. 2. Risk Factors. 3. Risk
Assessment. 4. Genetic Screening. 5. Genetic Counseling. QZ 202
032c 1998]
RC268.4.O34 1998
616.99'4042—dc21
DNLM/DLC
for Library of Congress   97-14958

The text of this book is printed on acid-free paper.
10 9 8 7 6 5 4 3 2 1

For Emily, Anna, Caroline, and Lily

Contents

Foreword

At mid-century, the signal discovery of the nature of DNA and the solution of the structure of this central molecule of life, set the stage for the most profound revolution in biology we have seen or are likely to ever see. The changes that these discoveries portend for medicine are profound. The DNA revolution is guiding us to a deeper understanding of health and disease with enormous implications for prevention and treatment. The ability to read and interpret an individual's genetic script will give us unprecedented tools for assessing risk and designing preventative interventions. That is the promise. Today, we find ourselves in the middle of change so rapid that it is, at times, dizzying. We follow each scientific breakthrough with the expectation that it is, as well, a medical breakthrough.

The discovery of specific genes whose alteration increases (or decreases) an individual's risk of cancer is a landmark in human medical science. It is a new field of discovery whose boundaries are yet to be explored. We currently estimate that 5 to 10 percent of all cancer arises in individuals who have inherited an altered form of a single gene and are members of families where multiple individuals carry greatly elevated risk of developing cancer. Thus, 50,000–100,000 new cases of cancer each year in this country can be traced to such inherited susceptibilities. The number of Americans who carry such genetic alterations may well be in the millions. These inherited susceptibilities have been identified because they are capable of conferring very high lifetime risks of developing cancer. The field of cancer genetics will undoubtedly grow beyond these so called high penetrance genes to encompass altered forms of many other genes that affect the metabolism of hormones, environmental agents and other fundamental cellular processes. Such genes give rise to less dramatic but clinically important elevated risks of cancer, often only in concert with specific exposures. Other genes will affect how individuals respond to specific therapies. Thus, the lessons we learn now from the study and care of cancer-prone families and the responsible genes, will provide both a testing ground and a model for the much more pervasive role of genetics that we expect in the future of cancer prevention and treatment.

The transition from an important scientific discovery to a beneficial medical or public health change is fraught with hurdles and challenges. These include:

1. Disseminating new knowledge based on real understanding to all those involved in delivering information and advising individuals about genetics and genetic testing.

2. Learning how to communicate the full range of issues associated with risk and what genetics and genetic testing mean—and what they do not mean—in order to aid in the decisions that individuals will make.

3. Incorporating new technologies for genetics into practice, including knowledge about the meaning of specific tests.

4. Linking new information about genetic tests to clinical decision-making by a better understanding of age-specific penetrance, as well as of the evidence for the efficacy of preventive, surveillance and therapeutic interventions. This includes awareness of the need to establish answers through research.

5. Assessing and being sensitive to the unique implications of genetic testing to the individual and the family, as well as the potential effects of laws and practices that might affect them.

Dr. Kenneth Offit's new book *Clinical Cancer Genetics* addresses all of these challenges with a lucidity and level of detail that will make it a widely used and valuable asset to those responsible for individuals with or at risk for cancer. Beginning with a superb explication of genetics, cancer genetics and familial cancer syndromes, Dr. Offit educates and informs. He confronts head on the misconceptions about strict and simplistic genetic determinants, and places the issue of inherited cancer susceptibility in the context of risk and probability—right where it belongs. The informed counseling model is reinforced with examples, and the full range of issues from communication to test interpretation and psychosocial dimensions are covered. While the science is in rapid flux, Dr. Offit finds his anchor in a clear designation of the basic principles of cancer genetics, of risk assessment, and of communication that will apply to our current and future discoveries.

Dr. Offit is one of the leading figures in clinical cancer genetics and his mastery of the field is well matched by his writing. This book is a welcome addition to the genetic revolution in cancer.

Richard D. Klausner, M.D.
Director, National Cancer Institute
Department of Health and Human Services
National Institutes of Health
Bethesda, Maryland

Preface

Physicians, nurses, and other health-care professionals have been called to serve on the front line of the genetics revolution in medicine. Provider organizations, patients, and their families are looking to those who deliver health care to control the most common and deadly human malignancies by utilizing genetic technologies. With tests for hereditary predisposition to cancer increasingly available, it has become apparent that knowledge of cancer genetics must now be accessible at the grassroots level of medical practice.

These developments are not a surprise. A need to "educate professionals about the known genetic basis of cancer" was recognized by J. Mulvihill and colleagues two decades ago. They realized that genetic knowledge could identify individuals who would benefit from preventive practices and early detection of cancer. A decade ago, a special conference at the National Cancer Institute reiterated the need for greater attention to genetics as a means for cancer control. It was admitted, however, that there was not "a sufficient number of persons with expertise in cancer genetics" to carry out this task.

The major impetus for expanding clinical cancer genetic services will be the demand. A recent March of Dimes survey of consumers found that 80% of people were willing to take a genetic test although 68% said they knew relatively little about genetic testing. Gene frequency estimates vary, but there are, at a minimum, hundreds of thousands of Americans with genetic susceptibilities to the common cancers of the breast, ovary, colon, or other sites. Genetic tests of patients already affected by cancer may help cancer specialists to individualize treatments and improve outcome.

In response to the need for increased genetics education, federal agencies and professional societies have undertaken to organize training programs in cancer genetics. These curricula will emphasize that, in ordering a genetic test, the clinician sets in mo-tion a chain of events that may have profound medical, psychological, and ethical consequences. Physicians who offer genetic tests to families, and the genetic counselors, nurses, psychologists, and other health-care providers who participate in this process, will be expected to be informed of the potential consequences. They will need to ensure that their interpretations of genetic tests are accurate, their assessments of cancer risk are appropriate, and their mode of conveying risk information is helpful and not counterproductive.

This book provides an introduction to the broad scope of cancer risk assessment and cancer genetic testing. It should serve as a practical guide to the literature linking clinical oncology, molecular genetics, epidemiology, psychology, ethics, and the law. It is intended for physicians, nurses, genetic counselors, and other health professionals who will be involved in cancer risk counseling and genetic testing.

The first three chapters outline the scope of clinical cancer genetics and the basic scientific concepts that underlie it. Chapters 4 and 5 review the most prevalent syndromes of cancer predisposition. Subsequent chapters address the use of quantitative methods in risk counseling, the methodologies of genetic testing, genetic testing of patients with cancer, reproductive risk counseling of cancer patients, and the special psychological, ethical, and legal challenges in clinical cancer genetics. Throughout the text, case examples are presented. Principles are emphasized rather than details of genetic models, which will continue to evolve with the rapid pace of scientific discovery.

The writing of this book has been an adventure as well as a discipline, and I am indebted to colleagues and family for providing both guidance and support. Dr. Paul A. Marks, President of Memorial Sloan-Kettering Cancer Center and Joan Marks, M.S., Director of the Graduate Program in Human Genetics at Sarah Lawrence College, had the prescience to anticipate the need for cancer genetic counseling, and encouraged me to develop the Clinical Genetics Service at Memorial Sloan-Kettering Cancer Center. I am especially grateful, too, to Dr. Lucio Luzzatto and Dr. R.S.K. Chaganti, distinguished geneticists, teachers, and founders of the Department of Human Genetics at our institution. Dr. Robert W. Miller, Dr. David Golde, Dr. John Mendelsohn, and Dr. Joseph Simone each played a personal role in helping to create the cancer genetic risk assessment program at Memorial. Dr. George Bosl, Dr. Sidney Winawer, and Dr. Larry Norton realized the importance of genetics in oncology long before the recent identification of adult cancer predisposition genes. I have been influenced by Dr. Francis Collins, Dr. Mark Skolnick, Dr. Henry Lynch, Dr. Mary-Claire King, and Dr. Fred Li who have provided both inspiration and counsel, and by Dr. Jessica Davis and Dr. Harry Ostrer, colleagues and friends.

The preparation of a multidisciplinary text requires a geneticist's eye for repetitive motifs and basepair mismatches. I thank Dr. John Mulvihill, Dr. Louise Strong, Dr. Judy Garber, Dr. David Goldgar, Dr. Steven Narod, Dr. Susan Neuhausen, Dr. Randall Burt, Dr. Tim Bishop, and June Peters, M.S. for their reading of portions of the manuscript. Genetic counselors Karen Brown, Bruce Haas, and Charlene Schulz drew on a considerable clinical experience in contributing cases, Heather Hampel, M.S., Dr. Mark Robson, and Dara Brener assisted in compiling the Appendices, and Amelia Panico utilized her creative skills in drafting the Figures. Colette Bean at John Wiley & Sons provided the editorial guidance and empathy that enabled me to stretch the scope of this text—as well as its deadlines. I am grateful to my wife, Emily Sonnenblick, M.D. for preparing a number of the radiographic cases, and to my mother, Avodah Offit, M.D. for her scholarly attention and timely counseling. Finally, I was motivated by students at the Sarah Lawrence Graduate Program in Human Genetics and the Cornell University Medical College. They provided the initial impetus and encouragement for this effort.

Introduction

The question, "Is cancer hereditary?" has been answered with a resounding "Yes." Molecular genetic discoveries now enable the physician to focus attention on individuals who are *positive* for germline mutations and to provide highly targeted screening and management recommendations. Conversely, individuals who are *negative* for the mutation may revert to the general population cancer screening risk and follow the American Cancer Society or National Cancer Institute surveillance recommendations. However, a litany of vexing questions emanates from these discoveries. How does one resolve the myriad of new and complex cancer genetic issues? In this comprehensive and elegantly written book, Kenneth Offit addresses these concerns with compassion and finesse.

Historically, segregation analysis of large and meticulously documented pedigrees showing familial cancer clusters and/or correlation of phenotypic stigmata (such as a colon carpeted with adenomatous polyps) led to a presumptive hereditary cancer syndrome diagnosis. More recently, the *sine qua non* for verifying genetic etiology has been at the molecular genetic level as evidenced by the following discoveries: 1) the identification of oncogenes, such as the *RET* proto-oncogene in the MEN2 syndrome; 2) the identification of tumor suppressor genes, such as the *APC* gene for familial adenomatous polyposis, the *RB* gene for hereditary retinoblastoma, and *BRCA1* and *BRCA2* for hereditary breast cancer; and 3) the finding of a new class of genes referred to as mutator genes or mismatch repair genes which are responsible for hereditary nonpolyposis colorectal cancer (HNPCC), namely *hMSH2, hMLH1, hPMS1,* and *hPMS2.* The mismatch repair (*MMR*) gene corrects base-pair mismatches that have the propensity to destabilize the genome. When post-replicative DNA repair occurs, such mismatch repair errors will predispose to recombination rates between homologous

DNA sequences, thereby further confounding the ability to maintain genomic integrity. Cancer may then ensue.

These molecular discoveries raise such questions as: How much of the total cancer burden is hereditary? (Perhaps all cancer is genetic when acquired somatic mutations are considered.) What is the impact of low penetrance genes on the total cancer burden? Who should pay for genetic counseling in the face of the often prohibitive expense of DNA testing? When should genetic counseling be provided, who should perform it, and how should it be done? What are the potential malpractice issues for a physician who fails to collect a sufficiently detailed family cancer history, who fails to perform DNA testing (as, for example, in the *RET* proto-oncogene in a patient from a MEN2 family), or who fails to advise patients of pertinent surveillance and management recommendations? Will insurance companies or employers discriminate against those who are harbingers of germline mutations? These issues are legion and interminable. Fortunately, many of these vexing concerns are addressed in this book.

Genetic counseling is mandatory *before* family members undergo DNA testing and again at the time of *disclosure* of results. The reason for this admonition is that patients need to understand fully the advantages and disadvantages of being tested for a genetic mutation. Knowing removes the uncertainty as to whether they do or do not carry the deleterious gene. If found to be positive, highly targeted surveillance and management recommendations can be made available in some but not all circumstances. The "down side" is the potential for experiencing fear, anxiety, apprehension, intrafamily strife, employer or insurance discrimination. Once armed with this pro and con information, the patient may decide to accept DNA testing, to defer it, or to reject it outright. Clearly, rejection is the patient's prerogative.

Following an excellent opening chapter surveying clinical cancer genetics and cancer risk counseling, the remaining nine chapters of this book cover hereditary and acquired risks for cancer, common as well as rare hereditary forms of cancer, the importance of quantitative methods in cancer risk assessment, laboratory methods for cancer genetic testing, management implications and reproductive counseling as well as the psychological, ethical and legal aspects of cancer risk counseling. A glossary of terms is also provided. Appendices contain information dealing with familial risk tables for common cancers such as breast and colon; they also offer practical materials for cancer genetic counseling, as well as a directory of laboratories that provide cancer genetic testing. Rich clinical genetic vignettes frequently elucidate the text. Each chapter has been written in a style that is easy to read, with up-to-date literature citations.

Dr. Offit addresses such controversies as non-directive genetic counseling vs. directive genetic counseling. He shows how and when directive counseling needs to be performed, for example, when recommending full colonoscopy as a screening procedure for patients at risk for HNPCC. Directive counseling is also indicated when advising prophylactic colectomy in familial adenomatous polyposis, or prophylactic total thyroidectomy for patients, including children, with MEN2a and 2b who are positive for the *RET* proto-oncogene. Clearly, these procedures are now an established part of the management of these hereditary cancer-prone syndromes. In contrast, recommendations for prophylactic surgery in the hereditary breast-ovarian cancer syndrome, and for prophylactic subtotal colectomy in HNPCC germline mutation carriers, remain controversial. In these particular situations a "non-directive" approach is prudent, as Dr. Offit points out, ". . . at least until the efficacy of these interventions has been established."

Genetic counseling extends even to complex pregnancy concerns. Advice is required when cancer chemotherapy or radiation has been administered either inadvertently or on a lifesaving basis during pregnancy. Dr. Offit's review of the literature on the pharmacology of anti-neoplastic agents during pregnancy shows that chemotherapy delivered in the first trimester increases teratogenic risk by 10–15% in some series. However, the older fetus is quite resistant even to the teratogenic effects of combination chemotherapeutic regimens. Radiation therapy of the 8–15 week fetus, even at low levels (10 cGy), may lead to diminished IQ. In cases of high-dose radiation, hydrocephalus and short stature may result.

Dr. Offit has provided oncologists, other physicians, genetic counselors, registered nurses, social workers, molecular geneticists and cancer genetic researchers an opus on cancer genetics and genetic counseling that is timely and long overdue. A practicing medical oncologist with intensive training in genetics and laboratory medicine, his extensive hands-on experience in the evaluation and management, including genetic counseling, of countless high-risk cancer patients, has been used to great advantage to educate readers to achieve insight into how to evaluate cancer genetic issues and how to provide genetic counseling. Virtually every aspect of the hereditary cancer genetic problem has been addressed in this book.

Henry T. Lynch, M.D.
Chairman and Professor, Department of Preventive Medicine
and Public Health Professor of Medicine
President, Hereditary Cancer Institute
Director, Creighton Cancer Center
Creighton University
Omaha, Nebraska

Clinical Cancer Genetics

1

Clinical Cancer Genetics and Risk Counseling

In his epic history of human knowledge, Charles Van Doren (1992) observed that there have been two periods of cataclysmic expansion of human understanding. The first was in and around Greece in the fourth century B.C. We are living through the second explosion of human knowledge today. Nowhere have the results of basic research been more evident than in the study of genetics. Scientific breakthroughs have made possible genetic engineering of organisms to produce needed substances, genetic cloning of entire animals, and genetic therapy of diseases. Rapid progress in understanding the genetics of cancer, the most deadly killer of humans, has resulted in a virtual revolution in the study of the molecular biology of malignant cells. Advances in cancer genetics have already been reflected in medical clinics and offices. The impact of genetics in cancer medicine has been felt in the three areas that currently define clinical cancer genetics: cancer genetic counseling, diagnostic cancer genetics, and prognostic cancer genetics.

Cancer genetic counseling has been energized by the recent development of genetic tests that pinpoint familial cancer risk. A range of health professionals, including genetic counselors, nurses, and physicians, provide cancer risk counseling. Advising cancer patients about reproductive risks after treatment has been included as part of oncologic care, and specialists in medical genetics or reproductive medicine are providing prenatal counseling. The use of genetic tests to diagnose cancers is increasingly included in clinical evaluations by pathologists and hematologists. Finally, many types of cancer specialists are incorporating cancer genetic tests that predict treatment outcome into the care of patients.

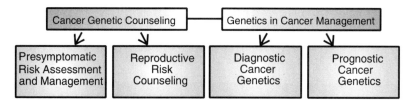

FIGURE 1-1 *The components of clinical cancer genetics.*

THE SCOPE OF CLINICAL CANCER GENETICS

Across the field of clinical cancer genetics, the current focus of attention is on presymptomatic risk assessment (Figure 1-1). Recent breakthroughs in the understanding of inherited cancer susceptibilities pose an immediate challenge to practicing genetic counselors, nurses, physicians, and other health professionals. Whether working in an academic setting, a community practice, or a managed care environment, healthcare providers have been asked to integrate genetics into the risk assessment and management of families with cancer.

Detection of an inherited genetic alteration can provide information about the risk of disease in members of the family as well as risk for those yet unborn. It can also give a strong clue about the clinical behavior of a newly detected cancer in an affected individual. As will be seen, the medical, social, and ethical implications of a genetic alteration in a tumor are vastly different from the implications of a similar alteration in one's inherited genetic makeup.

Cancer genetic counseling for the presymptomatic individual at hereditary risk for cancer has two components: risk assessment and counseling about behavioral, medical, and surgical options to decrease risk. This latter dialogue addresses such issues as lifestyle, diet, and occupational factors, as well as medical or surgical interventions. Although the distinction between genetic and nongenetic cancer risk counseling is useful conceptually, families seen in the office or clinic do not recognize such boundaries. Individuals are concerned about the bottom line—what can be done about risk, including dietary, lifestyle, hormonal, or other modifications, and the medical options for early cancer detection. Cancer genetic counseling is best considered as part of a process of cancer risk counseling that recognizes the interplay between environmental and genetic factors.

Because the scope of these issues is broad, a multidisciplinary approach is required. Certain aspects of cancer risk counseling can be provided, in some cases most effectively, by nonphysician specialists (Schneider, 1994). Genetic counselors and specially trained nurses are increasingly providing cancer risk counseling. Other aspects, particularly the discussion and planning for specific medical and surgical options, are more effectively presented by medical or surgical specialists. This chapter provides a framework for cancer risk counseling and its relationship to other aspects of clinical cancer genetics. Subsequent chapters provide specific data and methodology to assess cancer risk and to counsel families on options to reduce risk or detect cancers at a curable stage. The goal of this synthesis of genetic, epidemiologic, and medical information is to be client centered. The benefit of all predictive genetic testing and counseling rests on the informed decisions fashioned by the at-risk individual and the health-care provider.

SPECIAL CONSIDERATIONS IN CANCER GENETIC TESTING

The most powerful and most clinically challenging development in cancer risk counseling is the availability of testing for inherited mutations of cancer predisposition genes. For some hereditary cancer syndromes, the level of risk associated with specific mutations is well established. For other syndromes, precise estimates of risk are still being derived through research studies. Statements in the early 1990s by professional genetics societies sought to limit cancer genetic testing to research studies (e.g., the National Advisory Council for Human Genome Research, 1994). As an increasing number of cancer susceptibility genes were identified and characterized, guidelines for the responsible clinical translation of this information were developed by medical and surgical subspecialty societies (e.g., the Statement of the American Society of Clinical Oncology, 1996). Each of these guidelines emphasized that in the process of offering a predictive genetic test to a patient or family affected by cancer, the provider and the individual being tested must be prepared to deal with all the medical, psychological, and social consequences of a positive, a negative, or an ambiguous result.

The need to understand and effectively act on genetic information cuts across the fields of medical genetics, primary care medicine, oncology, public health, behavioral science, and public policy. A study of gastroenterologists, surgeons, medical geneticists, oncologists, and other physicians offering colon cancer genetic testing from one commercial laboratory revealed that almost a third of the providers misinterpreted the results. No one specialty group demonstrated any greater proficiency in interpreting genetic test results, and only 19% offered genetic counseling before the test (Giardiello et al., 1997). A genetic test of outstanding scientific interest is of little clinical value if the clinician is unable to interpret it, the patient afraid or unsure how to act on it, and the national health-care system unable to provide it without penalty or discrimination.

For these reasons, it is a central premise of this book that genetic testing should be offered in the context of a full discussion about the implications of possible results. Whether performed as part of a research study or as part of routine clinical care, genetic testing for inherited cancer risk requires careful informed consent (see Chapter 10). In many cases, the terms *pretest counseling* and *informed consent* are used interchangeably. However, cancer risk counseling is more than education about cancer risk in families (genetic risk assessment) and discussion of possible risks and benefits of genetic testing (informed consent). It also includes psychological support, guidance about medical options, and referral for medical or surgical means of early detection or prevention of cancer.

Cancer genetic testing is increasingly available for practitioners to offer patients as part of routine care. It is important to realize, however, that genetic testing, even for medical management, may not be required or desired. Just as the primary care physician can defer ordering a chest X ray and prescribe antibiotics based on physical findings, the counselor can motivate an at-risk individual to follow screening guidelines without recourse to complicated nucleic acid analysis. In other circumstances, DNA testing may be critical to the decision process. Through teaching and communication, a powerful new technology will be most efficiently and effectively applied to limit the human suffering that too often is associated with cancer.

THE CONTENT OF CLINICAL CANCER GENETICS CONSULTATIONS

The threshold for referral for consultation for cancer risk counseling varies according to the experience of the clinician. At present, most cancer risk counseling is provided by specialists in consultation liaison with referring practitioners. The composition, staffing, and support for these services vary widely. A survey of National Cancer Institute cancer centers revealed that only half of the centers offered any genetic services for familial cancer patients (Thompson et al., 1995). Thus, even at the largest academic programs, clinical expertise and experience in cancer genetic risk counseling may be limited.

Because of the multidisciplinary nature of cancer risk assessment, oncologists, geneticists, genetic counselors, nurses, psychologists, and other individuals specially trained in clinical cancer genetics can contribute to the management of at-risk individuals. The increasing commercial availability of genetic testing for susceptibility to common adult cancers, and incentives to include these services as part of managed care programs, will lead to increased efforts to train physicians and other health-care providers to deliver these services.

The clinical content of major areas of clinical cancer genetics is represented in Table 1-1. In practice, each of the areas identified in the table may be interrelated.

Assessment of Hereditary Cancer Risk and Options to Reduce Risk

A basic goal of cancer risk counseling is to derive and explain an individual's cancer risk in understandable terms. The polygenic and multifactorial nature of common adult cancers, which is discussed in subsequent chapters, is explained as an interplay between environmental and genetic factors that determine an individual's cancer risk. In the absence of clinical subspecialties in cancer genetics and epidemiology, it has been left to physicians to recognize inherited cancer syndromes and explain epidemiologic risk ratios in their daily practice. In the setting of family histories suggestive of a known hereditary cancer predisposition syndrome, Mendelian risk calculations, Bayesian adjustments, and quantitative risk counseling utilizing DNA markers (outlined in Chapter 6) are appropriate.

Cancer risk counseling is most frequently requested for families with the most common hereditary neoplasms: breast, ovarian, prostate, and colon cancers. For each of these malignancies, the threshold of family history for which counseling may be appropriate will vary according to the counseling resources available and the model for health care delivery in which counseling is offered. In general, counseling should be

TABLE 1-1 Scope of Clinical Cancer Genetics

1. Assessment of hereditary cancer risk and options to reduce risk:
   - Identification of hereditary syndromes in which susceptibility to cancer is a primary or secondary feature.
   - Determination of recurrence risks or risk of second tumors for affected individuals, risks to unaffected family members, options for genetic testing, pretest genetic counseling, posttest genetic counseling, options for screening and prevention, options for modification of risk, psychological support.
2. Genetic counseling for survivors of cancer, or for their families, regarding reproductive risks:
   - Postchemotherapy risks for sterility and possible teratogenic effects.
   - Options for prenatal diagnosis to determine genotype in families with known germline mutations of cancer predisposition genes (if ethically acceptable).
3. Interpretation of genetic tests for the diagnosis of malignancy:
   - Appropriate genetic tests to order, type of specimen required, and when best to obtain.
   - Interpretation of results, sensitivity, specificity, discrepancies with histologic diagnosis, types of confirmatory tests indicated.
4. Interpretation of genetic tests with prognostic utility for cancer patients:
   - Prognostic significance of cytogenetic or molecular assays, relationship of genetic markers to clinical prognostic factors, selection of therapeutic approaches based on prognostic markers.

offered to families with multiple cases of related cancers in several generations, multiple related cancers in the same individual, or cancers at an early age.

Medical geneticists and genetic counselors have developed a nondirective approach to counseling families faced with decisions regarding reproductive choices, or individuals considering genetic testing for late-onset disorders with limited therapeutic options. The goal of this approach is to avoid the imposition of the practitioner's personal preferences when medical options are not fully proven or are strongly influenced by religious beliefs. Although some aspects of cancer genetic counseling are shared with this model, there are significant differences. For a number of reasons, including the strong presumption of benefit of some cancer screening and early detection options, cancer genetic counseling may be more directive than reproductive counseling. In each of these circumstances, however, the counselor's role is to educate and enumerate options for patient and clinician, answer questions about what is known, and suggest appropriate referrals to help reach difficult decisions.

Indications for DNA Testing A common indication for referral for cancer genetic counseling is pretest evaluation for DNA testing for inherited cancer predisposition. Although limited to families that fit criteria for cancer family syndromes, genetic testing may also be appropriate for individuals with unusual clinical features, including very early age of onset, multiplicity of tumors, or certain congenital abnormalities. The most common indications for DNA testing and the specific genes with an associated cancer predisposition are listed in Table 1-2.

Some of the tests listed in Table 1-2 are still in transition from investigational to ac-

TABLE 1-2   Selected Indications for DNA Testing for Cancer Predisposition

Associated Cancers	Gene Test
Multiple cases of breast and/or ovarian cancer; commonly bilateral and at early age	*BRCA1, BRCA2*
Multiple cases of colon cancer, accompanied by other cancers of the uterus, ovaries, renal pelvis, and other sites	*hMSH2, hMLH1, hPMS1, hPMS2*
Childhood polyposis leading to colon cancer and other cancers	*APC*
Medullary cancer of the thyroid and other endocrine tumors	*RET*
Childhood sarcomas and breast cancer and other tumors in adults	*p53*
Familial retinoblastoma	*RB1*
Familial Wilms' tumor and associated syndromes	*WT1*
Renal cancer with retinal angioma and cerebellar hemangioblastomas	*VHL*
Multiple cases of malignant pigmented skin cancers (melanomas) or premalignant lesions (dysplastic nevi)	*CDKN2^{p16}, CDK4*

cepted clinical procedures. In the absence of federal guidelines, some state health departments have taken regulatory control over the definition of the investigational nature of some of these assays. For example, in New York State, tests are no longer considered "research" once results are shared with those undergoing the testing. For investigational assays, special licensing is often required for the laboratories providing these services to New York residents.

Current concerns about the widespread commercial availability of cancer susceptibility tests relate both to the clinical validity of the tests (see Chapters 6 and 7) and to the potential for misuse and misinterpretation of data. These concerns are also heightened by the enormous scale of the potential demand for these tests, the unproven nature of many of the medical options that may follow testing, and the lack of suitably trained clinicians to provide adequate informed consent and interpretation of results. To address these issues, the National Cancer Institute has moved toward putting in place national research protocols and educational programs. Professional societies and consumer groups have also stated policies aimed to facilitate the most responsible transition of cancer genetic testing from research trials to medical practice in the clinic or office.

Reproductive Risk Counseling

Young adults receiving curative treatments for leukemias, lymphomas, germ cell tumors, and some solid tumors are increasingly seeking consultation regarding reproductive risks and options. Unaffected family members also seek counseling regarding cancer risks for their unborn children. Considerable data exist pertaining to possible teratogenic effects of chemotherapy and radiotherapy (see Chapter 9). Less well-defined at present are the reproductive options following genetic testing for cancer risk. These include prenatal diagnosis of genotype and possible preimplantation diagnosis to select embryos which do not carry altered cancer predisposition genes. The appropriateness of these options which are, at present, no longer theoretical, will be defined by ethical as well as medical considerations. These issues must be anticipated by health professionals who will be asked to participate in this dialogue.

Diagnostic Cancer Genetics

Just as genetic markers may identify a susceptibility to cancer, they may also indicate the earliest stages in the evolution of common cancers. Thus, the patient with low red blood cell indices may be diagnosed as having a preleukemic state on the basis of a genetic study. The treatment of a child with a peripheral neuroectodermal tumor may depend on a cytogenetic evaluation. As a result of the rapid translation of basic genetic research, practicing cancer specialists are faced with a growing menu of diagnostic genetic tests to request and integrate into the management of patients. These issues are explored in Chapter 8.

The identification of a recurring genetic abnormality can be diagnostic of a tumor type, influence the treatment approaches chosen, or serve as a sensitive measure of disease in a biopsy or blood specimen. With expanding use of the polymerase chain reaction (Chapter 7), the sensitivity of cancer detection through blood or serum markers has increased dramatically. It is important to distinguish between molecular screening for presymptomatic cancers and genetic testing for inherited cancer risk. Cancer genetic specialists will continue to serve as a resource in the clinical application of current and emerging technologies of cancer genetic diagnosis.

Prognostic Cancer Genetics

The results of genetic assays performed on tumor specimens have been correlated with clinical features such as stage of disease, relapse rate, and survival after treatment. For some tumor types, including hematopoietic malignancies, neuroblastoma, and breast cancer, genetic assays already provide valuable predictive information that can be utilized to guide therapies. There is a continuing increase in the availability of genetic reagents and assays for the protein products of normal and altered cancer-related genes. These assays comprise a new class of prognostic markers. An emerging literature is defining genetic prognostic "panels," which represent the biological characteristics and clinical aggressiveness of a variety of common tumors. Clinical cancer geneticists will be called upon to guide clinicians regarding the indications and interpretation of genetic tests for patients already affected by cancer.

Therapeutic Uses of Cancer Genetics

One of the major benefits of the recent understanding of cancer genetics is the therapeutic application of this knowledge. At present, the major strategies of gene therapy

Case Example 1.1. In examining a 49-year-old woman, her primary care physician palpated a lump in the upper outer quadrant of her left breast. She was diagnosed with an invasive breast cancer involving two lymph nodes. The *HER2*/neu oncogene expression in her tumor was markedly elevated, as was the DNA index and other markers of tumor aggressiveness. Her oncologist was concerned because her mother died of breast cancer at an early age. After receiving counseling and testing, the woman was found to carry a mutation of the *BRCA1* gene. She was very concerned about her own prognosis and the cancer risk for her daughter, whom she desired to have tested.

Such a case illustrates the challenges of clinical cancer genetics. The prognostic significance of the elevated *HER2*/neu expression in the breast tumor was one of several factors leading to the choice of a more intensive adjuvant chemotherapy regimen (reviewed in Chapter 8). The *BRCA1* mutation is an inherited genetic change that has implications for the patient's risk for a second breast cancer, as well as subsequent ovarian cancer (reviewed in Chapter 4). Options for prevention or early detection of these tumors were integrated into her care. The patient decided to undergo prophylactic oophorectomy after the completion of her adjuvant chemotherapy. The *BRCA1* mutation identified in the patient will serve to inform the testing of her daughter, after full discussion of risks and benefits of testing.

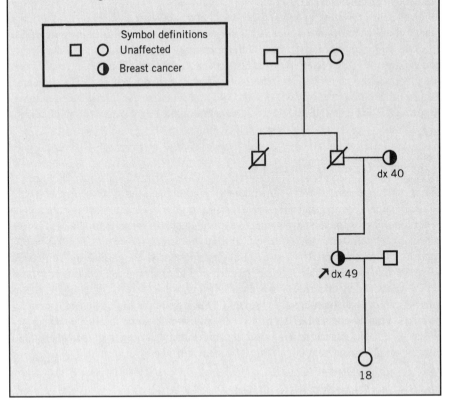

include: (1) transferring genes into tumors in order to augment antitumor immune responses; (2) transferring of genes into tumors in order to increase drug susceptibility; (3) transferring genes into normal cells to make them more resistant to drugs; and (4) replacing or inactivating cancer-associated genes. During 1997, about 100 clinical trials for cancer gene therapy were in place (Roth and Cristiano, 1997). Most trials were being conducted in severely ill patients, and only a few clinical responses had been observed. It seems certain, however, that the scope and number of trials will continue to grow as knowledge of the molecular basis of cancer increases. Although outside the current scope of clinical cancer genetics, research activities in gene therapy can be expected to be integrated into the future practice of cancer medicine.

*

Individual practitioners may not be able to address all of the components of clinical cancer genetics outlined previously. Their ability will depend, in large part, on their training and background and their access to specialized services. Because the major demand for cancer genetic counseling and testing will come from individuals at familial risk for the common cancers, presymptomatic genetic counseling and testing is the major focus of this volume. Questions about risks, benefits, and interpretation of genetic tests are commonly addressed to primary health-care providers as well as cancer specialists. A strategy to approach these questions has been developed by genetic counselors.

THE GENETIC COUNSELING MODEL

Genetic counselors are master's degree-level health-care professionals with training in both psychosocial and medical aspects of inherited diseases. The genetic counseling model was developed primarily in the prenatal and pediatric setting, but it is fully applicable to recurrence risk counseling for adult-onset disorders (Kessler, 1979). Whether provided by a genetic counselor, nurse, or physician, the content of cancer genetic counseling should be the same. In some instances, requests for counseling are driven by requirements for informed consent for genetic testing. If the individual chooses not to undergo DNA analysis, the basic elements of the cancer genetic counseling session listed in Table 1-3 are still relevant.

The most widely cited definition of genetic counseling, written 20 years ago by a joint committee of American and Canadian health professionals, described it as "a communication process which deals with the human problems associated with the occurrence, or risk of occurrence, of a genetic disorder in a family." This process involves "an attempt to help the individual or family (1) comprehend the medical facts . . . and the available management; (2) appreciate the way heredity contributes to the disorder . . . ; (3) understand the options for dealing with the risk of recurrence; (4) choose the course of action which seems appropriate . . . ; and (5) make the best possible adjustment to the disorder." (Ad Hoc Committee on Genetic Counseling, 1975).

In his historical essay on genetic counseling, Charles Epstein criticized aspects of

TABLE 1-3 Components of the Cancer Risk Counseling Session

1. Contracting
2. Baseline risk perception
3. Pedigree construction
4. Pedigree documentation
5. Medical history
6. Exposure history
7. Physical examination
8. Empiric risk assessment/genetic risk assessment
9. Options for early detection and prevention; specialty referrals
10. Options, risks, benefits for genetic testing; pretest counseling
11. Response to questions, support, and plans for follow-up

this definition, stating that "the emphasis on communication appears to separate counseling per se from the other aspects of what might be called the diagnosis, management, and prevention of genetic disorders." He disagreed with the false division between genetic counselors, concerned with communication and support, and medical geneticists (physicians), concerned with diagnosis and treatment (Epstein, 1979). Many of Epstein's admonitions are fully relevant today for clinical oncologists and primary care physicians. The goals of cancer genetic counseling are important components of all preventive oncology consultations, regardless of the graduate training of the provider. Cancer genetic counseling closely resembles its reproductive and pediatric counterparts with its emphasis on communication, risk assessment, guidance, and support. In contrast to most reproduction-centered genetic counseling, means of cancer prevention or eradication are often available. Environmental and behavioral factors, which may be modulated, also impact on cancer risk. For these reasons, cancer genetic counseling, defined earlier as part of the broader process of cancer risk counseling, fits into the context of preventive medicine.

Contracting

The initial phase of "contracting" is borrowed from the concept of the therapeutic contract in psychotherapy. It is a critical process of introduction and alliance between the counselor and the consultand (*proband*) and family members. *Proband* refers to the individual who seeks counseling and around whom the family tree is constructed. Not all probands are patients—they may be healthy individuals with no greater than average risks. (Many genetic counselors prefer the term *client,* but this may bring to mind fiduciary or legal relationships that are unappealing to many health-care providers.) In the process of contracting, the counselor elicits from the consultand and family members what they hope to learn from the visit, and then attempts to reconcile this with what can realistically be accomplished during the session.

If there are differences in expectations about the counseling session, it is best to address these up front. For example, some families may suspect that genetic information has already been learned from blood tests they have had in the past, while others will express fear that they have been referred by their physician to "get the bad news." Early clarifications and reassurances are an important part of contracting. An explanation of the process to be expected, with an emphasis on the goal of working together to reach decisions, sets a tone of openness and partnership.

Baseline Risk Perception

After contracting, and before the beginning of the process of information gathering, it is useful to ask the proband about his or her perceived cancer risk. This is often done by putting a mark on an analog scale from 0 (lowest risk) to 100 (highest risk). Such scales are often included in the precounseling questionnaires administered as part of research studies. If incorporated into a routine session, documentation of baseline risk perception can be enormously useful in later phases of counseling.

Pedigree Construction

Assembly of the pedigree information is often regarded by nongeneticists as an onerous task. Although family history is a part of the canonical ritual of the history and physical, this information is too often recorded as "family history positive" or "family history negative" on the admitting note. Indeed, a survey of teaching and nonteaching hospitals in the New York area found that family history information was completely missing in 37.5% of cases in hospitals without tumor registries and 12.5% of cases from hospitals with registries. Where family history information was recorded, it was often incomplete (David and Steiner-Grossman, 1991). In the context of a cancer genetic counseling session, the careful recording of the family history of cancer is, of course, paramount.

The full family structure, including all known relatives, should be represented on the pedigree. The symbols commonly used to construct pedigrees are shown in Figure 1-2, and the types of familial relationships are reviewed in Figure 1-3. In practice, it may be advantageous to send to the proband a family history questionnaire, which can be assembled into a working draft to be checked and updated during the interview. A

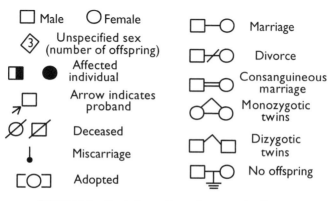

FIGURE 1-2 *Symbols used in pedigree construction.*

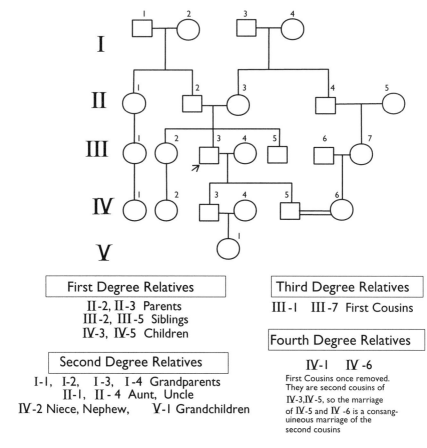

FIGURE 1-3 *Sample pedigree.*

number of software packages are available to record and graphically represent family history data (see Appendix B).

Information recorded in pedigree assembly includes the relative's name, age when affected, current age or age at death, type of cancer(s), and other medical conditions. Information on type of treatment and the hospital where the diagnostic biopsy was performed should also be obtained. Complete information is also obtained on all unaffected family members. Information on the unaffected family members is crucial in the analysis of patterns of inheritance. The process of pedigree ascertainment can also, understandably, be an emotional ordeal for the proband who may represent the "survivor" and chronicler of the family's hardships.

Pedigree Documentation

Pedigree documentation is a critical adjunct to taking the family history. To the greatest extent possible, this documentation should include obtaining of hospital records,

Case Example 1.2. A 54-year-old woman was strongly considering prophylactic oopho-rectomy because of a family history of breast and ovarian cancer in her mother. Review of the medical record revealed that the diagnosis of ovarian cancer in the patient's mother was not definitive. Slides and blocks were requested. It was possible to perform addition-al immunohistochemical studies and make the diagnosis of metastatic breast cancer. The prophylactic oophorectomy was canceled by the proband.

   This case emphasizes the importance of documentation of diagnoses. Breast cancer metastatic to ovaries is an uncommon but described phenomenon.

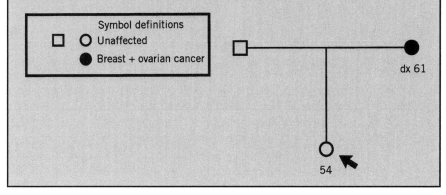

pathology reports, autopsy records, death certificates, and, in special circumstances, histologic sections or paraffin-blocks to confirm diagnoses. Death certificates general-ly underreport cancer-related mortality, listing cardiovascular causes as the immediate cause of most deaths. By far the most reliable sources of information are pathology records, which can usually be requested directly from the hospital where the individual received treatment.

   In a classic study by Love and colleagues at the University of Wisconsin, the histo-logic diagnosis of cancer was verified in 83% of first-degree relatives, but only 67% and 60% of second- and third-degree relatives, respectively (Love et al., 1985). Out-side of funded research studies, the logistical support for pathologic verification must come from the consulting family itself. Very often, a designated family member is willing to act as the facilitator and collector of records. These efforts can be aided by providing supporting documents and information, including release forms, slide re-quests, and lists of addresses of state agencies that may be of assistance. The costs of this effort, which are rarely prohibitive, are generally borne by the individual request-ing the documentation.

Medical History

The past medical and surgical history of the proband should be as complete as possi-ble, and should include reference to known preneoplastic lesions (e.g., polyps, dys-plastic nevi, *in situ* breast lesions). It is obviously desirable to include a special empha-sis on associations of congenital abnormalities and related medical conditions with the

Case Example 1.3. A 24-year-old woman sought counseling and genetic testing because of a family history of cancer. Her pedigree was significant for cases of chronic myelogenous leukemia, cervical cancer, lung cancer, choriocarcinoma, and Hodgkin's disease. All cases were confirmed by pathology records. The case of lung cancer occurred in a smoker. The choriocarcinoma occurred as a complication of a molar pregnancy.

This pedigree represents an abundant cancer family history but no diagnosis of a syndromic predisposition. Ages of onset are typical, there are no multiple cancers in a single individual, and the tumor types are not known to be associated. In this case, cancer genetic counseling served to reassure the family members. Clinical genetic testing for other than research purposes was not indicated.

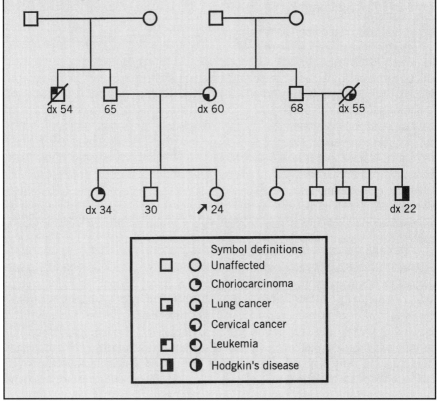

cancers reported in the family. Appendix A summarizes the major components of the cancer predisposition syndromes associated with each tumor by site. It may be helpful to refer to the relevant list of manifestations of syndromes for each component cancer. Thus, for example, in a family with multiple cases of colon cancer, past medical history of polyps, sebaceous cysts, epidermoid cysts, skin lesions (cafe au lait spots, melanin spots, etc.) may be the clue to a syndromic diagnosis. For the vast majority of common susceptibilities to breast, ovary, and colon cancer, the past medical history will be unrevealing and no congenital abnormalities will be evident.

Exposure History

As outlined in Chapter 2, an increasing number of chemical, occupational, or other environmental exposures have been associated with risks for specific cancers. Risk assessment should include an occupational and exposure history. For women, a detailed history of hormone use, as contraceptive agents or as part of replacement therapy, should be elicited. For individuals treated for cancer, details of doses and duration of systemic chemotherapy and radiotherapy are necessary to deduce secondary cancer risk.

Physical Examination

Considered part of a comprehensive medical evaluation, the type and scope of the physical examination conducted as part of a genetic counseling session will vary with the experience and background of the counselor. Targeted preventive oncology examinations can reliably be performed by trained nurses or other specialized personnel. Even for physicians, some aspects of the physical exam may be simple for one specialist but difficult for another. For example, the examination of the reconstructed breast or intestinal stoma may be unfamiliar to nononcologists, whereas medical geneticists may be most experienced in the identification of some of the rare congenital abnormalities. In some cases, it may be desirable to refer the relevant examination to the specialty cancer prevention clinic (e.g., gynecologic or ophthalmologic examinations).

For the most common hereditary cancer susceptibility syndromes associated with breast, colon, and skin (melanoma), a targeted physical examination of the head and neck and skin can exclude the rarer syndromes associated with physical stigmata (Table 1-4). The common cancer predisposition syndromes of adults are generally not associated with congenital abnormalities. However, a review of over 20,000 cases of malignancy diagnosed in children did reveal increased rates of congenital abnormalities among children with Wilms' tumor, Ewing sarcoma, hepatoblastoma, or gonadal tumors (Narod et al., 1997). Abnormalities of the eye, rib, and spine were most frequently encountered. The associations between cancer types and congenital abnormalities were quite rare, and were felt to be more useful as research opportunities than for clinical management, because of the lack of specificity in many of the associations observed (reviewed by Friedman, 1997).

Empiric Risk Assessment/Genetic Risk Assessment

As presented in Chapter 6, considerable empiric data are available to inform quantitative cancer risk counseling. Advantages of these data are that they are readily applicable to the majority of individuals with negligible or modestly increased risk for cancer based on pedigree analysis. The interest and ability of individuals to receive quantitative risk estimates vary greatly. In general, individuals prefer absolute risk information, comparing expected risks over the remainder of a lifetime with other common risks. More precise derivation of risks, utilizing Bayesian adjustments will become possible as DNA testing is gradually introduced. The methodology of these calculations is presented in Chapter 6.

TABLE 1-4 Stigmata of Selected Syndromes Associated with Susceptibility to Cancers

Syndrome	Major Cancer Risks	Selected Physical Findings
Cowden's syndrome[a]	Breast cancer	Facial papules, oral "cobblestone" papules, macrocephaly
Down syndrome	Acute leukemia	Characteristic facies, round head, congenital heart disease
Fanconi anemia[b]	Acute leukemia	Upper extremity malformations, increased skin pigmentation
Familial adenomatous polyposis (Gardner subtype)[c]	Colon cancer	Retinal pigmentation, sebaceous cysts, osteomas, impacted teeth, exostoses, desmoids, florid polyposis
Muir-Torre syndrome[c]	Colon cancer, skin tumors	Sebaceous adenomata, keratoacanthomata, basal cell carcinomas
Multiple endocrine neoplasia type 2b[d]	Medullary thyroid carcinoma, pheochromocytoma	Enlarged and nodular lips, Marfanoid habitus
Peutz-Jehger syndrome[c]	Breast, colon cancers	Dark spots on lips, perioral areas, buccal mucosa and extremities
Turcot syndrome[c]	Colon cancer, brain tumors	Polyps, cafe-au-lait spots, sebaceous cysts on skin
"WAGR"[d] syndrome (Wilm's tumor, aniridia, genitourinary abnormalities, mental retardation)	Wilms' tumor	Aniridia, genitourinary anomalies

[a]Discussed in Chapter 4, part A.
[b]Discussed in Chapter 3.
[c]Discussed in Chapter 4, part B.
[d]Discussed in Chapter 5.

The communication and explanation of genetic risks for cancer requires a review of basic concepts of Mendelian genetics as well as a simplified presentation of the two-hit hypothesis (Chapter 3). Although this presentation will vary according to the background and characteristics of the consultand (Pearn, 1973), it will be facilitated by prepared graphic or audiovisual aids. In many cases, there will be no evidence of inherited cancer predisposition and reassurance can be provided instead of quantification of increased risk.

Options for Early Detection and Prevention; Specialty Referrals

Perhaps the most challenging aspect of cancer risk counseling is the formulation and discussion of medical and surgical options to decrease the risk of cancer or to diagnose it at an early stage. In most cases, these options will include cancer screening by radiographic, endoscopic, or other means of physical examination or laboratory testing.

Although most of these options (e.g., mammography, colonoscopy) have been proved to be effective in the average-risk population, they are only presumed to be of benefit in the high-risk population. For these reasons, guidelines by expert panels are available, and individualizing of cancer screening programs is essential. The most dramatic option for cancer prevention, the removal of healthy organs, is now an established part of the management for some syndromes (e.g., familial polyposis, MEN2a), while it remains a controversial recommendation for other syndromes (e.g., breast/ovarian cancer syndrome). In these situations, a nondirective approach is needed until the efficacy of these interventions has been established. The details of these options are discussed in the context of the specific syndromes outlined in Chapters 4 and 5.

A major role of the cancer risk counselor is as triage coordinator for the at-risk family. For some syndromes, referral to a variety of surgical or medical subspecialists is called for (e.g., referral to both gastroenterologists and gynecologists for monitoring of women at risk for hereditary nonpolyposis colon cancer). The threshold for referral to medical and surgical specialists will depend on the level of training of the counselor and the counselor's willingness and ability to assume primary-care responsibilities. In many cases, the cancer risk counselor's most efficient role will be as a facilitator and coordinator, rather than a provider, of preventive oncology services.

Options, Risks, Benefits for Genetic Testing; Pretest Counseling

As genetic testing for cancer susceptibility has become more widely available, health professionals have been called upon to offer testing to family members. This discussion requires an educational effort to impart the potential impact of both a positive, negative, and ambiguous test result. The decision by the proband or family member to proceed with testing must follow a careful process of pretest counseling regarding the medical, psychological, and economic risks and benefits of testing (Chapter 10). The explanation of the potential impact of test results requires a familiarity with the technical specifications of the tests, their predictive value, and the various regulations that govern genetic testing for cancer predisposition. These issues are explored in later chapters, with a detailed list of the components for informed consent for genetic testing reviewed in Chapter 10.

Response to Questions, Support, and Plans for Follow-up

The level of detail requested by probands and family members in counseling sessions varies considerably. The enormous publicity given to genetics and biotechnology in the media has resulted in a generally high level of public interest. An understanding and ability to explain the basic concepts of the molecular biology and epidemiology of cancer is required in counseling sessions, and this forms the basis of the next two chapters. To be most effective, the cancer risk counselor should come prepared with illustrative charts and tables to communicate risk information and explain important genetic concepts. Equally important to the patient and the family, the counselor should be able to provide convenient referrals to pursue discussions of preventive trials, cancer screening, and surgical options. For those patients already affected by cancer and at risk for other tumors, a highly individualized approach to the discussion of these options is required.

The importance of individualized preventive oncology management has not yet been addressed by behavioral research. A randomized trial of flip-chart style educational approaches compared to counseling by oncology nurses failed to demonstrate a difference in knowledge of genetic testing acquired by subjects receiving either approach. Interestingly, neither approach had an impact on individual decisions to undergo breast cancer genetic testing (Lerman et al., 1997). However, the relevance of these findings to practice settings, where the pretest counselor may also be the health-care provider, remains to be established. Probably some combination of standardized educational materials combined with personalized medical care will be necessary to most effectively provide clinical genetic services.

Throughout these discussions, a sensitivity to psychological and ethical aspects of counseling is essential (Chapter 10). Although it is a truism that counseling should be "supportive," such an outcome may require preparation and considerable interpersonal skill. Awareness of differing cultural perspectives and a sensitivity to possible stigmas associated with cancer are prerequisites. Empathetic concern and understanding regarding the cancer-related experiences of the family can transform a painful emotional session into an opportunity for the family to feel empowered and reassured that they have taken the course best suited to their unique needs and concerns. In some circumstances, however, risk notification inevitably has a disturbing impact on families. Continued follow-up by the counselor after the session is the best way to limit the real potential for the adverse impact of the communication of inherited cancer risk. Ready access to liaison mental health professionals with experience in cancer genetics is a valued asset in cancer risk counseling.

RECORD KEEPING AND RECOVERY OF COSTS FOR CANCER GENETIC COUNSELING

It should be clear to the family member whether the preventive medicine recommendations discussed with him or her will be sent to the individual's physician, or any other health-care professional that the individual would like notified. For ethical and liability-related reasons it is important that the line of responsibility for medical follow-up care be communicated and carefully documented in the consultation note. It should also be stated in counseling sessions that communication of medical information to a referring physician will not include the results of genetic test results unless permission is obtained. In some states (e.g., New York), written releases for genetic test results are legally required. Discussion of other provisions pertaining to privacy of records (e.g., certificates of confidentiality, see Chapter 10) should be included as part of this aspect of the session.

It is also prudent for the health provider to document in consultation notes the limitations of the clinical information collected and the medical options discussed. If family history information was provided verbally and not verified by reports, that should be noted. It should be stated to family members that the interpretation of a pedigree may change dramatically after the change in health status of even one family member. The limited sensitivity and specificity of genetic tests employed should be explained and documented, and it should be understood that recommended measures for cancer screening or the age ranges chosen to begin screening do not guarantee that cancers will not occur. Documentation of discussion of Mendelian inheritance and what is known about risks of specific genetic changes should be included. Such documentation is consistent with basic rules of medical record keeping. It provides a record of the session that documents the medical care delivered.

In the United States, genetic counseling and testing for some heritable cancer syndromes have been reimbursed as part of the routine care (e.g., MEN2a), while for other syndromes these same services may be deemed "experimental." For the pediatric hereditary cancer syndromes, cost recovery for genetic services has been successfully achieved as part of the oncologic care of the proband. The same model may be utilized for the more common syndromes of adult cancer predisposition. The level of care of oncology visits may appropriately be extended by genetic counseling. Separate consultations by cancer specialists with expertise in cancer genetics are also reimbursable.

For patients already affected by cancer, genetic discrimination by insurance carriers may be perceived as much less likely due to age or other medically related issues (see Chapter 10). Cancer patients and cancer survivors may request that costs for genetic testing be recovered through their health plans. To the extent that clinical cancer genetics services relate to the continued oncologic management of the patient already affected by cancer, coverage for these services can be anticipated.

For the unaffected member of a family afflicted by the common adult cancers (breast, colon, prostate), prospects for recovery of costs for genetic counseling and testing are less certain. Because of fears about future discrimination (see Chapter 10), unaffected individuals may be loathe to submit insurance claims for genetic testing or counseling. The submitted charges for these services can be substantial, ranging up to thousands of dollars for some genetic tests and hundreds of dollars for one or more counseling sessions. Some managed care companies have concluded that the cost/benefit ratio for cancer genetic counseling and testing is favorable for certain conditions. Increasingly, HMOs and managed care plans are beginning to offer clinical cancer genetic services. Except for large academic centers, where some genetic services may be offered without a fee as part of funded research studies, the costs for genetic counseling and testing may be daunting. Even when clinical charges are reimbursed, the actual costs may not be fully recovered, due to the labor-intensiveness, time, and complexity of individual cases.

REFERENCES

Ad Hoc Committee on Genetic Counseling. 1975. Report to the American Society of Human Genetics. Amer J Hum Genet 27:240–42.

David KL, Steiner-Grossman P. 1991. The potential use of tumor registry data in the recognition and prevention of hereditary and familial cancer. NY State J Med 91:150–2.

Epstein CJ.1979. Foreword to Kessler S (ed) Genetic Counseling: Psychological Dimensions. New York: Academic Press, i–xiii.

Friedman JM.1997. Genetics and epidemiology, congenital anomalies and cancer. Amer J Hum Genet 60:469–73.

Giardiello FM, Brensinger JD, Petersen GM, et al. 1997. The use and interpretation of commercial APC gene testing for familial adenomatous polyposis. New Engl J Med 336: 823–7.

Kessler S. 1979. The processes of communication, decision making, and coping in genetic counseling. In Kessler S (ed) Genetic Counseling: Psychological Dimensions. New York: Academic Press, 35–51.

Lerman C, Biesecker B, Benkendorf JL, Kerner J, Gomez-Caminero A, Hughes C, Reed MM. 1997. Controlled trial of pretest education approaches to enhance informed decision-making for *BRCA1* gene testing. J Natl Cancer Inst 89:148–75.

Love R, Evans AM, Josten DM. 1985. The accuracy of patient reports of a family history of cancer. J Chron Dis 38:289–93.

Narod SA, Hawkins MM, Robertson CM, Stiller CA. 1997. Congenital anomalies and childhood cancer in Great Britain. Amer J Hum Genet 60:474–85.

National Advisory Council for Human Genome Research. 1994. Statement on use of DNA testing for presymptomatic identification of cancer risk. JAMA 271:785.

Pearn JH. 1973. Patients' subjective interpretation of risks offered in genetic counselling. J Med Genet 10:129–34.

Roth JA, Cristiano RJ. 1997. Gene therapy for cancer: what have we done and where are we going? J Natl Cancer Inst 89: 21–39.

Schneider K. 1994. Counseling about cancer: Strategies for genetic counselors. Dana-Farber Cancer Institute, Boston, MA.

Statement of the American Society of Clinical Oncology: Genetic Testing for Cancer Susceptibility (Offit K, Biesecker BB, Burt RW, Clayton EW, Garber JE, Kahn MJE, Lichter A, Lynch P, Watson MS, Weber BL, Wells SA) 1996. J Clinical Oncol 14:1730–6.

Thompson JA, Wiesner GL, Sellers TA, Vachon C, Ahrens M, Potter JD, Sumpmann M, Kersey J. 1995. Genetic services for familial cancer patients: A survey of National Cancer Institute cancer centers. J Natl Cancer Instit 87:1446–55.

Van Doren, C. 1992. A History of Knowledge. New York: Ballantine Books.

2

Hereditary and Acquired Risks for Cancer

CANCER AS A HEREDITARY DISEASE

The Greek philosophers of the fourth century B.C. did not anticipate the importance of hereditary factors in cancer. Democedes cured a woman of breast cancer with primitive surgery and Hippocrates described cancers of the skin, breast, uterus, and internal organs. However, the prevailing theory of the era was that cancer—and every other disease—was due to acquired defects. It resulted from deficiency or excess of blood, mucus, or bile. Galen (A.D.131 to 203), the founder of physiology and pathology, espoused theories of the origin of cancer that would remain for over a thousand years. Cancer, according to this humoral theory, was due to the concentration of black bile.

Although Galen described familial malignancies, cancer as a hereditary disease did not gain widespread attention until the eighteenth and nineteenth centuries, partly because of the notoriety of a number of well-known cancer families. Napoleon I's father, one brother, and two sisters died of stomach cancer, and the proband himself probably succumbed to linitis plastica, a virulent form of stomach cancer (Ewing, 1922). The most famous cancer family of the era was that of Madame Z, described in 1866 by the French physician Broca. In this family, 16 of 26 members—mother, children, and grandchildren—all who reached the age of 30, died of cancer of the breast or "liver" (most likely metastatic breast cancer) (Broca, 1866). Other large families with breast cancer were described by Korteweg and others. Paget described cancer of the uterus in a mother, daughter, and granddaughter, and felt that "it is hence certain that cancerous disease, or a tendency to it, is prone to pass by inheritance from parent to offspring" (cited in Ewing, 1922; Schneider et al., 1986).

The monk Gregor Mendel described the basic modes of inheritance in his pea garden in the 1850s, but his work was little known until its rediscovery in 1900. Examples of human diseases following Mendelian patterns of inheritance were soon observed, and some of these were cancer families. In the United States, Michigan pathologist Warthin reported the family of his seamstress, in which 17 of 48 descendants died of cancers largely of the colon, uterus, and stomach (Warthin, 1913). In virtually all of these cancer families, the inheritance of cancer appeared to follow the pattern of autosomal dominant inheritance described in Mendel's pea garden (Figure 2-1).

The Importance of Mendelian Inheritance in Human Cancer

In reviewing the concept of Mendelian inheritance as it applied to human cancers, Dr. James Ewing, consulting pathologist to Memorial Hospital, was unimpressed. He believed that the proportion of human cancers following a Mendelian pattern of inheritance was minuscule, and that other, more powerful factors determined cancer susceptibility. Writing in the 1922 edition of his *Treatise on Tumors,* he stated that "nothing about cancer is more generally accepted than its hereditary nature, and nothing is less satisfactorily proved. In the interests of the public," he wrote, "this doctrine ought to be combated" (Ewing, 1922). In a later edition, Ewing admitted that "there is among human beings a general susceptibility to tumors . . . but . . . as a rule, this susceptibility is negligible and the disease does not develop until other exciting factors, which are the real effective causes of the disease, are brought into play."

What is our current understanding of cancer as a hereditary disease? Each of the 2.3 million deaths due to cancer each year in the industrialized countries (500,000 in

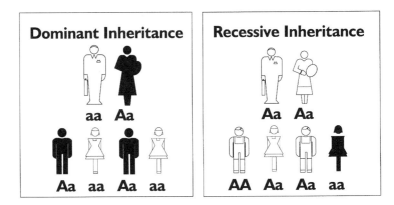

FIGURE 2-1   *Dominant and recessive inheritance of cancer susceptibility. Dominant traits (left) are those in which only one altered allele (A) is required to produce the disease. Since each child receives one of two alleles from the parent, there is a 50% chance that an affected parent would pass the altered (A) gene, and hence the trait, on to the child. In recessive traits (right), it is necessary for two copies of an altered gene (aa) to be present in order to express the features of the disease. If two parents heterozygous (carriers) for such an altered gene (Aa) have offspring, 50% will be "carrier" heterozygotes, 25% will be homozygous for the normal gene, and 25% will be homozygous for the altered gene. The homozygotes will show the disease features (phenotype). Darkened figures represent those with susceptibility to cancer, inherited as a result of dominant or recessive transmission.*

the United States) was genetic in origin, because every tumor resulted from genetic defects in the somatic tissue (bodily tissues such as lung, breast, prostate, etc.) that gave rise to the malignancy. In the majority of cases, the accumulation of genetic damage in these tissues appeared to be random and the tumors were termed *sporadic*. In some cases, however, all of the cells of the individual's body contained an inborn genetic defect, which increased the probability that certain tissues would become cancerous. This type of cancer susceptibility, present in the heritable genetic material (*germline*) of the individual, can be passed down from parent to child. That such cancer families exist was definitively demonstrated by Lynch and coworkers in the 1970s (Lynch, 1976). It is the relative contribution of hereditary cancer to the 2.3 million cases that was so difficult for Ewing to decipher, and which is still being defined.

Mendelian Patterns of Inheritance

Examples of human diseases that follow the simple Mendelian patterns of dominant, recessive, or sex-linked inheritance are well established. Examples include cystic fibrosis (recessive), the fragile X syndrome of mental retardation (X-linked), and Huntington disease (dominant). The identification of the genetic defects associated with these disorders provided extraordinary diagnostic tools. The notion that certain cancer susceptibilities also follow Mendelian modes of inheritance is now accepted. Most cancers are sporadic in nature, in that they do not follow clear patterns of inheritance and are presumed to be due to environmental or other causes. However, in some instances, families affected by certain cancers fit Mendelian patterns (Lynch, 1976). Subsets of patients with tumors of the breast, ovary, colon, endocrine organs, prostate, and other sites inherit susceptibilities to these cancers as part of dominant syndromes, whereas other syndromes follow recessive patterns (Table 2-1). In these families, the transmission of the cancers is referred to as *hereditary*. When the number and distribution of cancers is suggestive of a hereditary pattern of transmission, but the pattern is not definitive, the cancers are often referred to as *familial*.

Clusters of cancers in a family may also be due to environmental exposures or to chance. Finally, there are many Mendelian syndromes in which a susceptibility to cancer is a secondary feature. In these syndromes, which are included in Appendix A, cancers and noncancerous manifestations comprise the features of Mendelian syndromes.

Dominant Inheritance

In the Mendelian model, individuals have two copies (*alleles*) of a gene that determines a disease or physical trait. Different forms (alleles) of a gene may occupy a given genetic *locus,* or position on the chromosome. The genetic constitution of the individual is referred to as the *genotype,* and the expression of the physical, biochemical, or clinical characteristics of the trait is referred to as the *phenotype*.

Dominant traits are those in which only one altered allele is required to produce the disease (Figure 2-1). One manifestation of the trait may be susceptibility to cancer. Since each child receives one of two alleles from the parent, there is a 50% chance that an affected parent would pass the altered gene, and hence the trait, on to the child. This

TABLE 2-1   Selected Human Cancers Associated with Mendelian Syndromes

Cancers	Selected Syndromes
Dominant	
Breast/ovarian cancers	Breast/ovarian cancer syndrome
Colon cancer	Hereditary nonpolyposis colon cancer
	Familial adenomatous polyposis
Endocrine tumors	Multiple endocrine neoplasias
Melanoma	Dysplastic nevus syndrome
Prostate cancer	Hereditary prostate cancer
Renal cancer	Von Hippel-Lindau syndrome
Retinoblastoma	Hereditary retinoblastoma
Wilms' tumor	Hereditary Wilms' tumor syndromes
Basal cell skin cancers	Nevoid basal cell carcinoma syndrome
Recessive	
Acute leukemia and	Ataxia telangiectasia
non-Hodgkin's lymphomas	Fanconi anemia
	Bloom syndrome
Skin cancers	Xeroderma pigmentosum
X-linked	
Lymphomas	X-linked lymphoproliferative syndrome

pattern of inheritance results in multiple generations with the trait, with about half of individuals in each generation inheriting the susceptibility trait. An individual inheriting one copy of the altered gene from a parent is termed *heterozygous* for that genetic locus. The individual inheriting two copies of the altered gene, one from each parent, is termed a *homozygote.*

When speaking of women at inherited risk for breast and ovarian cancer due to, for example, alterations of the gene *BRCA1,* the term *BRCA1 heterozygotes* is more genet-

---

Case Example 2.1. A 20-year-old woman came for counseling regarding her risks for cancer. Her family history was significant for multiple cases of breast and ovarian cancer in both maternal and paternal lineages. No family members were alive for germline DNA testing. Both sets of grandparents were of Jewish Eastern European background.

Determination of Mendelian risk in this case must be based on the possibility of inheriting susceptibility gene mutations from both lineages. Given the high prevalence of founder mutations in the Ashkenazi Jewish population (see Chapter 4), it is possible that each side of the family could be segregating the same mutation, different mutations of the same gene, or different mutations of different genes. For the first two examples, the frequency of heterozygotes would be determined by:

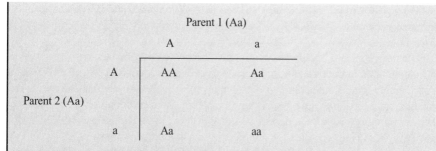

Parent 1 (Aa)

	A	a
A	AA	Aa
a	Aa	aa

Parent 2 (Aa)

Thus, there was a 75% probability that the offspring would inherit a dominant suscep-tibility allele from one of her parents.

If we assume that each parent was heterozygous for a different mutation of different genes, the rule of independent segregation would apply to the dihybrid cross. Thus, off-spring would be given by the cross Aabb × aaBb, with outcomes:

Parent 1 (Aabb)

	Aa	Aa	aa	aa
Bb	AaBb	AaBb	aaBb	aaBb
bb	Aabb	Aabb	aabb	aabb
Bb	AaBb	AaBb	aaBb	aaBb
bb	Aabb	Aabb	aabb	aabb

Parent 2 (aaBb)

Thus, 12/16 = 3/4 of the offspring would carry a dominant susceptibility allele from one or both parents.

In fact, at least one case of a homozygote for a *BRCA1* mutation, as well as cases of compound heterozygotes for different mutations have been reported (see Chapter 4). In both cases, the phenotypes were indistinguishable from the heterozygous phenotype.

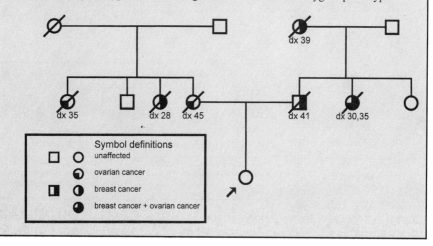

Symbol definitions
- □ ○ unaffected
- ◐ ovarian cancer
- ◑ breast cancer
- ◐ breast cancer + ovarian cancer

ically correct than the common appellation *BRCA1 mutation carriers.* Either of these terms is preferable to *BRCA1 carrier,* since all individuals carry two copies of the *BRCA1* gene.

The term *carrier frequency* is commonly utilized to describe the prevalence of specific mutations in the population. Because the carrier frequency of some mutations is sufficiently high in some ethnic groups, it may not be rare for individuals to inherit different mutations of the same gene from each parent. Such compound heterozygotes for *BRCA1* mutations have been described and appear to have a similar phenotype to other heterozygotes. Homozygotes for dominantly transmitted genes usually have more severe symptoms and signs of the disease compared to the heterozygote. This does not appear to be the case, however, in at least some hereditary cancer syndromes in which homozygotes may be indistinguishable from heterozygotes (e.g., Boyd et al., 1995).

In looking at pedigrees, the pattern of disease in multiple generations (*vertical transmission*) associated with dominant disorders may not be evident initially. This is due to age-at-onset considerations, i.e., the phenotype may not become manifest until later in life. On the other extreme, affected individuals may suddenly appear in a pedigree in the absence of affected parents or grandparents. New mutations must be considered in these cases. While the new mutation rate for some cancer predisposition genes (e.g., neurofibromatosis) is quite high, the rate for the more common cancer predisposition genes is still being determined. Since the reproductive *fitness* (probability of passing one's genes on to the next generation) of heterozygotes for most cancer predisposition genes is assumed to be normal, many cases will be due to inherited mutations.

In dominant disorders, there may be variable manifestations of the phenotype, referred to as *expressivity.* For example, there is a subset of individuals with familial adenomatous polyposis, in which the number of polyps is less than the minimum of 100 necessary to establish the diagnosis (see Chapter 5). *Penetrance* is defined as the proportion of individuals with a mutant allele who will express the associated trait. For a relatively penetrant trait like *APC*-associated colon cancer, virtually 100% of individuals who are heterozygotes will develop colon cancer in their lifetime. Expressivity

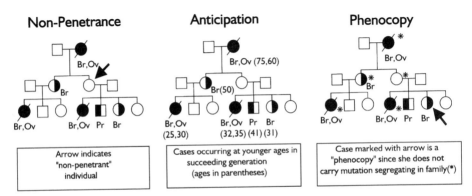

FIGURE 2-2 *Nonpenetrance, anticipation, and phenocopies in dominant syndromes. Br = breast cancer; Ov = ovarian cancer; Pr = prostate cancer*

of a gene in an individual should not be confused with the concept of penetrance of a gene in a population. In pedigrees, heterozygotes who have not developed a related cancer and whose children have inherited the altered gene are often termed *nonpenetrant* (Figure 2-2) To some extent, penetrance may be a function of how hard one looks for the phenotype. For example, it may be that tiny, undetectable cancers are actually present in a fraction of individuals thought to be nonpenetrant.

Pleiotropism refers to the many effects of a single genetic alteration. For example, alterations of a gene causing hereditary polyposis of the colon may also result in a variety of congenital abnormalities as well as susceptibilities to both upper and lower gastrointestinal tract neoplasms.

Recessive Inheritance

Although most cancer predisposition syndromes follow a dominant pattern of inheritance, there is also a group of recessive disorders. In these syndromes, it is necessary for two copies of an altered gene to be present (*homozygous state*) in order to express the features of the trait. If two parents heterozygous for such an altered gene have offspring, half will be heterozygotes, 25% will be homozygous for the normal gene, and 25% will be homozygous for the altered (cancer susceptibility) gene (see Figure 2-1).

In looking at pedigrees for rare, recessive cancer predisposition genes, common ancestors may result from marriage of related individuals (*consanguinity*). Consanguinity should be carefully sought in documenting pedigrees from such families. For example, in Bloom's syndrome, a disorder characterized by congenital abnormalities, chromosome fragility, and a tendency to develop a variety of cancers, consanguineous marriages between distant cousins were utilized to locate the gene. For at least one recessive cancer predisposition syndrome, the heterozygote frequency is so high that there may be no increased probability of consanguinity in the parents of the affected individual. It has been estimated that as many as 1% of individuals in the general population are heterozygotes for alterations of the *ATM* gene, which is associated with the ataxia telangiectasia trait in its homozygous state. The clinical features of this disorder and the possible susceptibility of heterozygotes to breast cancer are discussed in Chapter 4.

X-linked Inheritance

While infrequently encountered in cancer predisposition, sex-linked inheritance is described for other genetic disorders. An altered gene located on the X chromosome may be expressed in a dominant or recessive manner in females (XX), while such a mutation will always be expressed in the *hemizygous* males (XY). The Y chromosome appears to mediate few heritable disorders but carries the male sex-determining genes.

Non-Mendelian Inheritance

Most hereditary cancer syndromes fit patterns of Mendelian dominant inheritance. Several distinct patterns of non-Mendelian inheritance may be evident in cancer-associated pedigrees.

Sex influence in Mendelian disorders refers to the expression of a trait more commonly in one sex than another. For example, *BRCA2* heterozygotes, whether male or female, are both at increased risk for breast cancers, although this risk is substantially greater in females. In some cases there are different versions of a gene found at a given chromosomal location (locus). There may be one normal allele (wild-type), or many forms of normal alleles (*polymorphisms*). Sometimes there is different expression of

Case Example 2.2. A mother sought consultation regarding the age her 5-year-old son should start colonoscopy screening. During her own screening colonoscopy, recommended by her internist, she was found to have a focus of adenocarcinoma in a polyp at age 28. Her father was diagnosed with colon cancer after an employment physical revealed blood in the stool at age 36. Her grandmother died after presenting with metastatic colon cancer at age 60. The mother was worried about the early age of colon cancer occurrence in her family. She wanted to know if she should start screening her son immediately.

This family meets criteria for hereditary nonpolyposis colon cancer (HNPCC), a form of hereditary colon cancer discussed in Chapter 4. Colonoscopy screening should begin for her son at age 25. These conclusions are based on the median age of onset of colon cancer in HNPCC families (age 40–45) and observations regarding the timing of the adenoma-polyp sequence (see Chapter 4). As discussed in this chapter, the phenomenon of anticipation predicts an earlier age of onset in succeeding generations. However, it can also be explained by increasing intensity of screening, as evidenced in this family, over the course of time. For some genetic diseases (e.g., myotonic dystrophy), anticipation has a biological basis and must be considered in genetic counseling. For syndromes of predisposition to common malignancies such as colon cancer, guidelines concerning ages of initiation of screening have been based on analysis of penetrance of known mutations, where available, or data on age-of-onset of affected individuals in kindreds meeting accepted diagnostic criteria. Childhood colon cancer is not part of the typical pattern in HNPCC families.

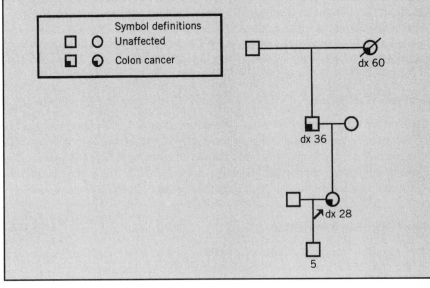

an allele, depending on from which parent the allele was inherited. *Genomic imprinting* refers to the different expression of genetic disorders depending on whether the gene was inherited from mother or father. In familial chemodectoma, a rare syndrome of head and neck cancers, the children of affected fathers but not of affected mothers appear to be at risk. In neurofibromatosis type 2, children of affected females show earlier and more severe symptoms than children of affected males. In multiple endocrine neoplasias (MEN), there appears to be an excess of affected female children of parents with MEN-associated cancers. Each of these patterns is consistent with genomic imprinting. Imprinting also appears to be a factor in the genetics of some sporadic tumors (e.g., osteosarcoma and rhabdomyosarcoma).

The concept of *anticipation* refers to the younger age or increased severity of a disease in successive generations. It has been observed in a number of nonmalignant dominant traits, for example, myotonic dystrophy, in which a genetic mechanism of unstable genetic elements (triplet repeats) has been shown to correlate with severity of disease. Anticipation may also be explained by a bias in ascertainment, where the youngest or most severe cases are noticed first, with milder disease discovered in the course of surveying prior generations. In addition, a *cohort effect* may result in the diagnosis of cases at earlier ages as exposure to other risk factors, detection technologies, or physician awareness change over time. Anticipation has been observed in some families with leukemia, as well as in ovarian cancer, but has not yet been clearly established in other cancer predisposition syndromes (Horwitz et al., 1996).

The concept of *somatic mosaicism* explains how, in a single individual, there can be genetically different cells. These differences may be due to a mutation in the embryo, leading to a patchy distribution of a clone of cells with the mutant genotype. The symptoms of the disease will also be patchy, i.e., observed only on some parts of the body. Such a distribution of abnormalities has been observed for some patients with new mutations of neurofibromatosis type 1. In families exhibiting *germline mosaicism* of a trait, there is the appearance of the trait in two or more siblings of unaffected parents. In this circumstance, a mutation presumably arose in the gonadal tissues (*germ cells*) of one of the parents (e.g., during embryogenesis of that parent). This mutation was then passed to multiple offspring. Germline mosaicism has important implications in counseling parents of a child with an apparently new mutation, because recurrence rate in a sibling may be greater than that expected in the general population. For example, in the absence of a family history of the disease, siblings of a child affected with bilateral retinoblastoma are at a greater risk for the disease. Germline mosaicism has been observed in families with retinoblastoma (Sippel et al., 1997).

Mendelian Inheritance in Man

The opening slide at Dr. Victor McKusick's annual review of mammalian genetics at the Jackson Labs in Bar Harbor, Maine, has traditionally been a picture of the first slim edition of his *Mendelian Inheritance in Man*. The most recent edition takes up two volumes, spans over 2000 pages, and has been transferred to an on-line database. A vital reference, it documents many conditions associated with an increased susceptibility to cancer. For the most part, however, these syndromes are quite rare and the susceptibility to cancer may be a secondary manifestation of a multisystem disorder. Other attempts have been made to catalogue Mendelian syndromes of cancer predisposition. A table of inherited disorders with their associated cancers is included as Appendix A. Documentation of the more common Mendelian syndromes of cancer predisposition comprise Chapters 4 and 5.

The Relationship of Genotype and Phenotype

Most human cancer susceptibility syndromes are *genetically heterogeneous,* which means that there are a number of distinct genotypes associated with similar phenotypes. Because of genetic heterogeneity, similar phenotypes may result from mutations in different genes (*locus heterogeneity*), or from different mutations within the same gene (*allelic heterogeneity*). For example, mutations in at least 5 genes can result in a syndrome of colon cancer susceptibility. The nature of both locus and allelic heterogeneity for the two major hereditary breast cancer genes is also a topic of considerable clinical significance because of the highly variable risk for ovarian cancer.

In addition to the heterogeneity considerations discussed previously, confusion in the interpretation of pedigrees associated with hereditary cancer syndromes may occur due to the existence of phenocopies. For high prevalence diseases, such as breast and colon cancer, sporadic cases (*phenocopies*) indistinguishable from other cases in the family but unrelated to those due to a genetic predisposition may exist (see Figure 2-2). As will be seen, the presence of phenocopies can cause serious overestimates in both risk and genetic linkage determinations.

A basic concept of population genetics that relates to the unusual prevalence of specific genotypes in a population is the notion of a *founder effect*. Founder effects produce a greater than expected frequency of a specific mutation in common descendants of an ancestor. This frequency results from chance genetic variations in small populations that have become amplified after migration of a founder carrying a specific mutation. The result is transmission of this mutation among the progeny of the founder, typically in a single ethnic group or geographic isolate, and a high frequency of a specific genotype associated with the phenotype. The classic example of this phenomenon is the high prevalence of a rare metabolic disease, porphyria, due to specific mutations in some South Africans. This phenomenon is explained by the historical observation that a number of founding Dutch settlers had this condition and passed specific mutations on to their descendants. As presented in Chapter 4, remarkable founder effects have been documented for breast and colon cancer among Jews of Eastern European ancestry and for colon and other cancers among a number of Scandinavian populations.

ACQUIRED RISK FACTORS FOR CANCER

An awareness of the environmental factors that caused cancer began to emerge at the same time as the hereditary susceptibilities and genetic origins of cancer were being appreciated. A new field of inquiry was spurred by the recognition of rare forms of oc-

Case Example 2.3. A 42-year-old woman came for counseling regarding a history of multiple cancers in her family. Her mother died at age 51 due to cancer of the larynx and her father had just been diagnosed with bladder cancer. She was concerned because her brother died of bladder cancer a few years ago. The proband's mother did not smoke. On questioning, the proband indicated that her siblings spent every summer during childhood and early adulthood working in her parents' tanning business in New England. The business was started by her paternal grandfather.

  The presence of horizontal transmission of a nonhereditary malignancy suggested the presence of a common occupational exposure in this family. The high risk of bladder and head and neck cancers associated with the leather industry is an association well known to epidemiologists, but was unknown to the proband or her physicians. It was recommended that she undergo surveillance urine cytologies and regular examination by an otolaryngologist.

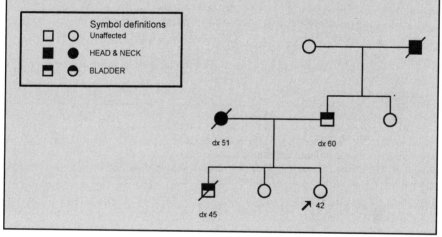

cupational cancers, and also by the obviously carcinogenic effects of ionizing radiation and certain industrial exposures in the latter half of the twentieth century. Simplified assays measured the ability of substances to cause mutations in bacteria, and these assays were used to set environmental standards to protect consumers. Experiments soon revealed that naturally occurring substances also contained significant quantities of DNA-damaging agents, suggesting that cancer risk might be dependent on differences in individual sensitivity to carcinogens as well as to the distribution of the carcinogens themselves.

The Epidemic Nature of an Environmental Cancer

Combinations of mutational assays, animal models, and epidemiologic studies established associations of specific environmental and lifestyle exposures resulting in increased risk for specific cancers (Tables 2-2 and 2-3). By far the most significant association on these lists relates to the cancer with the highest mortality rate in the United States.

TABLE 2-2   Suggested Dietary Risk Factors for Cancer

Dietary Factor	Cancer Risk	Comment
Fat	Colon	Correlation with red meat and animal fat
	Prostate	Correlation with red meat and animal fat
	Lung	Possible association
	Breast	Association unclear
Alcohol	Breast	Increased risk if in moderate to high amounts
	Colon	Increased risk if high amounts, also associated with low folic acid
Vitamin A/	Breast	May be protective
beta carotene	Lung	Lower risk with high fruits and vegetables; no protection from beta carotene or Vitamin A
	Prostate	Possible protection of high Vitamin A; no protection from beta carotene
	Head and neck	Retinoids are effective therapy in oral premalignancy; decreased second primary tumor rate
	All cancers in men	No effect of beta carotene on cancer incidence or mortality
Vitamins C and E		No proven effects on cancer risk currently known

Sources: Data from Willett WC: Diet and Cancer:what do we know now? Adv Oncology 1995; 11(4): 2–8; Hong WK, Endicott J, Itri LM et al. 13-cis-retinoic acid in the treatment of oral leukoplakia. New Eng J Med 1986; 315:1501–1505; Hong WK, Lippman SM, Itri LM et al. Prevention of second primary tumors with isotretinoin in squamous cell carcinoma of the head and neck. New Eng J Med 1990; 323:795–801; Hennekens CH, Buring J, Manson JE, et al. Lack of effect of long-term supplementation with beta carotene on the incidence of malignant neoplasms and cardiovascular disease. New Engl J Med 1996; 334:1145–9.

Cancer of the lung, unlike cancer of the breast, was unknown to Hippocrates. Astonishingly, this disease was not documented in humans until the later part of the nineteenth century. We now know that lung cancers are associated with respiratory exposure to carcinogens primarily in cigarette smoke. In 1988, lung cancer surpassed breast cancer as the greatest killer of American women. The proportion of human cancer deaths attributable to cigarette smoke dwarfs that of any other known human environmental exposure; it is estimated that 85% of the 170,000 lung cancer cases each year in the United States are attributable to smoking. When all smoking-related cancers are included, 30% of deaths from cancer in the United States are attributed to smoking. In addition, cigarette smoke is associated with more than 180,000 deaths from cardiovascular disease and 84,000 deaths from pulmonary diseases. Fortunately, cessation of smoking will reduce one's risk back to the baseline (population) cardiovascular risk in 5 years and to population lung cancer risk 10 years from time of smoking cessation. However, 46 million adults, 25% of the U.S. population, smoke. Although this percentage plunged during the 1970s and 1980s, it has remained steady during the 1990s. Six million teenagers and 100,000 children younger than age 13 smoke (data from Bartecchi, 1995).

Case Example 2.4. A 50-year-old woman sought counseling because of a history of multiple cancers in her family. Her sister was recently diagnosed with myelodysplastic syndrome. Her brothers died of acute myeloid leukemia and osteosarcoma at early age. Their mother died of lung cancer at age 82. The proband had complaints of joint pains, although her rheumatoid arthritis serologies were negative. Upon questioning, it was learned that their father owned a shoe store. During the 1950s the children would play "for hours" with a fluoroscopy unit that was in the shoe store. It was used to test the fit of customers' shoes. The proband remembered looking at her "hand bones" on several occasions.

The family was offered *p53* germline mutation testing as part of a research study (see discussion of variants of Li-Fraumeni syndrome in Chapter 5). Because of her age and disease-free status, the proband was reassured that she was unlikely to be a mutation-carrier even if a *p53* mutation was documented in her family. The review of the literature and available records revealed the most likely manufacturer of the fluoroscopy device and the associated radiation doses. The proband was reassured that the risk of transmission of cancer susceptibility to her children was small. It was recommended that MRI examinations of the affected extremities (hands and feet) be considered as surveillance for possible sarcoma, although such a strategy would be of no proven benefit.

This case represents a case of familial clustering possibly due to environmental or hereditary causes.

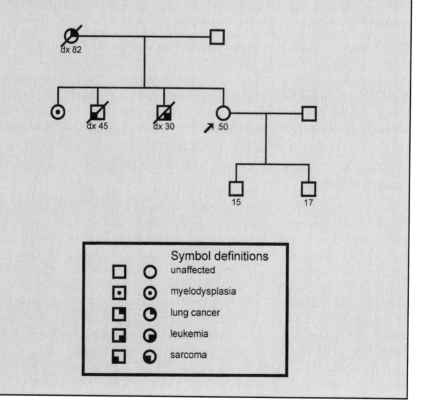

Symbol definitions

□ ○	unaffected	
▣ ◉	myelodysplasia	
◪ ◕	lung cancer	
◪ ◑	leukemia	
◪ ◐	sarcoma	

TABLE 2-3   Lifestyle and Occupational Risk Factors for Cancer

Exposure	Related Cancer
Tobacco smoking	Mouth, pharynx, larynx, lung, esophagus, stomach, pancreas, kidney, bladder
Betel nut chewing	Mouth
Sexual promiscuity	Cervix uteri
Arsenic (mining, pesticides)	Lung
Asbestos (shipyard/pipe insulation)	Lung, mesothelioma
Aromatic amines (dyes)	Bladder
Benzene (varnishes, other industrial uses)	Leukemia
Bis-ether	Lung
Shoe manufacture	Nasal cavity
Chromium (metal plating)	Lung
Hardwood manufacture	Nasal cavity
Hematite mining	Lung
Isopropyl alcohol manufacture	Para-nasal sinuses
Nickel refining	Lung, nasal sinuses
Benzidine, napthylamine (rubber industry)	Leukemia, bladder
Soots, tars, oils	Skin, lung, bladder
Vinyl chloride (PVC)	Liver (angiosarcoma)

Sources: After Doll R and Peto R. The Causes of Cancer. New York: Oxford University Press, 1981. Only those listed as with "sufficient" proof of causation are cited. Also Henderson B. Toward the primary prevention of cancer. Science 1991; 254: 1131–1137.

As a worldwide epidemic, smoking is growing, particularly in the developing countries. The epidemiologist Richard Peto has estimated that deaths due to smoking will increase from 2.5 million today to 12 million by the year 2050. The scope of this epidemic dwarfs that of AIDS and rivals that of the Great Plague of the Middle Ages.

The Relative Contributions of Hereditary and Acquired Causes of Cancer

Observations of large populations of individuals with cancer by Paget, Bilroth, Baker, Velpeau, Lichtenstern and many other investigators in Europe in the nineteenth and early twentieth centuries, and by Lynch and coworkers in the United States, revealed that 5–10% of cancers showed marked familial clustering suggesting hereditary cancer predisposition. Confirmation of these estimates would await the development of modern epidemiologic methodology in the late twentieth century. Epidemiologists have estimated that as much as 35% of cancers can be attributed to dietary risk factors, 5% to occupational exposures, and a few percent to radiation, viruses, and other known acquired risks. In view of the 30% of cancers attributed to smoking, one can put into perspective the 5–10% of cancers thought to be due to hereditary syndromes.

Even assuming the (conservative) estimate of 5–10% of cancers due to strong familial predisposition, the absolute number of cancers attributed to hereditary factors is substantial because the existing number of (*prevalent*) cancer cases due to hereditary causes is so great. As shown in Table 2-4, over 50,000 *incident* (newly diagnosed) cancers in 1997 were associated with hereditary factors. It is less known to the general public that there are in excess of 2 million survivors of breast cancer and over 1.5 million survivors of colon cancer alive in the United States (prevalent cases). Thus, one can infer that there are 175,000–350,000 prevalent hereditary malignancies, in addition to the incident hereditary cases. The data in Table 2-4 also underscore the relatively modest contribution of the hereditary cancer predisposition syndromes of children (e.g., retinoblastoma). However, it is important to note that the pediatric cancer predisposition syndromes served as a model for the discovery of the genes associated with the more common adult hereditary cancer predisposition syndromes.

Evidence for a larger hereditary component of common cancers emerged from a unique experiment of nature: the state of Utah. From the perspective of the population geneticist, Utah was a paradise. Virtually the entire population of the state could be traced back to a small number of European pioneers in the nineteenth century. Because of the prevailing practices of the Church of Latter Day Saints (the Mormons), careful attention was paid to genealogy. Even more interesting to geneticists, the early Mormons embraced polygamy; prior to 1890, 10–20% of male pioneers had multiple wives. Their leader, Brigham Young, had 29 wives. This practice resulted in large extended families (*kindreds*) and an abundance of meiotic events (children) from single founders. So great were the research opportunities posed by the Mormon genealogies, that a new wave of academic pioneers, led by Mark Skolnick, emigrated to Salt Lake City. They began to assemble a massive database that included 185,000 Utah families (1.5 million individuals) on a computer network. This Utah Genealogical Database was linked to the state cancer registry to create the Utah Population Database (Skolnick, 1980).

One product of the Utah genetic database was the calculation of a genealogic index or indices of familiarity, which could compare degree of relatedness between groups

TABLE 2-4   Incidence Rates for Hereditary Cancers in the United States

Cancer Type	Estimate of Hereditary Proportion	Incident Hereditary Cases/Year
Breast	10%	18,000
Ovarian	5%	6000
Colon	10%	15,000
Prostate	10%	25,000
Melanoma	10%	3000
Medullary thyroid	25%	125
Retinoblastoma	40%	70
Wilms' tumor	5%	25
Renal cell cancer (associated with von Hippel-Lindau syndrome)	rare (<1 in 36,000)	
Breast/sarcoma (associated with Li-Fraumeni syndrome)	rare	

of individuals in the state. Distantly related individuals might not even know one another, but the database could ascertain their common ancestors. Such individuals, living in different locations, eating different diets, having different occupations, could be linked by their common genes (Cannon-Albright, 1994). In this fashion, the genealogic index derived for common cancers reflected the degree of familiarity for each malignancy (Table 2-5).

The data in Table 2-5 confirm an increased familiarity (genealogy index) for common adult cancers of breast, ovary, colon, prostate, and malignant melanoma. Interestingly, the statistical measure of familial aggregation for some environmental cancers (e.g., lip cancer, lung cancer) appears higher than some cancers with known hereditary components (e.g., breast cancer). Other cancers not considered as commonly hereditary (e.g., testis, leukemia, brain) show marked familial aggregation.

The distinction between purely hereditary (germline) and acquired (somatic) forms of cancer is, of course, artificial. Cancer-causing chemicals and ionizing radiation damage the basic genetic elements of the cell. Most chemical carcinogens are subject to both hepatic activation and metabolism, and the phenotypes for these activities are also inherited. DNA damaging chemicals (*xenobiotics*) are detoxified by enzymes, which have been divided into two groups. The Phase I enzymes often create intermedi-

TABLE 2-5 Genealogical Index of Familiarity for Cancers by Site

Site	MRG
Testis	1.80
Lip	1.72
Thyroid	1.72
Melanoma	1.54
Leukemia	1.45
Myeloma	1.43
Connective tissue	1.40
Prostate	1.34
Brain	1.32
Colon	1.29
Lymphoma	1.29
Ovary	1.24
Lung	1.19
Breast	1.18
Stomach	1.18
Cervix	1.17
Rectum	1.11
Bladder	1.09

Source: From Table 2 in Cannon-Albright LA, Thomas A, Goldgar DE, et al. Familiarity of cancer in Utah. Cancer Res 1994; 54:2378–85.

Note: MRG = median of the distribution of the ratio of case:control genealogic indices of familiarity; only those sites for which p<.05 are shown.

ates, which are themselves potent carcinogens. The Phase II enzymes are true detoxifying agents, seeking to make the xenobiotics more water soluble so they can be excreted. Polymorphisms for the genes encoding these enzymes have been associated with risk for specific cancers. A list of selected enzymes that mediate sensitivity to carcinogens and associated cancer risks are listed in Table 2-6. As noted in the footnote to this table, studies of genetic metabolic polymorphisms and cancer risk have used a variety of methodologies to assess genotype and phenotype, with marked discordance in results.

The data in Table 2-6 may explain some of the familial clustering of environmental cancers (e.g., head and neck cancer) observed in the Utah genealogies. These traits may best be termed *polygenic* because there are multiple genetic determinants of the familial cancers observed. The multiple genetic determinants may include inherited susceptibilities to DNA damage by environmental agents, or ineffective DNA repair after the damage is done. Alternatively, these traits may be viewed as *multifactorial,* i.e., due to a combination of both inherited genetic as well as nongenetic factors. Other multifactorial human disorders include diabetes and heart disease, in which genetic as well as environmental factors determine risk of the disease.

TABLE 2-6 Selected Xenobiotic Metabolizing Enzymes with Known Genetic Polymorphisms and Associated Cancer Risks

Phase I Metabolism	Phase II Metabolism
Oxidation	*Conjugation*
• Cytochrome p450 　*CYP1A1* (aryl hydrocarbon hydroxylase)(**L**) 　*CYP2D6* (debrisoquine hydroxylase)(**L**)(**Br**)(**Bl**) • Alcohol and aldehyde dehydrogenase	• Glutathione-S-transferase 　*GSTM1* (**L**)(**Co**)(**St**) • N-acetyl transferase 　*NAT1* (**Bl**) 　*NAT2* (**Bl**)(**Co**)(**Br**)
Hydrolysis	*Methylation*
• Epoxide hydrolase	• O,N,S, methyltransferase
Radical scavengers	*Sulphation*
• Superoxide dismutase	• Sulphonotransferases
	Glucuronidation
	• UDP glucuronyl transferase

Sources: Data from Smith CAD, Smith G, Wolf LR. Genetic polymorphism in xenobiotic metabolism. Eur J Can 1994; 30A(13):1921–35; d'Errico A, Taioli E, Xiang C, Vineis P. Genetic metabolic polymorphisms and the risk of cancer: a review of the literature. Biomarkers 1996; 1:149–173; Rebbeck TR, Blackwood MA, Walker AH et al. Association of breast cancer incidence with NAT2 genotype and smoking in BRCA1 carriers. Am J Hum Genet 1997; 61:242 (abstr).
Notes: Cancer risks shown in bold: L= lung cancer; Br = breast cancer; Bl = bladder cancer; Co = colon cancer; St = stomach cancer.

REFERENCES

Bartecchi CE, MacKenzie TD, Schrier RW. 1995. The global tobacco epidemic. Scientific American May: 272:44–51.

Boyd M, Harris F, McFarlane R, Davidson HR, Black DM. 1995. A human *BRCA1* gene knock-out. Nature 375:541–2.

Broca P. 1886. Traite des tumeurs. Paris, France: Asselin.

Cannon-Albright LA, Thomas A, Goldgar DE, Gholami K, Rowe K, Jacobsen M, McWhorter WP, Skolnick MH. 1994. Familiality of cancer in Utah. Cancer Res 54:2378–85.

d'Errico A, Taioli E, Xiang C, Vineis P. 1996. Genetic metabolic polymorphisms and the risk of cancer: a review of the literature. Biomarkers 1:149–173.

Ewing J. 1922. Neoplastic Diseases: A treatise on tumors. Philadelphia: W. B. Saunders Co., 17, 18, 19, 105–8.

Horwitz M., Goode EL, Jarvik GP. 1996. Anticipation in familial leukemia. Am J Hum Genet 59:990–98.

Lynch HT. 1976. Cancer Genetics. Springfield, Ill.: Charles C Thomas Co.

Schneider NR, William WR, Chaganti RSK. 1986. Genetic epidemiology of familial aggregation of cancer. Adv in Cancer Research 47:1–36.

Sippel KC, Fraioli RE, Smith GD, Schalkoff ME, Dryja TP. 1997. Frequent somatic and germi-line mosaicism in retinoblastoma: relevance to genetic counseling. Am J Hum Genet 61:75 (abstr).

Skolnick MH. 1980. The Utah genealogical data base: a resource for genetic epidemiology. In Banbury Report No. 4: Cancer Incidence in Defined Populations (eds. J Cairns, JL Lyon, and MH Skolnick) Cold Spring Harbor Laboratory Press, New York: 285–97.

Warthin AS. 1913. Heredity with reference to carcinoma as shown by the study of the cases examined in the pathological laboratory of the University of Michigan, 1895–1913. Arch Intern Med 12:546–55.

Willet WC. 1995. Diet and cancer: What do we know now? Adv Oncology 11:3–8.

3

Cancer as a Genetic Disorder

The discussion of the results of a genetic test or the meaning of a diagnosis of a hereditary cancer predisposition syndrome requires a general knowledge of cancer genetics. In offering patients test results concerning possible myocardial damage or counseling patients about the risk of a sexually transmitted disease, the health professional can draw on a substantial education in physiology and infectious disease. However, most of what we know of the molecular genetics of cancer was discovered relatively recently, and health professionals may have only a superficial understanding of the meaning of specific mutations or the way in which genetic defects cause cancer.

This chapter outlines the current understanding of the genetic basis of cancer and describes the major classes of cancer-causing genes that have relevance to clinical practice today: oncogenes, tumor suppressor genes, and DNA-damage response genes (reviewed by Cavenee and White, 1995; Hartwell and Kastan, 1994; Weinberg, 1991, 1996; Rabbitts, 1994; Krontiris, 1995; Latchman, 1996; Malkin and Portwine, 1994). *Oncogenes* are genes, normally involved in cell growth and proliferation, that cause cancer when they are overexpressed, amplified, or mutated. *Tumor suppressor genes,* on the other hand, normally regulate cell growth, and only result in malignant progression when their negative regulatory controls are impaired. Recently, a third group of genes involved in regulating DNA repair has been implicated in hereditary human cancers. This class of DNA damage response genes shares many of the features of tumor suppressor genes.

As depicted in Figure 3-1, the three types of genes can be thought of as acting at different phases of the dividing cell. The oncogenes act as accelerators of growth during the G1 or growth phase of the cell cycle. The suppressor genes act as stop signals before the S or synthesis phase of the cycle. The third class act as repairmen, identifying and fixing DNA mismatches following DNA replication, just before the chromosomes condense in G2 phase for mitosis (M). When individuals are born with muta-

Cell Cycle

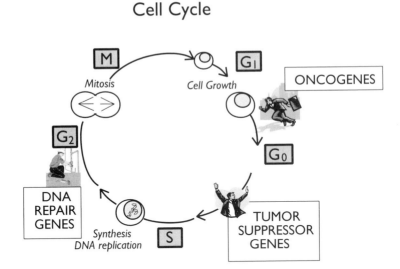

FIGURE 3-1 *The major classes of cancer-causing genes. Oncogenes act to accelerate cells during the G1 or growth phase of the cell cycle, whereas tumor suppressor genes normally act as breaks against cell growth and proliferation, with a check point just before DNA synthesis begins in S phase. A third class of repair genes fix DNA mismatches after synthesis and DNA replication.*

tions of a gene in one of these three groups, they are susceptible to one or more types of cancer.

THE MOLECULAR BASIS OF HUMAN DISEASES

The experiments proving that nucleic acids were the vehicles of hereditary information were carried out by Avery, MacLeod, and McCarthy in 1944. They showed that an extract containing nucleic acids could change a colony of bacteria from "rough" to "smooth" coat variety. These early experiments in bacteria established the foundation for modern molecular genetics, but it took many years to determine the way in which genetic information was stored in nucleic acids.

During the 1950s and 1960s, it was discovered that nucleic acids were composed of long chains of nucleotides. Each nucleotide was composed of a nitrogenous base, a sugar molecule, and a phosphate molecule. If the sugar moiety contained ribose, the acid was called *ribonucleic acid* (RNA). If the sugar was deoxyribose, the acid was called *deoxyribonucleic acid* (DNA). The nitrogenous bases include purines and pyrimidines. The purines are adenine (A) and guanine (G), and the pyrimidines are cytosine (C), thymine (T), and uracil (U). Thymine is found only in DNA and uracil only in RNA.

The contribution of Watson and Crick in 1953 was to propose a structure for DNA that explained how it carried genetic information and how it reproduced itself during cell division. They proposed that the DNA molecule was composed of two nucleotide chains arranged in a double helix. The double helix was held together by hydrogen bonds between complementary bases A—T and G—C. The bases at the center were attached to the backbone of the molecule, consisting of sugar and phosphate molecules. The orientation of the two chains was determined by whether a 5′ or 3′ carbon atom in the sugar was at the end, with the two strands running in opposite (antiparallel) directions (Figure 3-2). This complementarity offered a ready mechanism for replication, because each chain could serve as the template for the generation of a "daughter" strand.

Since there are 20 amino acids in various proteins and only 4 nucleic acid bases, it was deduced that a sequence of 3 bases (a codon) would be necessary to specify a distinct amino acid. This would yield 4^3 (64) combinations, although only 20 are needed. Because of the excess of combinations, some amino acids are coded for by several triplet sequences (resulting in redundancy or *degeneracy* of the code).

Genetic information is communicated from DNA to *messenger RNA* (*mRNA*) by the process of *transcription,* and the mRNA is *translated* into an amino acid sequence to make a protein. Translation takes place in cytoplasmic ribosomes outside of the nucleus. The mRNA is translated to protein by *transfer RNA* (*tRNA*), which recognizes specific amino acids and incorporates them into the growing polypeptide chain.

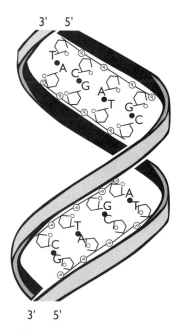

FIGURE 3-2 *Structure of DNA. The DNA molecule is composed of two nucleotide chains arranged in a double helix. The double helix is held together by hydrogen bonds between complementary bases A—T and G—C. The bases at the center are attached to the backbone of the molecule, consisting of sugar and phosphate molecules. The orientation of the two chains is determined by whether a 5′ or 3′ carbon atom in the sugar is at the end, with the two strands running in opposite (antiparallel) directions.*

Gene Structure

Most DNA (80%) does not code for proteins. Some of this DNA codes for the various RNAs, and some is clustered around centromeres (satellite DNA). For most DNA the function is not known. Even within genes, there are noncoding DNA sequences (*introns*), between the translated portions (*exons*) (Figure 3-3). RNA transcription from DNA may be initiated by TATA and CAT boxes, located on the 5' side of genes. The 100-300 base pair promoter region contains TATA and CAT boxes as well as regions rich in the paired nucleotides cytosine and guanine (CG islands). Other sequence elements, called *enhancers*, may be located a significant distance from the gene and act to stimulate transcription. During transcription, the precursor RNA from the exons is spliced together, removing the intronic sequences. Messenger RNA'S also have a string of adenosines at their 3' end that seems to play a role in transport out of the nucleus.

Identification of New Genes

In order to screen a cancer predisposition gene for mutations, it is necessary to know its precise sequence. The various methodologies for identification of the sequences of disease-causing genes marked the high point of the "recombinant DNA revolution" in the 1980s. Two basic strategies of isolating (cloning) genes have been used. The first approach looks for expression of the gene at the mRNA level. If the target gene is expressed in high quantity in a specific tissue, the mRNA can be converted into double

"Typical" Gene

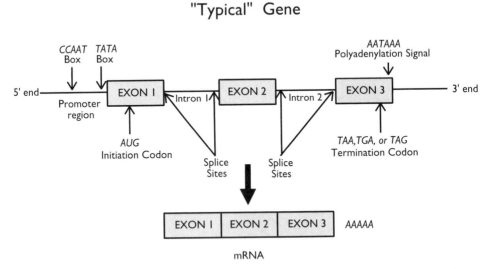

mRNA

FIGURE 3-3 *Gene structure. Genes are composed of noncoding DNA (introns), between the translated portions (exons). Transcription from DNA may be initiated by TATA and CCAAT boxes, which lie in promoter regions of the gene. Toward the end of the gene are sequences encoding the poly A tail of the protein. Transcription ends with a termination codon in the DNA. During transcription, the precursor RNA from the exons is spliced together to form messenger RNA (mRNA) that will be translated into protein.*

stranded DNA (called complementary DNA or cDNA) by the enzyme reverse transcriptase. This technique was utilized to clone the gene for hemoglobin. Alternatively, if the amino acid sequence of a protein can be derived using the genetic code, a synthetic DNA molecule (oligonucleotide) can be matched to the predicted sequence. Even if the amino acid sequence is not known, antibodies to the protein can be generated and used to "pull out" ribosomes in the process of making the protein. These ribosomes will have some partially translated mRNA in them, which can then be used to generate the clone.

A second set of cloning strategies was initially termed *reverse* genetics because it assumed no prior knowledge of the protein structure, or any biochemical understanding about the basis of a disease. Now referred to as *positional* gene cloning, these strategies aim to locate the position of disease-causing genes. Two techniques are employed: physical mapping and genetic mapping. Physical mapping in cancer genetics has been aided by the many structural chromosomal abnormalities that have pinpointed the locations of cancer-causing genes. Genetic mapping, utilizing genetic material from large families affected by cancers, has recently had resounding success in identifying a number of important cancer susceptibility genes. As is shown in the next section, the strategies employed to identify cancer predisposition genes have combined both physical and genetic mapping approaches.

Mutations

Mutations are changes in the DNA sequence. Mutations can affect even a single base pair of a DNA molecule, producing disastrous consequences on the corresponding protein. If the single base pair (point) mutation results in another triplet that codes for the same amino acid (due to degeneracy), there will be no effect. This may occur in a quarter of all mutations. Alternatively, the mutation may result in the substitution of an incorrect amino acid (*missense mutation*) which may cause reduction or loss of function of the protein. In about 2% of point mutations, a premature "stop" signal (*nonsense mutation*) is generated, causing termination of the peptide chain. Alternatively, there may be the insertion or deletion of one or more bases that will shift the reading frame of the triplet sequence (Figure 3-4). These *frameshift* mutations result in an abnormal, often unstable, mRNA. As shown in Figure 3-4, frameshift mutations often occur in sequences where there are repeats, for example, the AG in the 185delAG, or the run of C's in the 5382insC mutation of *BRCA1*. These repetitive patterns may lead to slipping of the template strand of DNA and a resulting deletion or insertion of a base pair. Mutations may also occur in the promotor, or enhancer sequences, resulting in altered levels of structurally normal protein. Mutations may also occur in the intron/exon splice sites. Finally, mutations in the polyA tail can influence the stability of the mRNA, which can also lead to decreased protein synthesis.

Of the various types of mutations described, missense mutations pose the greatest diagnostic challenge. The question arises whether the missense mutation is a normal polymorphism observed in the general population or a disease-causing change. When the function of the gene is known, it may be possible to devise a functional assay to deduce whether the observed mutation will inactivate the normal protein. In the absence

Deletions

◉ (truncating)
BRCA1   normal   5' .....ATC TTA GAG TGT CCC..... 3'
185delAG   mutant   5' .....ATC TTA GTG TCC C....ter 3'

◉ (in-frame deletion)
MLH1   normal   5' .....T GAA GAA GAA G...............3'
ΔK617   mutant   5' .....T GAA GAA G........................3'

Insertion

BRCA1   normal   5' .....AAT CCC AGG ACA GA.......3'
5382insC   mutant   5' .....AAT CCC CAG GAC AGA....3'

Single base pair substitution

◉ missense

CDKN2   normal   5' .....C GAT GTC TCA CG..............3'
val 118asp   mutant   5' .....C GAT GAC TCA G...............3'
(V118D)

◉ splice donor site

hMLH1   normal   5' ......A TCG gtaagt............3'
IVS15+1G→A mutant   5' ......A TCG ataagt...........3'

FIGURE 3-4 *Examples of pathogenic mutations in cancer predisposition genes. Key: upper case nucleotides (A,T,C,G) correspond to exons; lower case to introns. In the 185delAG BRCA1 mutation, there is deletion of two base pairs in codon 23, at nucleotide 185. This causes a stop signal to occur in codon 39. In the in-frame deletion in exon 18 at codon 616-618 of hMLH1, there is the deletion of one amino acid spacer that results in changes in the functional conformation of the hMLH1 polypeptide. The insertion C mutation of BRCA1 at nucleotide 5382 in codon 1756 results in a stop signal in codon 1829. The missense mutation at nucleotide 371 in codon 118 of CDKN2 results in the substitution of a valine by an aspartic acid. The substitution of an adenine for a guanine at the splice donor site for exon 15 (in intervening sequence (IVS) 15) of the hMLH1 gene leads to the deletion of the entire exon.*

of functional assays, indirect means are often employed to make this determination. The presence of the mutation in control panels of normal volunteers and the lack of association of the mutation with affected members within families constitute two lines of evidence against the deleterious role of a particular missense mutation.

The identification of specific mutations cited in clinical or research reports follows certain conventions (Beaudet and Tsui, 1993). An understanding of this nomenclature is important both to decipher laboratory reports and to explain findings to patients and their families. Keys to the genetic code and alphabetical abbreviations for amino acids are provided in Table 3-1.

A mutation is described according to its type and location within the gene. One method of finding the mutation is by the exon and codon location where it occurred. Thus, for example, one of the common mutations causing breast cancer susceptibility occurs in the 23rd codon, which is in the second exon of the *BRCA1* gene. This mutation is a frameshift mutation and is written 185delAG, signifying that at the 185th nucleotide, a deletion of an adenosine and a guanine occurred. (In fact, depending on where the first nucleotide is counted, the deletion occurs at the 187th nucleotide of the normal sequence, leading some laboratories to refer to this mutation as "187delAG".) If more than two nucleotides are deleted, the number of nucleotides is written instead. Thus 926ins11 means that at the 926th nucleotide an insertion of 11 additional nucleotides occurred. If exactly three nucleotides are deleted, the symbol "delta" (Δ) is utilized followed by the single-letter symbol for the amino acid that is deleted. This is called an *in frame* deletion, because the order of the following nucleotides is not al-

TABLE 3-1   Genetic and Alphabetic Code for Amino Acids

First Base	Second Base				Third Base
	U	C	A	G	
U	UUU phe	UCU ser	UAU tyr	UGU cys	U
	UUC phe	UCC ser	UAC tyr	UGC cys	C
	UUA leu	UCA ser	UAA stop	UGA stop	A
	UUG leu	UCG ser	UAG stop	UGG trp	G
C	CUU leu	CCU pro	CAU his	CGU arg	U
	CUC leu	CCC pro	CAC his	CGC arg	C
	CUA leu	CCA pro	CAA gln	CGA arg	A
	CUG leu	CCG pro	CAG gln	CGG arg	G
A	AUU ile	ACU thr	AAU asn	AGU ser	U
	AUC ile	ACC thr	AAC asn	AGC ser	C
	AUA ile	ACA thr	AAA lys	AGA arg	A
	AUG met	ACG thr	AAG lys	AGG arg	G
G	GUU val	GCU ala	GAU asp	GGU gly	U
	GUC val	GCC ala	GAC asp	GGC gly	C
	GUA val	GCA ala	GAA glu	GGA gly	A
	GUG val	GCG ala	GAG glu	GGG gly	G

Note: Abbreviations for amino acids:

ala (A)	alanine	gln (Q)	glutamine	leu (L)	leucine	ser (S)	serine
arg (R)	arginine	glu (E)	glutamic acid	lys (K)	lysine	thr (T)	threonine
asn (N)	asparagine	gly (G)	glycine	met (M)	methionine	trp (W)	tryptophan
asp (D)	aspartic acid	his (H)	histidine	phe (F)	phenylalanine	tyr (Y)	tyrosine
cys (C)	cysteine	ille (I)	isoleucine	pro (P)	proline	val (V)	valine

tered. Thus, a frequent mutation causing cystic fibrosis is called ΔF508, signifying a three base pair deletion encoding phenylalanine at codon 508.

If the resulting frameshift results in a termination signal, the amino acid in which the termination occurs may also be noted. For example, 926ins11→ter301 means that an 11 nucleotide insertion resulted in a termination or truncation of the protein at the 301st amino acid. For missense and nonsense mutations, the description generally includes the normal (wild-type) amino acid, the affected codon, and the altered amino acid (or "ter" if the mutation results in a termination). Thus, arg1443gly and glu1541ter signify the substitution of a glycine for an arginine at the 1443rd codon, and a mutation resulting in a stop signal at the 1541st codon, respectively. Increasingly, the single-letter codes for the amino acid are utilized, with X signifying a change to a stop codon (nonsense mutation). For example, the arg1443gly would be R1443G, and glu1541ter would be E1541X.

Splice site mutations are noted by a + or − sign that indicates the location of the mutation relative to the beginning or end of the exon. Some authors note these mutations as IVS (intervening sequence), while others use the nucleotide position, followed by + or − and the type of substitution, deletion, or insertion. For example, the mutation IVS15+1G→ A of the *hMLH1* gene is illustrated in Figure 3-4. This mutation occurs one nucleotide into intron 15 of the gene.

Amino acid polymorphisms may be described with a slash between the benign alleles, and DNA polymorphisms with a slash between the nucleotide variants. For example, a common polymorphism in exon 16 of *BRCA1* is M1652I, which may also be written as 5075G/A.

Once a cancer predisposition gene is isolated, there begins the process of describing the mutations that can affect it. Human diseases may have very different patterns of causative mutations at the molecular level (*genetic heterogeneity*). From the diagnostic point of view, it is obviously desirable if all cases of the disease are due to a specific mutation. This is true, for example, in sickle cell anemia, where a single missense mutation in codon 6 of the gene encoding hemoglobin results in all known cases of the disease in humans. For some of the common cancer predisposition syndromes, there are over a hundred discrete mutations associated with the same disease phenotype.

THE DISCOVERY OF TUMOR SUPPRESSOR GENES

The existence of tumor suppressor genes was predicted in 1971 by Dr. Alfred Knudson (Knudson, 1971). His two-hit model for retinoblastoma, and the subsequent model for Wilms' tumor by Knudson and Strong, explained the pattern of inheritance of cancers in these families. In these syndromes, the tumors occur at early age and are commonly bilateral. Retinoblastoma, a tumor of the retinal tissue of the eye, is observed in multiple family members about 40% of the time. Children with a family history of retinoblastoma tend to be younger when they develop the disease and are more likely to have both eyes affected. Alfred Knudson, a mathematically inclined geneticist and pediatrician, devised a model to account for these observations.

According to the Knudson model, individuals could be born with a predisposition to cancer inherited in Mendelian dominant fashion from the parent (see Figure 3-5). In order to develop cancer, however, there would have to be a second hit causing an alteration in a second gene in the cancerous tissue. The model explained why a child born with the first hit inherited in all of the cells of the body (including both retinas) would be more likely to get cancer in both eyes and at an earlier age. Another child, born without the first hit would develop cancers at a later age, and only in one eye, as the likelihood of the independent origin of both events in each eye during the limited developmental period of cell division would be infinitesimally small.

The Knudson model combined the concept of dominant inheritance of a susceptibility gene with a recessive mechanism of cancer development at the cellular level. The cellular event was recessive because both copies of the susceptibility allele needed to

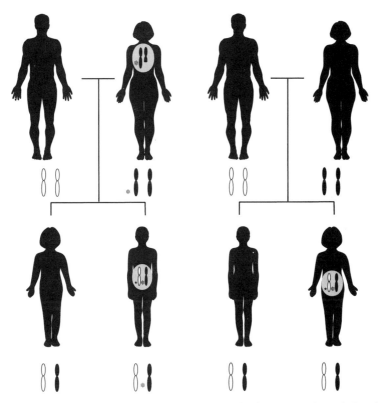

FIGURE 3-5 *The Knudson two-hit model. Inherited genetic changes are shown below the figures, while genetic changes in tumors are shown in circles inside the figures. In each tumor there are two hits or alterations of genes. In the family on the left, some individuals are born with one genetic hit already present in every cell of their body. These families will develop tumors more frequently and at an early age. The mother has an inherited mutation and has a missing segment of a chromosome in her tumor (the second hit.) Her son has the mutation he inherited from her plus a second mutation in his tumor. In the family on the right, the child was not born with an inherited predisposition to cancer, however both hits occurred in her tissues and a tumor developed.*

be altered for the phenotype to be expressed. If both alleles needed to be knocked out in the cell, it was logical to think of their normal function as cancer-preventing genes. In this way, Knudson's model anticipated a future discovery (tumor suppressor genes). Convincing evidence for tumor suppressor genes came from Stanbridge's observation that normal cells could actually suppress the malignant phenotype when mixed with cancerous cells of the same species in fusion experiments. Stanbridge's observations gave rise to the notion that so-called suppressor genes were defective in the cancerous cells (Stanbridge, 1976).

As was the case with the first oncogenes, the cloning of the tumor suppressor genes associated with a pediatric cancer syndrome was prompted by a cytogenetic observation. The syndrome was hereditary retinoblastoma, which had served as the example for the Knudson model. In a patient with hereditary retinoblastoma, a specific chromosomal deletion was observed in the "normal" circulating blood cells. Unlike chromosomal translocations, in which all of the rearranged material was accounted for, DNA was missing from the deleted chromosome. It was realized that a deletion could signify one of the hits in Knudson's two-hit model. A deleted region on the long arm of chromosome 13 in the normal lymphocytes of an individual as well as in a retinoblastoma tumor hinted at where to search for the gene. For the isolation of the *RB1* gene, the strategy taken was one of reverse genetics or linkage analysis, based on families with multiple cancer occurrences.

The method of genetic linkage analysis took advantage of the phenomenon of *recombination* that normally occurs during meiosis. Genetic recombination forms the basis for the genetic diversity within species. During recombination, new combinations of genes result from *crossing over* of homologous portions of the chromosome during meiosis. *Linkage* is defined as the tendency for two markers (alleles) close together on the same chromosome to be transmitted together through meiosis. Linkage is thus a statistical measurement of the frequency of recombination. Genetic distance is measured as the genetic length of a chromosome over which, on average, one recombination event is observed per meiosis. This unit is called the *Morgan* and is equal to about 100 million basepairs (see also Chapter 6). DNA markers closely linked to the disease gene are analyzed to observe if they cosegregate with the disease phenotype in a family (Figure 3-6).

By utilizing molecular markers around the region of deletion seen in the patient affected by retinoblastoma, it was possible to identify those markers that most frequently coincided with the affected family members. In isolating the *RB1* gene, Friend and coworkers were aided by the tight linkage of the esterase D gene to the retinoblastoma trait in families. Chromosome "walking" from this marker was a key element in the cloning strategy. In addition, the search was aided by the observation of a homozygous loss at this locus in a retinoblastoma tumor. Approaches to positional cloning, similar to those for *RB1*, have proved successful for a number of common cancer susceptibility genes (Table 3-2). Both of the major susceptibility genes for breast and ovarian cancer, *BRCA1* and *BRCA2,* were characterized by classical positional cloning techniques. In the case of *BRCA2*, as in *RB1*, the identification of a homozygous region of deletion in a tumor served as the key to recognizing the region of interest.

Recent technical advances have made available hundreds of highly polymorphic

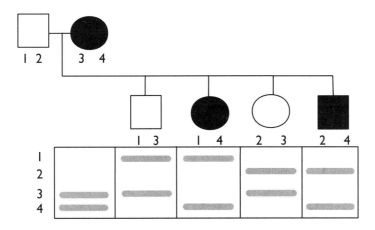

FIGURE 3-6 *Linkage analysis using DNA markers. Haplotypes are shown below the corresponding member of the pedigree. The 4 allele cosegregates with the disease phenotype (blackened circles and squares).*

markers scattered throughout the human genome that can be used in linkage studies. In addition, progress in the mapping of genes, due to the Human Genome Project, has made it possible for investigators to search directly for mutations of known candidate genes in the region defined by linkage studies. This was the strategy for the identification of the *CDKN2/p16* gene identified by studies of families with hereditary melanoma. Such "candidate gene" strategies were also utilized in the identification of *RET* gene mutations in multiple endocrine neoplasia 2a, mutations of the human *PTCH* homologue in Gorlin syndrome, and for some of the genes associated with hereditary colon cancer. With the faster-than-predicted progress of the Human Genome Project, its director, Francis Collins, has predicted that candidate gene analysis will come to dominate gene discovery in the next century (Collins, 1996).

The Function of Tumor Suppressor Genes

Unlike oncogenes, in which a single mutation may result in a cancer-causing gain of function, a loss of function of both copies of a tumor suppressor gene is generally required to induce cancer. The protein products of tumor suppressor genes would therefore be expected to inhibit cellular growth. Although the products of the tumor suppressor genes have been less well studied than their proto-oncogene counterparts, a number of observations about their function have emerged.

The protein products of some tumor suppressor genes localize to the nucleus and interact with proto-oncogene products. At least three tumor suppressor genes, including *RB1*, *WT1*, as well as *p53*, encode *transcription factors*. Transcription factors regulate other genes. However, the mechanisms of action of transcription factors vary. RB1 protein binds another transcription factor (E2F) and prevents it from stimulating other

TABLE 3-2   Three Classes of Cancer Predisposition Genes

Gene	Syndrome
Tumor suppressor genes associated with cancer predisposition	
APC	Familial adenomatous polyposis
VHL	von Hippel-Lindau syndrome
WT1	Wilms' tumor syndromes
RB1	Hereditary retinoblastoma
NF1	Neurofibromatosis 1
NF2	Neurofibromatosis 2
p53	Li-Fraumeni syndrome
p16/CDK4	Hereditary melanoma syndromes
PTCH	Nevoid basal cell carcinoma syndrome
MEN1	Multiple endocrine neoplasia 1
BRCA1[a]	Breast ovarian cancer syndrome
BRCA2[a]	Breast ovarian cancer syndrome
DNA damage response genes associated with cancer predisposition	
hMSH2	Hereditary nonpolyposis colon cancer
hMLH1	Hereditary nonpolyposis colon cancer
hPMS1	Hereditary nonpolyposis colon cancer
hPMS2	Hereditary nonpolyposis colon cancer
ATM	Ataxia telangiectasia[b]
XPA,C,D,F	Xeroderma pigmentosum
BLM	Bloom syndrome
Oncogenes associated with cancer predisposition	
RET	Multiple endocrine neoplasia 2, familial medullary thyroid cancer
MET	Familial papillary renal carcinoma syndrome

[a]Show features of tumor suppressor genes as well as interactions with *RAD51* DNA repair gene (see text).
[b]May be associated with radiation sensitivity when a heterozygous mutation is present.

genes, including *MYC*. Both the *WT1* and the *p53* gene product bind directly to DNA.

Surpassing the *RAS* oncogene and *RB1* as the most frequently mutated gene in human cancers, *p53* functions as "the guardian of the genome" (reviewed in Chang et al., 1995; Weinberg 1993, 1996). It allows cells to divide only if DNA is undamaged. Thus, a functioning *p53* serves as a check against a cancerous cell with mutations in its DNA. A defective *p53* allows the abnormal cell to proliferate. The *p53* gene performs its guardian role by binding to DNA, resulting in the expression of genes that inhibit cell growth and in expression of the *BAX* gene, promoting senescent cell death (apoptosis). Mutations of *p53* prevent it from binding DNA. The mutant p53 protein may also bind with normal *p53*, preventing the normal gene product from binding DNA. Finally, normal *p53* can be inactivated by overexpression of the *MDM2* oncogene, commonly observed in soft tissue sarcoma.

In contrast to *p53*, which stimulates inhibitory genes, the *WT1* gene product binds to DNA and is thought to function as a transcriptional repressor. It is believed that *WT1* directly inhibits expression of growth promoting genes, including a number of growth factors and their receptors. Thus, a mutation in *WT1* would result in enhanced expression of these genes. The model is made more complex, however, by the observation that, at least in vitro, *WT1* also binds with the p53 protein.

Although *p53* is the most frequently mutated gene in human tumors, it is relatively rarely inherited in a mutated state. When an individual is born with one altered copy of *p53*, that individual is predisposed to the development of sarcomas, breast cancer, and certain other tumors (see Chapter 5). Similarly, individuals born with mutations of *RB1* develop eye tumors, and also sarcomas. The reasons for these tumor specificities, and the relationship to the function of tumor suppressor genes, are not yet understood.

Tumor Suppressor Genes and the Cell Cycle

The identification of susceptibility genes for familial melanoma, a deadly form of skin cancer, focused clinical interest on the mechanisms of cell cycle control. Based on 11 large kindreds, it was possible to map a melanoma susceptibility gene, *MLM,* to a 2 centiMorgan region on chromosome 9p. Combining deletion mapping in tumors and a candidate gene approach, the gene *CDKN2* was identified. Familiar to students of the cell cycle, *CDKN2* was known to encode the p16 protein. As shown in Figure 3-7, p16 functions to specifically block the cyclin D1-CDK4 complex. This complex is one of the earliest cyclin-dependent kinase complexes of the cell cycle.

As the cell transitions from G1 to mitosis, each of the *cyclins* are briefly expressed, in the order cyclin D,E,A, and B. A succession of *kinase* units (called *cyclin-dependent kinases* or CDKs) are expressed along with the cyclins: CDK4 with the D cyclins early

---

Case Example 3.1. A woman came for consultation, referred by her clinician because of concern about cancer risk in her children. In the course of her postoperative recovery after a resection of a colon tumor at a teaching hospital, her physician was informed of genetic abnormalities identified in her tumor specimen. Mutations of the *APC* and *p53* genes were noted in her tumor. Her physician was concerned about risks of colon cancer and other risks in her children.

This case is illustrative of the potential for miscommunication that may occur when research genetic testing of tumors becomes confused with genetic testing performed to determine familial cancer risk. In this case, there were no germline mutations of *p53* or *APC,* since normal fibroblasts from the patient were used as controls in the experiments performed. There were no family history or physical findings suggestive of Li-Fraumeni syndrome or familial adenomatosis coli, discussed in Chapters 4 and 5. The acquisition of genetic changes such as *APC* or *p53* mutations as "secondary" abnormalities is a feature of the multi hit theory of the genetic origin of tumors. Such genetic changes may have prognostic significance for the affected patient (Chapter 8), but they are not transmitted to the next generation since they are not present in the germline.

Cell Cycle

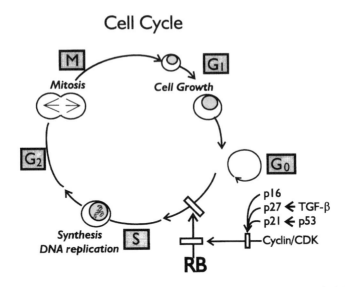

FIGURE 3-7 *Tumor suppressor genes and the cell cycle. The* p16, p27, *and* p21 *proteins specifically block the cyclin-CDK complexes that normally phosphorylate the RB protein, allowing the cell to progress past G1 in the cell cycle. The* p53 *protein induces* p21, *and* TGFβ *protein induces* p27. *Mutations in these genes remove the inhibitory pressure on the cyclin dependent kinases, allowing them to phosphorylate RB, removing its block on cellular proliferation. Mutations of RB1 directly act to remove the ability of RB protein to arrest cells in G0, and allow for cellular proliferation (see text).*

in the cycle as a response to growth factors, CDK2 with cyclins E or A during DNA replication, and CDC2 with cyclins A and B during mitosis. The cyclin-CDK complexes phosphorylate the *RB1* protein, allowing the cell to progress past G1 in the cell cycle. In addition to the inhibition of CDK4 by p16, the p27 and p21 proteins serve as CDK inhibitors. The pathways for control of these inhibitory proteins are under active inquiry (Hartwell and Kastan, 1994).

A number of cyclins have been implicated as oncogenes (e.g., cyclin D2 in mantle cell lymphoma, cyclin D1 and E in breast and other cancers). Thus far, germline mutations of only one CDK inhibitor (*CDKN2*/p16) has been implicated as a tumor suppressor gene associated with an hereditary cancer predisposition syndrome (melanoma). However, other tumor suppressor genes interact with these proteins. These include *p53* induction of p21, and *RB1*, which is the target of an activated cyclin-dependent kinase. Both *RB1* and *p53* bind the SV40 large T antigen, and have been shown to be interrelated in the complex web of cyclin-dependent kinases that regulate progression of cells through the cell cycle. The large T antigen is also part of a critical pathway in viral carcinogenesis. These observations unite the concepts of tumor suppressor genes and cell cycle control. The elucidation of the genetic mechanisms of cell cycle control has also provided a novel and exciting model for cancer therapies directed at modulating progression of malignant cells through the cell cycle.

DNA DAMAGE RESPONSE GENES

Mutations in a distinct group of genes implicated in human cancer share a phenotypic feature: defective repair of DNA damage and a susceptibility to a range of tumor types. The first group of syndromes of deficient DNA repair is associated primarily with skin and hematologic malignancies and displays the typical patterns of inheritance of autosomal recessive disorders. A second group of DNA repair deficient syndromes is associated primarily with an increased risk for colon cancer, and more closely resembles the features of cancer susceptibility syndromes due to inherited mutations in tumor suppressor genes.

Autosomal Recessive Cancer Predisposition Syndromes Associated with Deficient DNA Repair

There was solid clinical evidence that defective repair of genetic damage could result in an increased susceptibility to cancer. This evidence was supplied by a number of well-characterized but rare clinical conditions associated with chromosomal instability following DNA damage. These conditions, Fanconi anemia, Bloom syndrome, ataxia-telangiectasia, and xeroderma pigmentosum, were all associated with increased rates of cancers. In Fanconi anemia, a sensitivity of cells to small concentrations of DNA cross-linking agents was used as a diagnostic test for the condition. In ataxia-telangiectasia, repair of DNA damage by ionizing radiation was found to be defective. In Bloom syndrome, chromosome instability was also observed. In xeroderma pigmentosum, the tissue of sun-sensitive individuals exhibited deficient excision-repair of DNA damage due to ultraviolet radiation. These individuals commonly developed skin cancers.

Single genes or, in the case of Fanconi anemia and xeroderma pigmentosum, multiple genes, have recently been identified and associated with these disorders. While the precise functions of *ATM, BLM, FAA, FAC, XPA,* and *XPC* are being studied, the association of their gene products with repair of DNA damage was instrumental in their identification.

As a group, these conditions are rare, ranging from 1 in 40,000 for ataxia-telangiectasia to 1 in 360,000 for Fanconi anemia. Nonetheless, they represent models for cancer susceptibility. Of broader concern, it is possible that seemingly unaffected heterozygotes for these recessive conditions might be at risk for environmentally induced DNA damage. For example, some investigators recommend that ataxia-telangiectasia heterozygotes avoid exposure to diagnostic X rays. Conclusive evidence for the public health importance of these theories will await clinical trials, which have recently become possible because of the isolation of the genes associated with each of these disorders.

DNA-Repair Deficiencies Associated with Hereditary Nonpolyposis Colon Cancer

The observation that hereditary forms of a common adult-onset cancer were due to defects in genes involved in DNA repair expanded the public health implications of this mechanism of cancer susceptibility. In 1993, as part of a massive study involving investigators on several continents, a hereditary form of colon cancer was found to be linked to genetic markers on the short arm of chromosome 2 (reviewed in Service, 1994; Marra and Boland, 1995). The genetic markers utilized in this study were *microsatellite* probes that detected variations in naturally occurring repetitive elements in DNA.

It is believed that there are over 100,000 short runs of six or less base pair microsatellite sequences in the human genome. These sequences vary from one individual to the next (i.e., are polymorphic). Differences in the "DNA fingerprint" pattern of repeats allowed the identification of maternal and paternal alleles in linkage analysis. An unexpected finding in genetic studies of the colon cancers from these families was an exaggerated pattern of "laddering" of short sequences of DNA in the tumor samples. It was as if the DNA replication machinery momentarily got stuck, resulting in long strings of repeats where only a few such repeats would normally be found.

The observation of an apparent instability of the microsatellite probes (microsatellite instability) in hereditary colon cancers was of great interest to researchers. A group of geneticists interested in DNA repair in bacteria and yeast postulated that faulty DNA mismatch repair genes, which were very closely conserved between bacteria, yeast, and mammals, were to blame for the strings of repeats seen in the colon tumors. It was the function of these housekeeping genes to clean up those inevitable mismatches of single base pairs and short mismatched loops in newly synthesized DNA that accompanied cell division and DNA replication. It seemed simplistic to assume that such defects could be implicated in the pathogenesis of a common human cancer. Surprisingly, some of these genes, homologues of the *mutL* and *mutS* DNA repair genes in bacteria and yeast, were found to be mutated in families with multiple cases of colon and endometrial cancer. This observation provided the molecular explanation for the cancer family syndrome originally described by Warthin and Lynch and known to clinicians for decades.

Confirmation soon emerged that many of the families meeting strict criteria for hereditary nonpolyposis colon cancer (see Chapter 4) demonstrated linkage to 2p or 3p, sites of the human *mutS* and *mutL* homologues (hence termed *hMSH2* and *hMLH1*), or to three similar genes (see Chapter 4). While colorectal tumors, whether sporadic or hereditary, rarely showed loss of heterozygosity at these loci, the second hits predicted by the Knudson model were observed as somatic mutations in the hereditary colon tumors. The genes associated with this syndrome are listed in Table 3-3. It has recently emerged that the tumorigenic effects of *BRCA* mutations are mediated through a gene involved in control of DNA recombination, *RAD51* (see Chapter 4). Thus, a mechanism for hereditary breast and ovarian cancer may also involve defective DNA replication.Unlike the typical tumor suppressor genes, mutations associated with the human *mutS* and *mutL* homologues, and possibly the *BRCA* genes, may result in the more rapid accumulation of mutations of other tumor suppressor genes, as well as the third major group of cancer-causing genes, the oncogenes.

TABLE 3-3 Classes and Selected Examples of Oncogenes in Human Cancers

Gene	Description	Example of Cancer with Altered Oncogene or Oncoprotein
1. Growth factors		
SIS	Platelet-derived growth factor	Astrocytoma, breast cancer
INT-2	Fibroblast-growth factor related	Glioblastoma, breast cancer
HST	Fibroblast-growth factor related	Glioblastoma, gastric cancer
2. Protein tyrosine kinase receptors		
ERBB1	Epidermal growth factor receptor	Squamous cell carcinomas, astrocytoma, melanoma
ERBB2 (*HER2*/neu)	Epidermal growth factorlike receptor	Breast, ovarian, gastric adenocarcinomas, lung cancer
FMS	Colony-stimulating-factor receptor	Ovarian cancer
RET	Truncated receptorlike protein	Thyroid cancer
ROS	Insulin receptor	Breast cancer
TRK	Truncated receptorlike protein	Thyroid cancer
3. Protein tyrosine kinase, not receptors		
ABL	Membrane/cytoplasmic/nuclear	Chronic myeloid leukemia
SRC	Membrane-associated	Colon carcinoma
LCK	Membrane-associated	Colon carcinoma, lung cancer
FES	Membrane-associated	Lung cancer
4. Signal transducers		
HRAS	Membrane associated GTPase	Colon, lung, pancreatic cancer, melanoma
KRAS	Membrane associated GTPase	Acute leukemia, thyroid, lung, colon cancer
NRAS	Membrane associated GTPase	Genito-urinary cancer, thyroid, melanoma
BRAF		Gastric carcinoma
5. Nuclear transcription factors		
c-MYC	Helix-loop-helix	Lymphoma, lung, breast, ovarian, colon cancer
N-MYC	Helix-loop-helix	Neuroblastoma, small cell lung cancer
L-MYC	Helix-loop-helix	Lung cancer
SCL/TAL-1	Helix-loop-helix	T cell acute leukemia
E2A	Helix-loop-helix	Acute lymphocytic leukemia
FOS	Leucine zipper	Lung cancer
JUN	Leucine zipper	Lung cancer

(continued)

TABLE 3-3 (continued)

Gene	Description	Example of Cancer with Altered Oncogene or Oncoprotein
ATF-1	Leucine zipper	Malignant melanoma
CHOP	Leucine zipper	Myxoid liposarcoma
HLF	Leucine zipper	Pre-B leukemia
PBX	Homeobox	Acute lymphoblastic leukemia
HOX11(TCL3)	Homeobox	T cell acute leukemia
AML-1	Rhd motif	Leukemia
REL	Nfκb like	Lymphoma
ETS	3 Tryptophan DNA binding domains	Leukemia
MYB	*ETS* like	Lung cancer
ERG	*ETS* like	Malignant melanoma
FLI-1	*ETS* like	Ewing sarcoma/PNET
TTG-1	LIM motif (two cys-his motifs)	T-cell leukemia
TTG-2	LIM motif	T-cell leukemia
BCL-6	Zinc finger	Lymphoma
PML	Zinc finger	Promyelocytic leukemia acute myeloid leukemia
ETO	Zinc finger	Acute myeloid leukemia
MLL	Zinc finger	Mixed lineage leukemias and lymphomas
EVI-1	Zinc finger	Acute myeloid leukemia

Sources: Data complied from Vile, RG (ed). Introduction to the Molecular Genetics of Cancer. New York: John Wiley & Sons, 1992; Cowell, JK (ed). Molecular Genetics of Cancer. Oxford: Bios, 1995; Kurzrock R, Talpaz M (eds). Molecular Biology in Cancer Medicine. New York: Oxford University Press, 1995; and on-line databases.

ONCOGENES: THE COLLISION OF CANCER CYTOGENETICS AND TUMOR VIROLOGY

The description of cancer-causing genes, called oncogenes, in the 1980s was the culmination of efforts from two distinct schools within the broad field of human cancer genetics. These disciplines, cancer cytogenetics and tumor virology, had evolved separately since 1900. Their collision gave birth to a new understanding of the etiology of common cancers.

Cancer Cytogenetics

The birthdate of cancer cytogenetics is widely cited as 1914, the year the German cytologist Theodur Boveri speculated that cancer was due to abnormalities of the chromosomes in cells. Technical limitations in human cytogenetics were finally surmounted over 50 years later with the development of techniques to stain the chromosomes.

One of the first applications of this new level of resolution was to identify rearrangements (translocations) of portions of chromosomes in human cancers. The first genetic abnormality associated with a human tumor was a reciprocal exchange of material between the long arms of chromosomes 9 and 22 observed by Rowley and co-workers in a patient with chronic myeloid leukemia.

Another reciprocal translocation, involving the long arms of chromosomes 8 and 14 was observed in a deadly lymphoid tumor (Burkitt's lymphoma). As cytogenetic studies of the common tumors of breast, colon, and prostate became possible, other types of cytogenetic abnormalities were observed to be even more common than the translocations. These abnormalities were caused by deletions, insertions, and other structural changes of chromosomal material. Although the biological meaning of chromosomal alterations was unclear at the time, their diagnostic and clinical significance was obvious. Soon after the original reports, cytogenetic methods constituted diagnostic tests in many academic laboratories. This pattern of rapid translation from the basic laboratory to the bedside would become a theme for the cancer genetic discoveries that followed.

The Viral Theory of Cancer and the Discovery of Oncogenes

At about the same time in the early part of the century that Boveri posed his genetic theory of cancer, Peyton Rous reached a milestone in his quest to prove that cancer was, in fact, an infectious disease. In a classic application of Koch's postulates, Rous proved that, at least in chickens, the cause of cancer was a transmissible agent. The field of tumor virology, which sprang from the work of Peyton Rous, became one of the most active areas in the molecular genetics of cancer for many decades. A number of transmissible tumor types were identified in birds, cats, and rodents. In most cases, the transmissible agent identified was a simple type of virus containing only single stranded RNA.

The life cycle of the newly discovered RNA viruses was an extraordinary example of biological parasitism. The invading RNA virus came equipped with the minimal machinery to copy its genetic material to DNA, but relied on its host for everything else. The viral DNA would integrate into the host's genome. In so doing, it not only took control of the host, "transforming" it to a cancerous cell, but also manufactured for the virus new proteins to allow it to infect other cells. The viral DNA-making enzyme was termed a *reverse transcriptase*. These discoveries gave rise to a new concept in cancer genetics: the *viral oncogene*—or cancer-causing gene in viruses. The first of the viral oncogenes to be identified, v-src, was the transmissible agent causing tumors in chickens sought for by Rous many years earlier.

Despite these discoveries, there was scant evidence by the 1970s of a contagious pattern for common human cancers. Tumor virologists such as Robert Gallo comprised a small but steadfast group espousing the view that viral mechanisms held a key to the understanding of cancer.

A significant advance in both cancer cytogenetics and tumor virology came with the discovery in 1982 that the genetic counterpart of a viral oncogene was localized to the breakpoint of a chromosomal translocation in a human tumor. The tumor was a

Burkitt's lymphoma. A human version of the viral oncogene v-myc (which caused leukemia in chickens) was mapped to chromosome band 8q24. This was precisely the site that was involved in a translocation with another site, 14q32, as shown by cytogenetic analysis of tumor cells a decade earlier. The partner site, 14q32, was the location of the gene that encoded a key region of the immunoglobulin molecule. The translocation thrust together the human *MYC* gene and the immunoglobulin gene control region (Figure 3-8). In this process, the expression of the *MYC* gene was greatly enhanced, resulting in rapid cell growth and malignant proliferation.

From these observations, it was now apparent that (1) counterparts to the viral oncogenes existed in the normal human genome, and (2) these proto-oncogenes in humans, if disrupted by chromosomal translocation, could lead to cancerous change. Continued investigations established the role of proto-oncogenes in normal control of cellular processes, including growth and proliferation. It was not surprising that the viruses utilized such important genes in their life cycle. In so doing, however, they also indicated to cancer geneticists those genes in the normal human complement that could play a role in malignant transformation.

During the decade following the discovery of *MYC* activation in human lymphomas, human counterparts of over a dozen other viral oncogenes were implicated in common malignancies. Following Koch's postulates, it was shown that mutated proto-oncogenes could transform cell cultures to a malignant phenotype in transfection experiments. As additional proto-oncogenes were discovered, it became clear that there were ways they could be activated other than chromosomal translocations. A single mutation in a coding sequence of the proto-oncogene could induce cancers via a mutated oncoprotein. Alternatively, a mutation in a promotor or enhancer region could result in vastly increased expression of a structurally normal protein product. Whatever the mechanism of oncogene activation, two general principles emerged: (1) alteration of only one of the two copies of the gene was necessary (dominant expression) and (2) the result of the genetic alteration was a gain of function.

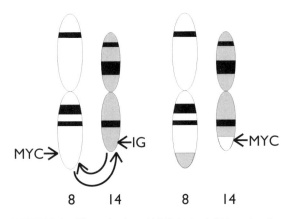

FIGURE 3-8   *The activation of* MYC *in the 8;14 translocation.*

The Function of Oncogenes

Over the past decade, a numbers of models have been devised to link together the functions of the known human oncogenes (reviewed in Krontiris, 1995). These models shared many features. They involved the recognition of external factors that stimulated cell growth and internal factors that conveyed this signal to the nucleus of the cell. These models stimulated basic research on the genetic mechanisms of cell growth and differentiation. They also offered the promise to shape a new approach to cancer therapies. For these reasons, the general features shared by these models are described here.

The products of oncogenes can be thought of as falling into four main classes. These include molecules that serve as intercellular signals for cell growth, membrane receptors for these growth factors, intracellular messengers of the growth and proliferation signals, and nuclear factors that activate DNA replication or transcription (Figure 3-9). Alterations of genes from each of these classes have been associated with different types of human malignancy (see Table 3-1).

The conveying or transduction of signals between the various members of the family of proto-oncogene products is accomplished by proteins called kinases. The kinases transfer phosphate groups from ATP to the side chains of proteins that contain tyrosine, serine, and threonine. After phosphorylation, the shape of the protein is changed, resulting in an enzymatic activity that makes it, too, a kinase. In addition, the change in conformation may expose binding sites for other proteins to aggregate.

The process of signal transduction begins with the binding of, for example, a growth factor to a growth factor receptor. In some instances, this results in the pairing (*dimerization*) of the receptor with another receptor. In the process, each receptor phosphorylates the other, opening up a number of new binding sites. Binding sites are located in a portion of the molecules that protrude into the cytoplasm. Here, other proteins are phosphorylated. Some of these proteins, called *adaptors,* in concert with other proteins, activate the third class of oncogene products, the *signal transducers.* The best studied of these signal transducers is the product of the *RAS* oncogene.

The ras protein is activated by hydrolyzing guanosine triphosphate (GTP) to guanosine diphosphate (GDP). It is therefore called a GTPase or G protein. The Ras product is assisted, and also regulated, in this process by other proteins. Activated Ras protein results in a cascade of activation of other proteins, including Raf, mitogen-activated protein kinase (MAPK), and extracellular signal-regulated kinase (ERK). ERK activates transcription factors, including the *FOS* and *JUN* oncogene products, which join and bind DNA near the *MYC* gene. This results in activation of *MYC*, which itself is a transcription factor that activates other genes. Among the genes activated by *MYC* is the gene encoding cyclin D1, which initiates progression of cells through the cell cycle.

Alterations of transcription factors, through chromosomal translocation and other mechanisms, are an increasingly documented mechanism of tumorigenesis. The transcription factors have been divided into a number of classes based on their structural organization (motifs) (Table 3-3). They include the group of helix-loop-helix gene products, which share a common amino acid motif involved in DNA binding and/or protein interaction; the homeobox-containing genes, which share a homology to

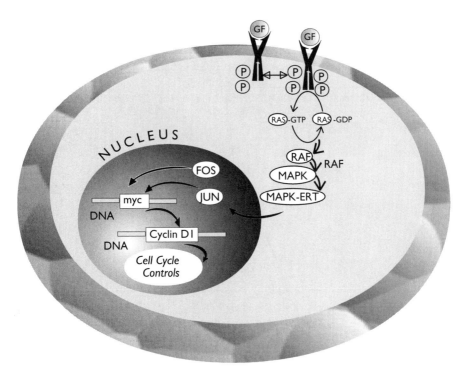

FIGURE 3-9 *Pathways of signal transduction by the products of proto-oncogenes. Signal transduction begins with the binding of a growth factor (GF) to a growth factor receptor, which may result in pairing (dimerization), shown by arrows between receptors. Phosphates from binding sites in the cytoplasmic portion of the receptor cause the Ras protein to be activated by hydrolyzing guanosine triphosphate (GTP) to guanosine diphosphate (GDP). Activation of Ras protein results in a cascade of activation of other proteins, including Raf, mitogen activated protein kinase (MAPK), and extracellular-signal regulated kinase (ERK). ERK activates transcription factors, including FOS and JUN,* which join and bind DNA near the MYC *gene. This results in activation of* MYC, *which activates the gene encoding cyclin D1, which initiates progression of cells through the cell cycle. Upregulation at any point along this pathway will result in a net gain of function and increased cellular proliferation.*

homeotic genes originally identified as regulating temporal and spatial aspects of development of other organisms; and leucine zipper or zinc finger-containing genes, based on common amino acid residues that bind DNA.

For each group of growth factors and receptors there may be shared or distinct protein tyrosine kinases associated with the intracytoplasmic signalling pathway. This sharing includes a large family of nonreceptor type kinases related to the *SRC* family of genes that are also involved in signal transduction. The complexity of this system suggests its vulnerability to perturbations resulting in neoplastic proliferation. Mutations of the *RAS* gene are among the most common genetic abnormalities in human cancers, observed in about a third of tumors. In addition, alterations in other genes encoding proteins in the signal cascade can result in tumorigenesis. These observations emphasize the potential diagnostic role of genetic alterations as markers of the malignant process. They also suggest a strategy for future cancer therapies targeted to the various components of the pathway. For example, inhibitors of specific tyrosine kinases, or competitive binding of receptors, could modulate signal transduction and shut down proliferation of cancerous cells.

Viral Causes of Cancer

The demonstration that retroviral mutants of human proto-oncogenes could transform cells was impressive but still did not prove that viruses caused cancers in man. By the 1980s, evidence was at hand implicating viruses in at least some human cancers. The viruses identified, however, were not the retroviruses associated with known oncogenes. The cancer-associated viruses included papillomavirus, linked to cancers of the reproductive organs; hepatitis virus, linked to liver cancer; and Epstein-Barr virus, linked to cancer of the nasopharynx and some lymphomas (Table 3-4). These viruses injected DNA, not RNA, directly into cells, and their genes bore no resemblance to their human counterparts.

At least one retrovirus was included on the list of human cancer viruses. Associated with a form of human adult leukemia, HTLV1 bore no resemblance to any known human genes (zur Hausen, 1991).

The mechanisms behind the carcinogenicity of the DNA viruses remained poorly understood. Unlike the acutely transforming retroviruses, the DNA viruses seemed to require other exposures, other genetic events, or immunosuppression of the host, in order to transform cells. The best studied of the DNA viruses was one that induced tumors in monkeys but not in man. The SV40 virus encoded a protein, the large T antigen, which perturbed the cell cycle components that regulate the growth and proliferation of cells. In so doing, the virus was rewarded with many new cells to infect. For the host cell, the result of these viral manipulations was indefinite cell growth, the first step in malignant transformation.

The elucidation of the effects of SV40 proteins on cell proliferation seemed a relatively arcane area of cancer genetics in the 1970s. By the 1990s, this model had provided a critical connection to tumor suppressor genes, because, as we have seen, the *RB1* gene product was also found to bind with the large T antigen. Thus, cell cycle control could be deregulated directly due to mutation of *RB1* or through binding of *RB1* by SV40-associated antigens. The human papilloma virus also acts by inactivat-

TABLE 3-4   Viruses Linked to Human Cancers

Virus	Human Cancer
Human papilloma virus	Cervical, other squamous cell carcinoma
Hepatitis B virus	Liver cancer
Epstein Barr virus	Nasopharynx cancer, Burkitt's lymphoma, posttransplantation polyclonal lymphomas
Human T-Lymphocytic Virus I	Adult T-cell leukemia/lymphoma

ing tumor suppressor genes. The proteins encoded by HPV 16 and 18 are called E7 and E6. These proteins bind and inactivate *RB1* and *p53*, respectively.

THE UNIFYING MODEL FOR GENETIC AND ENVIRONMENTAL CAUSES OF CANCER: THE MULTISTEP MODEL FOR GENETIC ALTERATIONS IN CARCINOGENESIS

Although a number of tumor suppressor genes were found to be altered in a variety of human tumors, there remained little explanation for the tumor specificity and species specificity of either the tumor suppressor genes or the DNA mismatch repair genes. A number of conundrums remained to be deciphered. For example, homozygous deletion of the *RB1* gene was found in human retinoblastoma but was also observed in pituitary tumors in mice. Somatic mutations of *RB1* were, however, among the most common genetic alterations found in a broad spectrum of human tumors. Of these, only sarcomas were observed with increased frequency in individuals with germline *RB1* mutations. The frequency of *RB1* mutations in sporadic tumors was surpassed only by that of the most frequently mutated gene in human cancers, *p53*. Persons born with germline mutations of the *p53* tumor suppressor gene developed cancers at an early age, but these individuals did not develop colon cancer. Colon tumors, however, were frequently characterized by acquired *p53* mutations. Individuals with germline mutations of a gene ubiquitously expressed in a number of tissues, *APC,* also predominantly developed colon cancer.

Presumably, the explanation for these observations lay in the concept of the multigenic pathogenesis of these tumors, and gene–gene as well as gene–environment interactions which could mediate phenotypic expression. Although now referred to as the Vogelgram, the multistep genetic model of carcinogenesis was developed several decades before the 1990 model for colon cancer progression described by Dr. Bert Vogelstein at Johns Hopkins (Fearon and Vogelstein, 1990). In 1952, Armitage and Doll derived a six-hit genetic model of tumor progression, based solely on statistical models of age and cancer death rates (Armitage and Doll, 1954). In the context of colon cancer, Vogelstein and colleagues observed that deletions of *APC* were present in about 30% of premalignant polyps (adenomas), but were no more frequent in the invasive cancers. In contrast deletions in the regions of 17p and 18q were seen in 75% of carcinomas, but few adenomas. Mutations of *RAS* genes were observed in over half of the adenomas with areas of carcinoma. This model (Figure 3-10) linked alterations of oncogenes (*RAS*) with those of putative tumor suppressor genes (*DCC,DPC4, JV18-1* at 18q and *p53* at 17p) as part of a continuum of events from premalignant to frankly malignant lesions (Figure 3-9).

Although mutations of tumor suppressor genes are considered a critical component of the multistep model, it is difficult to reconcile how two separate hits could occur with such high frequency during tumor progression as predicted by the Knudson model. One answer could be the subsequent loss of the remaining allele, consistent with observations of cytogenetic deletions. This additional event could take place separately, as a result of subsequent damage. Another answer lay in the unusual biology of

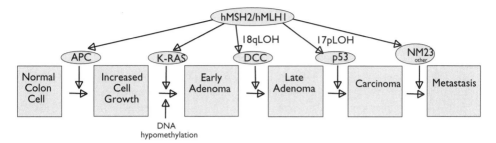

FIGURE 3-10 *The multistep model of colon tumorigenesis (Vogelstein). Deletions of APC, present in about 30% of premalignant polyps (adenomas), are among the early stages in the malignant transformation of colon tumors. APC mutations may also be inherited, resulting in predisposition to colon cancer. APC mutations are followed by mutations of RAS genes, observed in over half of the adenomas with areas of carcinoma and deletions of genes on 18q and 17p, including alterations of DCC and p53, in the later stages of carcinogenesis. Inherited mutations of genes such as hMSH2 and hMLH2 cause global genomic instability and increase the mutation rates for other genes.*

genes such as *p53*, for which, as we have seen, small amounts of mutated protein can recruit and bind up the wild type protein in a dominant negative fashion. This model explains experiments in which mutant *p53* was able to transform cells that still expressed some endogenous wild-type protein. It also explains how a single hit to *p53* or *APC* could result in loss of function of the wild-type protein. Finally, mutations in the setting of hereditary cancer syndromes might increase the mutation rate for *p53*, as well as other tumor suppressor genes and oncogenes.

Following the description of the Vogelgram, at least nine other genes were implicated in the pathogenesis of colorectal cancers. As refined by Kinzler and Vogelstein in 1996, genes such as *APC* (and *NF1, RB1, VHL*) could be thought of as gatekeeper genes in specific tissues (colonic epithelium, Schwann cell, retinal cell, and kidney cells, respectively) (Kinzler and Vogelstein, 1996). When mutated, these genes cause a permanent imbalance of cell division over cell death in specific tissues. Mutations of other genes (e.g., *RAS*) are necessary for malignant progression, but by themselves could not lead to a sustainable neoplastic growth in the absence of a mutated gatekeeper. In this model, mutations of the DNA mismatch repair genes represent more of a susceptibility state than a transforming event. Mutations in critical oncogenes and tumor suppressor genes would be more likely to occur in the repair-deficient cells. In the case of hereditary nonpolyposis colon cancer (HNPCC), mutations of the *mutS* and *mutL* homologues were found to increase mutation rates for other genes by two to three orders of magnitude. A gene encoding an important inhibitor of epithelial cell growth, for example, was frequently mutated in colon tumors with deficiencies in DNA repair (Parsons et al., 1995). Thus, *APC* mutations lead to a more rapid initiation of tumors due to loss of gatekeeper function, while mutations associated with HNPCC result in a global acceleration of tumor progression due to enhanced mutation rates (Kinzler and Vogelstein, 1996).

Two other common cancer predisposition genes, *BRCA1* and *BRCA2*, share some features with the DNA repair genes of HNPCC. For both groups of genes, as with *WT1*, mutations are infrequently observed in sporadic, nonfamilial tumors. *BRCA1* and *BRCA2* both interact with *RAD51,* a gene which in yeast and mammals repairs double strand DNA breaks and is involved in recombination-linked repair (Sculley et al., 1997; Sharan et al. 1997). Mice that lacked *BRCA2* expression were hypersensitive to radiation, probably due to deficient DNA repair. The C-terminal end of the the *BRCA1* gene shows similarities to a number of proteins implicated in DNA damage response (Bork et al., 1997). Thus, mutations of the *BRCA* genes may not cause cancer directly, but may act to increase genome instability, leading to mutations of other cancer-causing genes (Kinzler and Vogelstein, 1997).

Multistage models of genetic events accompanying malignant progression have now been devised for a number of human cancers, including cancers of the colon, bladder, head and neck, kidney, lung, brain, blood-forming cells, and skin. In many tumors, the patterns of genetic events are similar, suggesting that it is the accumulation of commonly altered genes that is associated with such clinically important events as tumor spread and metastases. These late genetic events, as explored in Chapter 8, have provided the best candidates for prognostic markers of disease outcome. In many cases these progression-associated genetic markers, such as mutations of *RB1* or *WT1*, are the same alterations seen as early changes in inherited cancer syndromes. When observed as "later events" in hematopoietic tumors, and certain solid tumors, these genes have been associated with clinical outcome and may play important roles as prognostic markers (see Chapter 8).

The multistep model of tumor progression brings together concepts of the environmental and genetic interactions of cancer development and progression, because external agents may act by causing DNA damage. The appeal of this model from the perspective of preventive medicine is its emphasis on the early genetic events in cancer cells, which in some cases may be due to inherited cancer susceptibilities. The clinical goal in these circumstances is to detect the inherited predisposition in order to guide preventive efforts, or to detect the malignant clone early enough so that it can be eradicated before too much damage is done.

REFERENCES

Armitage P, Doll R. 1954. The age distribution of cancer and a multi-stage theory of carcinogenesis. Br J Cancer 8:1–12.

Beaudet AL, Tsui LC. 1993. A suggested nomenclature for designating mutations. Human Mutation 2:245–48.

Bork P, Hofmann K, Bucher P, Neuwald AF, Altschul SF, Koonin E. 1997. The superfamily of conserved domains in DNA damage-responsive cell cycle check point proteins. FASEB J 11:68–76.

Cavenee WK, White RL. 1995. The genetic basis of cancer. Scientific American; March 272: 72–9.

Chang F, Syrjanen S, Syrjanen K. 1995. Implications of the *p53* tumor suppressor gene in clinical oncology. J Clin Oncol 13:1009–22.

Collins F. 1996. Positional cloning moves from perditional to traditional. Nature Genet 9: 347–50.

Cowell JK (ed). 1995. Molecular Genetics of Cancer. Oxford: Bios.

Fearon ER, Vogelstein B. 1990. A genetic model for colorectal tumorigenesis. Cell 61:759–67.

Hartwell LH, Kastan MB. 1994. Cell cycle control and cancer. Science 266:1821–8.

Kinzler KW, Vogelstein B. 1996. Lessons from hereditary colorectal cancer. Cell 87:159–70.

Kinzler KW, Vogelstein B. 1997. Gatekeepers and caretakers. Nature 386:761–2.

Krontiris TG. 1995. Oncogenes. New Engl J Med 333:303–6.

Knudson AG Jr. 1971. Mutation and cancer: statistical study of retinoblastoma. Proc Natl Acad Sci 68:820–3.

Kurzrock R, Talpaz M (eds). 1995. Molecular Biology in Cancer Medicine. New York: Oxford University Press.

Latchman DS. 1996. Transcription-factor mutations and disease. New Engl J Med 334:28–33.

Malkin D, Portwine C. 1994. The genetics of childhood cancer. European Cancer 30A:1942–46.

Marra G, Boland CR. 1995. Hereditary nonpolyposis colorectal cancer: the syndrome, the genes, and historical perspectives. J Natl Cancer Inst 87(15):1114–25.

Parsons R, Myeroff LL, Liu B, Wilson JK, Markowitz SD, Kinzler KW, Vogelstein B. 1995. Microsatellite instability and mutations of the transforming growth factor beta type II receptor gene in colorectal cancer. Cancer Res 55:5548–50.

Rabbitts TH. 1994. Chromosomal translocations in human cancer. Nature 372:143–9.

Sculley R, Chen J, Plug A et al. 1997. Association of BRCA1 with Rad51 in mitotic and meiotic cells. Cell 88:265–75.

Service RF. 1994. Stalking the start of colon cancer. Science 263:1559–60.

Sharan S, Morimatsu M, Albrecht U et al. 1997. Embryonic lethality and radiation hypersensitivity mediated by Rad51 in mice lacking BRCA2. Nature 386:804–10.

Stanbridge EJ. 1976. Suppression of malignancy in human cells. Nature 260:17–20.

Vile RG (ed). 1992. Introduction to the Molecular Genetics of Cancer. New York: John Wiley & Sons.

Weinberg RA. 1993. Tumor suppressor genes. Science 254:1138–45.

Weinberg RA. 1996. How cancer arises. Scientific American; September: 275:62–70.

zur Hausen H. 1991. Viruses in human cancers. Science 254:1167–73.

4

The Common Hereditary Cancers

Because of their high prevalence in the United States and Western countries, breast, prostate, and colon cancers have been the targets of special efforts at prevention and early detection. This chapter focuses on the epidemiologic, pathologic, and genetic features of these tumors and associated predisposition syndromes. Ovarian cancer tends to be overrepresented in families with either hereditary breast or colon cancer. For this reason, the common hereditary syndromes of ovarian cancer predisposition are also included.

The information in this chapter constitutes one element of the essential background for cancer genetic counseling of families. Additional elements, relating to methods of counseling, including psychological and ethical aspects, are outlined in the following chapters.

PART A: BREAST CANCER SYNDROMES

This section addresses breast cancer syndromes, whereas the next section focuses on hereditary ovarian cancer syndromes. The two cancer types are often, but not always, observed together in affected families. For this reason, and because of the different strategies for detection, they are discussed separately. In addition, Appendix A comprises a list of less common hereditary syndromes in which both breast and ovarian cancer may be a feature.

CLINICAL AND EPIDEMIOLOGIC FEATURES

One in nine American women who live to age 85 will develop breast cancer during their lifetime. Over 180,000 women are diagnosed with breast cancer each year, and 46,000 die of the disease. Only about 3000 cases will be diagnosed in women age 30 or younger. Breast cancer occurs rarely in males, with about 1000 cases per year diagnosed in the United States.

The 1 in 9 risk in the United States is double what it was in 1940 and has been rising steadily. A dramatic increase in breast cancer incidence in the late 1980s (an increase of 4% in 1987) was thought to be due to the impact of mammography. Even taking this into account, there has been a steady increase in breast cancer rates over the past 50 years (Marshall, 1993).

One of the benefits of the newer methods of diagnosis has been the shift in size of tumors at time of diagnosis (Miller et al., 1993). The incidence of large tumors, greater than 3 cm, has actually decreased since 1982. The type of breast cancers that have been increasingly diagnosed are the stage 0 *in situ* carcinomas. These tumors are treated surgically with or without radiation therapy. Stage I invasive tumors, which are less than 2 cm without lymphatic involvement, are treated surgically by lumpectomy, staging axillary lymph node dissection, and radiation therapy. This continues to be the practice for stage I patients with low proliferative index, positive estrogen receptors, or other favorable prognostic markers. Based on the results of clinical trials over the past decade, adjuvant chemotherapy is given for stage I patients with adverse prognostic markers. Adjuvant chemotherapy is the rule for all patients with stage II disease (tumors less than 5 cm in diameter with positive lymph nodes, or tumors more than 5 cm with negative lymph nodes). Patients with stage III disease, by virtue of lymph nodes fixed to one another or to other structures, or tumor size greater than 5 cm with positive nodes, are generally managed with induction chemotherapy followed by surgery if possible. Patients with metastatic disease (stage IV) receive systemic chemotherapy and/or radiotherapy on a palliative basis, or high dose chemotherapy and autologous bone marrow (or stem cell) infusion in an attempt to ablate the disease (Helzlsouer, 1995; Roy, 1995).

Newer diagnostic methods and the impact of modern chemotherapy have been reflected in mortality figures. Deaths due to breast cancer remained steady at a rate of 27 per 100,000 over 40 years. From 1989 until 1993, however, there was a 5% decrease in mortality. There are now over 2 million breast cancer survivors in the United States.

Risk Factors

By far the most significant risk factor for breast cancer is age. Risk increases steadily with age. Knowledge of this fact, however, is inversely correlated with age (Figure 4-1) (Breslow and Kessler, 1995).

The breast cancer incidence in North America and northern Europe is greater than the rate in most Asian and African countries. Since migrants from low-risk countries assume the higher U.S. risks after only one or two generations, it has been assumed that diet is an important environmental risk factor for breast cancer. Western diets are

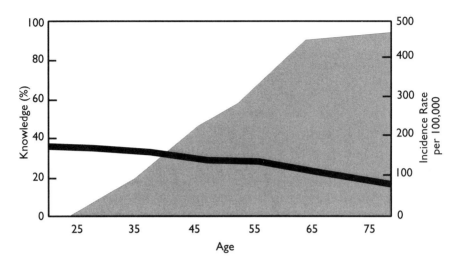

FIGURE 4-1   *Breast cancer rates and age of onset The incidence of breast cancer increases steadily with age (grey shaded area), from about 100 cases per 100,000 at age 35 to almost 500 cases per 100,000 by age 75. Knowledge of the association of breast cancer risk with age (dark line) decreases from 35% of those surveyed around age 30 to 16% by age 75 (Data from Breslow and Kessler, 1995).*

much higher in fat than Asian diets. However, epidemiologic analysis has thus far failed to demonstrate a clear association of fat in the diet and breast cancer risk, at least within the ranges that are consumed by average Americans. The most persuasive evidence for this comes from 120,000 nurses who have been participating in a large prospective trial started in 1976. In the Nurses Health Study, there was no association between varying fat consumption and risk for breast cancer (Willet et al., 1992; Helzl-souer, 1995). However, high levels of body fat were associated with breast cancer risk in postmenopausal women (de Waard et al., 1977). It is known that body fat produces estrogen, and this fact is believed to be the postmenopausal body fat–breast cancer link. Similarly, in women who exercise, estradiol and progesterone secretion is de-creased, possibly accounting for the 40% reduction in breast cancer risk among women exercising at least 4 hours a week (Thune et al., 1997).

Early studies by MacMahon and others established menstrual and reproductive his-tory as important risk factors for breast cancer. Increased risks were associated with early age of menarche, late age at first pregnancy, and nulliparity. A woman who had her first child before the age of 18 had only a third the lifetime breast cancer risk of a women who delayed childbirth until after 30 (MacMahon et al., 1973; Trichopoulos et al., 1968). Nulliparity or age of birth of first child after 30 also increased risk for intra-ductal breast cancer (Kerlikowske et al., 1997). The presumed explanation for these observations was that the continual episodic release of estrogen and progesterone each month served to stimulate breast proliferation, increasing the chances for expansion of a cancerous clone. Breast cancer rates increased in North America over the past 200 years as the age of menarche shifted from age 17 to the current 12.8 years of age. In China, where breast cancer is much less frequent than in North America, the age of menarche is, on average, 17 years (Marshall, 1993).

Surgically induced menopause (e.g., by oophorectomy) before age 35 decreases breast cancer risk by a third. Metanalyses by Grady and others have shown that post-menopausal administration of unopposed estrogen for 15–20 years will increase breast cancer risk as much as 40–50% (Grady and Ernster, 1991). Data from the Nurses Health Study have shown that this increase in breast cancer risk is the same even if opposed (estrogen plus progestin) replacement is prescribed (Colditz et al., 1995).

The association of oral contraceptive use and risk for breast cancer has been controversial. For women older than 45–50 years, there was no significant increase in risk when three case-control and three cohort studies were analyzed. There did appear to be an increased risk on the order of 36% for women younger than 45 years who had taken oral contraceptives for 10 years (Pike et al., 1993).

Other than estrogen, there are few known environmental risk factors for breast cancer. A number of studies have demonstrated that a high alcohol consumption increases risk. Recent consumption of three or more drinks a day doubled risk, while remote alcohol use (between ages 16–29) had no such effect (Longnecker et al., 1995). Interestingly, alcohol use increased total and bioavailable estrogen levels in premenopausal women, offering a possible explanation for the epidemiologic findings (Reichman et al., 1993).

Relatively little is known about environmental exposures and breast cancer risk. Radiation exposure in excess of 1–3 Gy, for example, in the setting of curative radiation therapy for Hodgkin's disease, is associated with an increased risk for breast cancer. Risk was increased only when radiation exposure occurred before the age of 40–45, and that risk increased with higher doses (Boice et al., 1992). Diagnostic radiation exposure is of very low dose, in the range of .00015 Gy for a mammogram. It has been estimated that less than 1% of breast cancers in the United States are due to diagnostic X-ray exposure (Evans et al., 1986). There may be an increased risk associated with radiation exposure for the .5–1% of the population believed to carry mutations for the *ATM* gene, as discussed in the section on hereditary syndromes.

Recent attention has focused on chemical and other exposures associated with breast cancer risk, particularly organochlorine pesticides (e.g., DDT and its major metabolite, DDE) or polychlorinated biphenyls (PCBs). A reason for this attention has been the observation of increased breast cancer rates in certain geographical regions of the country (e.g., the Northeast). However, epidemiologic studies have concluded that differences in breast cancer rates could largely be accounted for by differences in known risk factors. For example, nearly twice as many women from the northeast United States delayed childbearing until the 30s, compared to women from the southern United States. This may help explain the increased incidence of breast cancer in this region (Sturgeon et al., 1995). Epidemiologic studies of pesticide exposures and breast cancer risk have been contradictory, with no clear associations thus far proved (MacMahon, 1994). Further epidemiologic studies are in progress to examine these issues, including a large case-control study on Long Island in New York.

PATHOLOGY

To the pathologist, breast cancer is a generic term that encompasses a number of distinct clinico-pathologic entities. As more is known of the genetic etiology of these tumors, correlations with histologic and clinical features will be defined. Because the clinical implications of different histologic types of breast cancer comprise a significant aspect of risk counseling, a summary of the most common subtypes of breast cancer is presented here.

More than 90% of breast tumors arise in the epithelial cells that line the secretory ducts of the breast. At the initial stages, breast tumors begin as anaplastic proliferations within the ducts themselves, causing plugging of the lumina with the neoplastic cells. If the tumor remains within the confines of the ductal basal membrane, it is termed *noninfiltrating* (noninvasive) or *intraductal carcinoma* (in situ), often abbreviated as *DCIS*. These tumors do not invade surrounding stroma, and, in general, have a low likelihood of axillary node involvement and an excellent prognosis (Simpson and Page, 1995).

Until the advent of widespread screening mammography, *in situ* or noninvasive breast cancers were quite rare. They constituted only a few percent of all breast cancers. These tumors generally presented as palpable masses, caused by dilatation of the involved duct and periductal fibrosis. This pattern has shifted dramatically, with most *in situ* cancers now diagnosed by mammography.

In a large national mammography trial, almost a third of all cancers detected by mammography were noninvasive. Generally presenting as microcalcifications, the decision whether to biopsy or observe proves to be a difficult choice for radiologists and patients. Certain patterns, for example, more than five small calcifications in a linear or branching pattern, are considered highly suspicious. There remains significant variability in radiographic interpretation depending on the experience of the observer (Kopans 1994b). Even in the most experienced radiologist's hands, however, only 15–25% of suspicious lesions prove to be malignant.

A rare subtype of intraductal tumors are the *papillary carcinomas* in which the intraductal growth is papillary in configuration, caused by a piling up of pleomorphic duct epithelial cells. The *comedo carcinoma* subtype of intraductal carcinomas have a more solid pattern of growth with central detritus. Material can actually be extruded from the ducts with slight pressure, hence the appellation. These comedo DCIS tumors are thought to be more aggressive biologically, as shown by labeling index and a more malignant cytologic appearance. The comedo type DCIS also demonstrate higher levels of *HER2/* neu oncogene expression (van de Vijver et al., 1988). In the solid type of DCIS the tumor cells fill the ducts and lack significant necrosis.

In situ carcinomas can also arise in the lobule, and, on some occasions may extend into the terminal ducts. This is termed *lobular carcinoma in situ* or LCIS. When the degree of involvement of the lobules and terminal ducts is less extensive, i.e., less than 50% of the lobule, pathologists often call the lesion *atypical ductal hyperplasia.* LCIS generally is diagnosed as an incidental finding of a biopsy showing a benign lesion and accounts for only about 10% of abnormalities identified and localized by mammography. It cannot be palpated and hence is never diagnosed as a gross lesion. The diagnosis of LCIS presents a vexing problem for the clinician because of the high rate of relapse after biopsy and the risk of contralateral disease. Recurrence rates of 10% to 20% have been reported after excision with follow-up of 2 to 5 years. Half of these recurrences were invasive breast cancers. With longer follow-up (up to 24 years), it is believed that 20–30% of patients with LCIS will develop an invasive carcinoma.

The risk for breast cancer following the diagnosis of LCIS is about the same in both breasts. A rate of approximately 20% was reported at 24 year follow-up of a study at Memorial Hospital (Rosen et al., 1978), although the rate of contralateral recurrence after 16 years was somewhat lower in another study of over 200 patients (Haagensen et al., 1981). The proportion of cases of infiltrating lobular type was between 25% and 36% in these two studies. Thus, LCIS was viewed as a sensitive marker of increased breast cancer risk. Most surgeons now elect close surveillance, although mastectomy and extensive contralateral biopsy, or bilateral mastectomy remain options. As noted, the risk is elevated for invasive as well as *in situ* lobular tumors in the contralateral breast.

When the tumor extends through the basement membrane of the duct it is termed *infiltrating ductal.* The most common type of breast cancer is an infiltrating ductal carcinoma in which no special type of histologic structure is apparent. These tumors generally do not reach large size, are quite firm (and used to be termed *scirrhous*) but may metastasize to axillary lymph nodes. A rare variant of infiltrating carcinoma is *medullary carcinoma,* which accounts for about 6% of all breast cancers. These tumors lack the firm fibrous tissue of the other subtypes and grow to a soft brainlike consistency. The tumor is characterized by sheets of large cells with pleomorphic nuclei, and by infiltrating lymphocytes. This latter component was believed to give this tumor a better prognosis, even in the presence of axillary metastases. Medullary cancers appear to be more common in younger patients. *Mucinous* or *colloid carcinoma* accounts for 3% of breast tumors and tends to occur in older women. It grows in gelatinous masses and may contain lakes of amorphous mucin, in which float cells with glandular features. The prognosis for these tumors is good, with lymph node metastases less common. *Tubular* carcinomas account for only 1% of cases, and despite a more aggressive appearance of the cells, this type also appears to share a more favorable prognosis than other infiltrating tumors (Robbins, 1979).

A distinct form of invasive breast cancer that arises from the terminal ductules of the breast lobule is *lobular carcinoma,* which accounts for about 5% of mammary tumors. These tumors are rubbery and poorly circumscribed. The neoplastic cells are small and commonly arranged in single-file through the fibrous matrix or in concentric rings around normal ducts.

Paget's disease of the breast accounts for about 2% of breast cancers. It is a special type of ductal cancer that arises in the main excretory ducts, involving the nipple and areola. It commonly occurs in the setting of a history of eczematoid changes over many years, although most commonly the infiltrating ductal carcinoma antedates the skin complaints. The hallmark lesion is invasion of the epidermis by malignant cells, an event accompanied by a somewhat less favorable prognosis. Another type of breast cancer involving the skin, *inflammatory breast cancer,* has a poor prognosis because of the more aggressive natural history of this subtype. Poorly differentiated neoplastic cells invade not only skin but also the subdermal lymphatics causing obstructive lymphangitis and clinically apparent induration of the skin of the breast.

HEREDITARY SYNDROMES

Frequency of Hereditary Syndromes

Approximately 5–10% of breast cancer demonstrates clear patterns of dominant transmission. Several decades of epidemiologic studies demonstrated a two- to threefold increase in risk of breast cancer in first degree relatives of affected individuals (Cannon-Albright et al., 1991). When observed in families, breast tumors tended to occur at a younger age and were more frequently bilateral.

Breast cancers were also observed with other tumors. The reported association of breast and ovarian cancer by Lynch and Krush in 1971, was confirmed by many others. Associations between breast and prostate cancer were also reported (Cannon et al., 1982; Tulinius et al. 1992; Anderson and Badzioch, 1993). A 1994 study based on the Utah genealogy confirmed a 1.2 relative risk for breast and prostate carcinoma, but also found statistically significant links between breast and colon, thyroid, and lymphoproliferative malignancies (Goldgar et al., 1994).

Genetic epidemiologic analyses suggested an autosomal dominant pattern of susceptibility to breast cancer in the families studied (Cannon et al., 1986). In a study of breast cancer cases and controls, a gene frequency of .0003 was derived for gene(s) conferring susceptibility to breast cancer (Claus et al., 1991). This corresponds to a carrier frequency of 1 in 152 (as will be derived in Chapter 6). An English study based on families of patients with breast or ovarian cancer revealed a gene frequency of .0006 (carrier frequency of 1 in 833), whereas an analysis based on families of ovarian cancer patients gave an intermediate value of .0014 (1 in 345 carrier frequency) (Ford and Easton, 1995; Whittemore et al., 1997). These predictions will be tested by direct measurement of mutations in the general population.

Syndromes of breast cancer susceptibility have been linked to mutations of several genes, including *BRCA1* and *BRCA2*. There are a smaller number of cases with germline mutations of *p53*, and other genes not yet fully characterized (Miki et al., 1994; Wooster et al., 1995; Malkin et al., 1990). A polymorphism in *CYP17*, a cytochrome p450 enzyme involved in estrogen metabolism, has been correlated with a slight increase in risk for advanced breast cancer (Feigelson et al., 1997). Mutations of *BRCA1, BRCA2, p53, PTEN* (Cowden syndrome) and *AR* (androgen receptor) have been documented in families, but additional genes (e.g., *BRCA3*) have not been fully characterized. The relative proportion of hereditary families with these mutations remains to be determined. Predictions based on linkage studies suggested that about 40% of breast cancer kindreds were linked to *BRCA1*, 35% to *BRCA2*, and the remainder were linked to *BRCA3* and other genes (Wooster et al., 1994; Easton et al., 1993).

The proportion of breast cancer families linked to *BRCA3* or other genes may be higher than originally projected. Of 124 families with breast cancer, only 9 (7%) had *BRCA1* mutations, although 18 of 45 families with both breast and ovarian cancer had *BRCA1* mutations (Couch et al., 1997). An analysis of 23 families revealed that more than 20% failed to show mutations of *BRCA1* or *BRCA2* (Rebbeck et al., 1996). An-other series of 23 families with site-specific breast cancer (3 cases diagnosed before age 60 with one diagnosed before age 45), revealed that only 8 (34%) had mutations of *BRCA1* or *BRCA2* (Serova et al., 1997). Mutations in the *BRCA1*-associated gene *BARD-1* have been observed in rare familes with breast, ovarian, and uterine cancer (Bowcock et al., 1997). In addition to *BRCA3,* there may be other *BRCA* genes to ac-count for the remaining hereditary families.

Frequency of Cowden's Syndrome and Other Syndromes of Breast Can-cer Susceptibility

Clinical definitions of Cowden's syndrome (aka Cowden dis-ease) have recently been broadened to include a number of possibly related features (Nelen et al., 1996). As originally defined, in Cowden's syndrome there is dominant in-heritance of multiple hamartomatous lesions, including papillomas of the lips and mu-cous membranes and acral keratoses of the skin (Starink, 1984). The oral mucosal papules take on a cobblestone appearance, and there are rough-surfaced facial papules, called trichilemmomas. Expression of the disease is variable, but the penetrance of the skin manifestations has been reported as high as 100% by age 20. It has been proposed that a normal physical examination of the head and neck of the young adult can ex-clude this diagnosis. Hamartomas of the breast and intestines, as well as the skin and oral mucosa, have been described. Breast cancers in Cowden's syndrome occur at ear-ly age, with average age at 38 in one series and 46 in another (Schrager et al., 1997). It has been estimated that half of patients with Cowden's syndrome will develop breast cancer, although most patients will demonstrate a spectrum of benign breast disease, including ductal hyperplasia, intraductal papillomatosis, adenosis, lobular atrophy, fi-broadenomas, or fibrocystic changes (Schrager et al., 1997). Thyroid cancer has also been reported.

Patients with manifestations of Cowden disease and Lhermitte-Duclos disease (LDD) are affected by megalocephaly, epilepsy, and dysplastic gangliocytomas of the cerebellum (Padberg et al., 1991). It was proposed that Cowden disease and Lhermitte-Duclos disease represented a single entity (Padberg et al., 1991). A locus for Cowden disease was mapped to 10q22-3 (Nelen et al., 1996). The diagnostic criteria for Cow-den disease utilized in these studies, summarized in Table 4-1, were broader than those originally proposed. Mutations of a candidate gene, *PTEN,* mapped to 10q22-23, were observed in four of five Cowden disease kindreds (Liaw et al., 1997). Nonsense muta-tions were associated with macrocephaly in two cases; all affected individuals in the five families demonstrated trichilemmomas, regardless of the type of mutation ob-served. Thyroid tumors, adenomas, and goiter were also observed.

A number of less common Mendelian syndromes are associated with breast cancer risk (Appendix A). Muir-Torre syndrome, reviewed in Part C of this chapter, is charac-terized by both benign and malignant tumors of the breast, along with tumors of the skin and digestive and genito-urinary systems. Individuals with Peutz-Jegher syn-drome, described in Part C of this chapter, are also considered to be at increased risk for breast malignancies; a review of the literature revealed 16 such cases, commonly characterized by bilateral disease at median age of 35 years (McLemore et al., 1997). Based on epidemiologic studies, Swift predicted that the .5–1% of the population who

TABLE 4-1   Clinical Features of Cowden's Syndrome

Pathognomonic Criteria

Facial trichilemmomas[a]
Acral keratoses
Papillomatous lesions
Mucosal lesions

Major Criteria:

Breast cancer
Thyroid cancer (especially papillary type)
Macrocephaly (97th percentile)
Lhermitte-Duclos disease[b]

Minor Criteria:

Thyroid lesions (goiter)
Mental retardation (IQ <75)
Gastrointestinal hamartomas
Fibrocystic disease of the breast
Lipomas
Fibromas
Genitourinary tumors or malformations

Diagnosis

Pathognomonic skin features
or
2 major criteria
or
1 major and 1 minor criteria
or
4 minor criteria

Source: Nelen MR, Padberg GW, Peeters EAJ et al. Localization of the gene for Cowden disease to chromosome 10q22-23. Nature Genet 1996; 13:114–116.
[a]Six or more papules, three or more trichilemmomas
[b]Megalocephaly, epilepsy, and dysplastic gangliocytomas of the cerebellum.

are heterozygotes for ataxia telangiectasia have a fivefold increased risk for breast cancer. This could account for 3.8–18% of sporadic breast cancers in the United States (Swift et al., 1991). Ataxia telangiectasia homozygotes are affected by cerebellar ataxia, oculocutaneous telangiectasia, radiation hypersensitivity, as well as lymphoid, hematopoietic, and other solid tumors.

In Li-Fraumeni syndrome, early onset breast cancer occurs along with soft-tissue sarcomas, osteosarcoma, leukemia, brain tumors, adrenal cortical tumors, and other cancers (see below). Rarely, a typical breast-ovarian kindred may be found to have a germline *p53* mutation (Jolly et al., 1994). A separate syndrome of breast cancer predisposition is associated with inheritance of the constitutional chromosomal translocation t(11;22)(q23;q11) (Lindblom et al., 1994). Very few such cases have been documented. Another rare breast cancer susceptibility syndrome is characterized by mutations of the androgen receptor gene (*AR*) at Xq11.2-12. This syndrome is also characterized by partial androgen insensitivity (Wooster et al., 1992; Lobaccaro et al., 1993).

Frequency of BRCA and Other Mutations in Early-Onset Disease

BRCA1 mutations were relatively infrequent, even in women with early-onset breast cancer. Series of breast cancer patients diagnosed before the age of 30–35 revealed that about 8% of these women harbored germline *BRCA1* mutations (Fitzgerald et al., 1996; Langston et al., 1996). About the same percentage of women with breast cancer before the age of 45 who also had a first degree relative with the disease had *BRCA1* mutations (Malone et al., 1996a). Of 73 women with breast cancer diagnosed before the age of 33, 2 had *BRCA2* mutations and 9 had *BRCA1* mutations, as detected by a "truncated protein" assay (described in Chapter 7) (Krainer et al., 1997). In comparison, germline *p53* mutations, were noted in only 1 of 126 breast cancer patients diagnosed before age 41 (Sidransky et al., 1992). This patient's mother had premenopausal bilateral disease, and her grandmother had both colon and breast cancer at late age. The proband subsequently developed a melanotic spindle-cell carcinoma of the mediastinum. Analysis of 401 women with early-onset breast cancer demonstrated an *ATM* mutation frequency of only 0.5% (Fitzgerald et al., 1997). Analysis of 38 breast tumors not selected by age failed to document even a single mutation of the *ATM,* whereas at least one would have been expected to show this mutation given prior estimates of the gene frequency and the prevalence of heterozygous mutations in unselected breast cancer patients (Vorechovsky et al., 1996).

Risks Associated with Hereditary Breast/Ovarian Cancer

Breast and Ovarian Cancer Risk   The initial estimate of the risk conferred by a common breast cancer susceptibility gene was 67% by age 70 (Claus et al., 1991). This population-derived estimate was based on an analysis of a large number of younger women with breast cancer in an epidemiologic ascertainment. A similar analysis based on ovarian cancer cases revealed a penetrance of 69% by age 70 (Whittemore et al., 1997). Other estimates of the cancer risks associated with mutations of *BRCA1* and *BRCA2* were based on retrospective studies of families selected because of the occurrence of early-onset breast or ovarian cancer, which may have resulted in an overestimate of these risks.

For families with multiple cases of breast or ovarian cancer, it remains appropriate to utilize the risk estimates based on the retrospective (linkage) studies derived from similar families. These studies associated mutations of *BRCA1* and *BRCA2* with early onset disease, with a median age of onset around 45 years. Estimates of the lifetime risk for breast cancer were as high as 90% in families segregating mutations of either of these two genes. Based on the estimates from 214 17q-linked kindreds, the project-

Case Example 4.1. A 30 year old Ashkenazi Jewish woman desired genetic testing for breast cancer susceptibility. Her grandmother was diagnosed with ovarian cancer at age 50, but the proband's mother was alive and well at age 60 without evidence of cancer. The proband tested positive for a truncating mutation of *BRCA1* (5382insC) and wanted to know what her risk of breast cancer was. In view of studies citing a lesser penetrance for mutations detected in the "general population," a 40–60% risk for breast cancer by age 70 was cited (see text and Struewing et al., 1997). As part of a research protocol, full genotyping of the mother revealed her to be germline, while the father was carrying the mutation.

This case indicates the potential limitations of penetrance calculations derived from studies in which full genotyping was not performed. In this pedigree the grandmother most likely represents a "phenocopy" (see Chapter 3). The cumulative probability for breast cancer among heterozygotes is variable among families. Penetrance may vary according to other genetic or environmental factors.

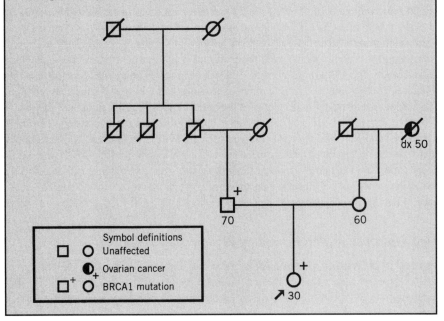

ed risk for either breast or ovarian cancer by age 50 was 59%, and by age 70 the risk was 82% (confidence intervals 64–91%) (Easton et al., 1993). The breast cancer risk by age 70 was 87% (CI 51–95%) in 33 families demonstrating linkage to *BRCA1* (Ford et al., 1994).

The relative risk for breast cancer in *BRCA1*-linked families compared to the general population was relatively high. In the general population, the cumulative incidence of breast cancer by age 50 was 2%, compared to over 50% in the *BRCA1*-linked kindreds. Lifetime cumulative probability of ovarian cancer was 1–2% in the general population, compared to 63% (CI 25–82%) in *BRCA1*-linked kindreds (Easton et al.,

1995). In the study by Easton et al., and a prior study (Ford et al., 1994), it was possible to estimate the risk for a subsequent ovarian or contralateral breast cancer in *BRCA1*-linked individuals already affected by breast cancer. These estimates of risk for contralateral breast cancer were 50% by age 50 and 64% by age 70. In comparison, the risk for contralateral breast cancer in a woman who had breast cancer in the general population was 0.4–0.7% per year. In a *BRCA1* heterozygote already affected by breast cancer, the risk of an ovarian cancer was 29% (CI 16–40%) by age 50 and 44% (CI 28–56%) by age 70 (Ford et al., 1994).

Clinic-based or population-based series documented a lower penetrance for some mutations (Oddeux et al., 1996; Krainer et al., 1997), or suggested lower penetrance because of the detection of mutations in individuals with minimal family histories of the disease (Malone et al., 1996; Struewing et al., 1997; Levy-Lahad et al., 1997). The observation of germline mutations in individuals with no family history of the disease (Langston et al., 1996; Neuhausen et al., 1996a; Malone et al., 1996; Struewing et al., 1997) raised the question of a lower penetrance in a subset of families.

The cumulative probability of breast cancer for carriers of either of two *BRCA1* mutations or one *BRCA2* mutation in a population-based series of Jewish individuals in the Washington, D.C. area was 56% by age 70 (confidence interval 40–73%) compared to the 85% derived from linkage-based ascertainments (Struewing et al., 1997) (see Table 4-2). The results of the Washington study came as a surprise to many and raised the issue of the limitations of "gene-based statistical prophecies" (Healy, 1997). However, as indicated previously, the confidence intervals for the initial linkage-based estimates were broad, and actually overlapped with the estimates derived from the Washington study (Easton, 1997). Breast cancer risks in some large families were closer to 70% (Ford and Easton, 1995). Penetrance estimates made on a clinic-based ascertainment of families revealed a 64% risk for breast or ovarian cancer by age 70 (Levy-Lahad et al., 1997).

TABLE 4-2 Cumulative Risk of Breast Cancer for the General Population, *BRCA1* Heterozygotes in Families with Multiple Cases of Breast or Ovarian Cancer, and Individuals in the Ashkenazi Jewish Population Analyzed for Specific *BRCA* Mutations

Age	General Population	*BRCA1* Heterozygotes in High Risk Families	*BRCA2* Heterozygotes in Selected Families	BRCA Heterozygotes in General Population (Ashkenazi Jews)
40	0.005	0.16	0.14	0.14
45	0.01	0.42		0.30
50	0.02	0.59	0.32	0.33
55	0.03	0.72		0.46
60	0.04	0.77	0.53	0.53
65	0.06	0.80		0.58
70	0.07	0.82	0.67	0.56
75	0.09	0.84		0.63
80	0.10	0.86	0.77	0.61

Sources: Data from Easton et al., 1993 and Ries et al., 1990 and cited in King et al., 1993; Figure 1B in Struewing et al., 1997; Schubert et al., 1997.

This range of reported penetrance functions may be mediated by other genetic, hormonal, or environmental factors. Indeed, one model suggested the existence of different alleles of *BRCA1* with differing risks for ovarian and breast cancer (Easton et al., 1995). Such considerations must be taken into account in the counseling of families. Until the precise impact of these modifying factors are elucidated, it seems prudent to tailor risk counseling to the pedigree (Easton, 1997). The counselor should reserve the higher range of risk figures in Table 4-2 for families with evidence of a "high penetrance" dominant susceptibility, while utilizing the lower range of risks for heterozygotes whose family history is not known or shows evidence of nonpenetrance.

Colon, Prostate, and Pancreatic Cancer Risks   In addition to breast and ovarian cancer risks, increased relative risks for colon and prostate cancers were observed in selected kindreds. Families with few ovarian cancers tended to have the excess in colon cancer, although this finding was only a trend. The risk for colon cancer was 4.0, translating to a 6% risk by age 70. The relative risk for prostate cancer in males was 3.33, corresponding to an 8% risk by age 70 (Ford and Easton, 1995). These absolute risk figures may be misleading because both colon and prostate cancer are less common in Great Britain. For example, the threefold increase in prostate cancer risk in the *BRCA1*-linked families (8% risk) is about equal to the risk for prostate cancer in the general U.S. population.

The excess risk for prostate cancer but not colon cancer was confirmed in studies of founder *BRCA* mutations in ethnically homogeneous populations (Struewing et al, 1997). An increased prevalence of cases of pancreatic cancer was noted in a series of 220 Ashkenazi Jewish families with specific *BRCA* mutations (Tonin et al., 1996). When 39 pancreatic tumors from Ashkenazi Jewish individuals were analyzed for a specific *BRCA2* mutation found in approximately 1% of Jews in the general population, four cases (10%) demonstrated mutations. This corresponded to a relative risk for pancreatic cancer of 8.3 and a cumulative risk to age 75 of 7% (CI 1.9–19%) (Ozcelik et al., 1997). This compared to 0.85% risk for pancreatic cancer in the general population.

BRCA2-Associated Risks   Male breast cancer appeared more often and ovarian cancers less often in *BRCA2*-associated families, although male breast cancer was also observed in a *BRCA1*-linked kindred (Wooster et al., 1994; Struewing et al., 1995b). The breast cancer risk for a male carrier of *BRCA2* mutations was estimated to be 6% by age 70. In a study of 50 male breast cancer cases in one series, 14% demonstrated a *BRCA2* mutation (Couch et al., 1996a). In this study, 80% of the cases had a family history of breast cancer. In a series of 54 male breast cancer cases unselected for family history, 2 (4%) had *BRCA2* mutations (Friedman et al., 1997). Interestingly, in both studies, there were mutation-negative cases of male breast cancer in the setting of a family history of breast cancer, suggesting the presence of genes other than *BRCA2* that confer susceptibility to male and female breast cancers.

Breast cancer risk in *BRCA2*-linked kindreds appeared similar to *BRCA1*-linked kindreds (Wooster et al., 1995). However, one *BRCA2* mutation showed a lesser cumulative risk for early-onset breast cancer (Oddeux et al., 1996), and this observation was later confirmed by other investigators (Krainer et al., 1997; Schubert et al., 1997). Although the lifetime breast cancer risk for *BRCA2* heterozygotes was 80%, the risk by age 50 was only 32%, compared to 59% in high risk *BRCA1*-linked families (Table 4-2), suggesting that *BRCA2* mutations conferred only 1/3 to 1/10 the risk of early-onset breast cancer, compared to *BRCA1* mutations (Oddeux et al., 1996; Krainer et al., 1997). Compared to *BRCA1* heterozygotes, the overall (lifetime) risk of breast cancer in heterozygotes for a specific *BRCA2* mutation did not appear lower in a population-based study (Struewing et al., 1997). However, this finding was not supported in another series, which demonstrated a significantly lower penetrance for a cohort heterozygous for a *BRCA2* mutation (Levy-Lahad et al., 1997).

The clinical significance of these differences in cumulative risk between studies remains unclear. Even assuming the lowest risk estimates for *BRCA* heterozygotes, a 40–50% lifetime breast cancer risk is greater than that of any other known risk factor. The increased risk for ovarian cancer in *BRCA2* heterozygotes was greater than originally predicted from linkage studies, and this is a major focus of concern in clinical risk counseling. As is further elucidated in the next section, ovarian cancer risk in heterozygotes was estimated to be less than 10% by age 70 in the initial linkage series (Ford and Easton, 1995). However, ovarian cancers were observed in about 20% of the families described when direct *BRCA2* mutation testing was available (Tavtigian et al., 1996). As presented in the next section, there is some evidence that ovarian cancer risk is increased in cases in which the *BRCA2* mutation occurs in a 3.3 kb region in exon 11, between nucleotides 3035 and 6629 (Gayther et al., 1997).

Modifiers of Cancer Risk   The magnitude and nature of the increased ovarian cancer risk in both *BRCA1* and *BRCA2* heterozygotes remains a topic of critical importance. Mutations in the 3′ portion of the *BRCA1* gene (exons 13 to 24) were associated with a lesser number of ovarian cancer cases, compared to breast cancer cases in a European series of 32 families (Gayther et al., 1995). However, this observation was not evident when data from a number of centers were combined (Shattuck-Eidens et al., 1995), and this effect is likely to explain a relatively small proportion of the observed variation in ovarian cancer cases within these families.

As mentioned previously, genotype-phenotype analysis of mutations from 25 families with *BRCA2* mutations suggested an association of ovarian cancer risk with a region in the middle of exon 11 (Gayther et al., 1997a). A review of an additional 45 families confirmed a three times greater risk of ovarian cancer for families with *BRCA2* mutations in this region (Gayther et al., 1997a). However, exon 11 is also the largest exon in the gene; hence the numbers of families with mutations in this region may be overrepresented in studies. The finding was of borderline statistical significance in other series (Serova-Sinilnikova et al., 1997).

In an analysis of 307 *BRCA1* heterozygotes, the lifetime risk of ovarian cancer increased from approximately 38% in *BRCA1* heterozygotes with common alleles of the *HRAS1* variable number of tandem repeat polymorphism, compared to 60% in *BRCA1* mutation carriers with one or more rare *HRAS1* VNTR alleles (Phelan et al., 1996). Rare *HRAS* alleles were also more common (62% vs 17%) in *BRCA1* heterozygotes with breast cancer compared to heterozygotes without breast cancer (Garcia-Foncillas et al., 1997). Although the mechanism of this gene–gene interaction remains unclear, analysis of other modifying genes, as well as hormonal and other environmental factors, may shed light on the highly variable range of breast and ovarian cancer risk observed among families with identical *BRCA1* mutations. Polymorphisms of genes involved in estrogen metabolism, as well as some of the xenobiotic metabolic genes mentioned in Chapter 3, have also been correlated with risks for breast or ovarian cancer (Feigelson et al., 1997). The magnitude and mechanism of these modifying effects is not sufficiently understood at present to allow use of these data in clinical counseling.

In linkage studies, young age of onset and bilateral disease were characteristic of both *BRCA1* and *BRCA2*-associated families. However, it remained unclear as to the factors that could modify penetrance of these mutations. Analysis of a large *BRCA1*-linked Utah kindred did not reveal an obvious effect of parity or age at first birth in affecting breast cancer risk (Goldgar et al., 1994). In a study of 28 *BRCA1*-linked families containing 333 women, mutation carriers with less than three pregnancies had twice the risk of developing breast cancer compared to those with three or more pregnancies (Narod et al., 1995). In this study there was no effect of age at first birth or age at last birth as it affected breast cancer risk in *BRCA1* heterozygotes. There may have been an increased risk of breast cancer in women with *BRCA1* mutations born more recently, compared to older women with the same mutation. Evidence of such a cohort effect was found in one large *BRCA1*-linked family, in which the age of onset was 40 years in individuals born after 1930, compared to 51 years for those born before 1930 (Narod et al., 1993).

The cohort effect was also confirmed in a larger study. Only 12% of *BRCA1* mutation carriers born before 1930 had developed breast cancer by age 40, compared to 42% of women born more recently (Narod et al., 1995). Earlier detection in the younger patients was excluded by review of medical records (Narod et al., 1993). These results were consistent with anticipation (see Chapter 2), or with an interaction of genetic susceptibility with an unidentified environmental risk factor of increasing frequency. As noted at the beginning of this chapter, an increase in incidence of breast cancer had been observed in the general population during this same time interval. It is also possible that these observations may have been due to increasing hormone use in the recent cohorts.

Clinico-Pathologic Features of Hereditary Breast-Ovarian Cancer Syndrome

Prior to the identification of *BRCA1* and *BRCA2,* numerous studies examined associations between a family history of the disease and histologic features. These studies found that medullary, lobular (both invasive and *in situ*), and tubular carcinomas appeared to be more common in those with a family history of breast cancer (Lagios et al., 1980; Rosen et al. 1982; LiVolsi et al., 1982; Lynch et al., 1984; Marcus et al., 1994; Claus et al., 1993). Initial reports of *BRCA1*-linked cases confirmed an association with medullary subtype (Lakhani et al., 1997) or "medullary features" in *BRCA1*-linked tumors (Marcus et al., 1996). Tubular carcinoma was less common in *BRCA2*-

Case Example 4.2. Three sisters ages 31, 33, and 36 came in for genetic counseling because of a family history of breast cancer. Their mother and maternal aunt were both affected at an early age with breast or ovarian cancer. They were of Ashkenazi Jewish background. The youngest sister had multiple biopsies because of fibrocystic disease. Her most recent biopsy revealed a focus of lobular carcinoma *in situ*. After being informed of the risks for ipsilateral and contralateral breast cancer associated with the diagnosis of LCIS, the 31-year-old sister was considering her screening options. She desired genetic testing but was only able to afford screening for the most common mutations in Ashkenazi Jews. She was found not to carry the 185delAG, 5382insC *BRCA1* or 6174delT *BRCA2* mutations, and opted for close breast surveillance. She understood that the breast cancers in her family could still be associated with another mutation of *BRCA1* or *BRCA2* or with mutations in another gene.

A year later, her sisters contacted her and requested a meeting with her genetic counselor. They questioned whether they should help their sister pay for full *BRCA1* and *BRCA2* sequencing. Instead, as part of a research study, the counselor was put in touch with the mother and obtained her consent to perform genetic testing. A 6174delT *BRCA2* mutation was detected. The sisters were offered definitive genetic testing to establish their risk.

This case reinforces the rule that genetic testing of families should begin with an affected member. In this case, the LCIS in the sister represented an indicator of increased risk for breast cancer, but one not related to the hereditary cancers in this family.

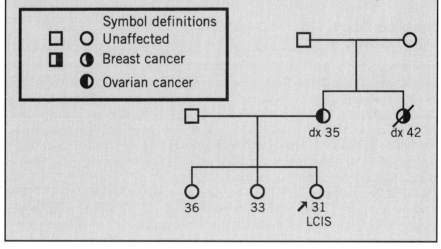

linked cases (Lakhani et al., 1997). In general, less tubule formation was noted in both *BRCA1* and *BRCA2*-linked tumors, although the *BRCA2*-linked tumors did not share the pleomorphism or higher mitotic index noted in the *BRCA1*-linked group (Lakhani et al., 1997). In another study, *BRCA1*-linked tumors were of higher grade and were more frequently negative for estrogen and progesterone receptors (Johannsson et al., 1997). Interestingly, tumors with *BRCA1* or *BRCA2* germline mutations had a higher frequency of specific somatic genetic alterations, consistent with the observation of a distinctive pathway of progression for these tumors (Tirkkonen et al., 1997).

Family history of breast cancer is also an important risk factor for intraductal breast cancer (Kerlikowske et al., 1997). There has been relatively little analysis of the association of DCIS and *BRCA1*-linked breast cancer. Indeed, in most studies, cases of DCIS were not counted as "affected." In some of the early families studied, observed cases of DCIS were not linked to *BRCA1* (e.g., IARC family 107). In one study of over 100 *BRCA1* linked cases, areas of DCIS were underrepresented compared to controls (Lakhani et al., 1997). An analysis of eight ductal tumors containing areas of DCIS revealed loss of heterozygosity in 17p13 (the region of *BRCA1*) in over half of cases, with one case showing this same pattern in adjacent normal tissue (Deng et al., 1996). The finding of similar genetic alterations in malignant and premalignant tissue is consistent with the multiple-hit model of carcinogenesis (Chapter 3).

It was observed that *BRCA1*-associated tumors displayed features suggestive of a more aggressive phenotype, including a higher proportion of cells in S phase, and other indices of higher histologic grade (Bignon et al., 1995; Jacquemier et al., 1995; Marcus et al., 1996; Eisinger et al., 1996; Lakhani et al., 1997). Thus, the relative paucity of noninvasive tumors in the hereditary group may be due to their more "aggressive" natural history. Alternatively, studies of large numbers of noninvasive breast cancers may show similar proportions associated with germline mutations. The need for these studies is paramount, because of the potential prognostic implications of mutation detection in this subset of affected women (Offit, 1996a).

Hereditary Predisposition to Breast Cancer in Ashkenazi Jews and Other Populations

As introduced in Chapter 3, numerous "founder" mutations have been documented for human hereditary disorders. These ancestral mutations have predominantly been identified in geographically isolated populations. Founder mutations of *BRCA1* and *BRCA2* are listed in Table 4-3. In Canada, common origin (haplotype sharing) of two *BRCA1* mutations was observed in breast and ovarian cancer families (Simard et al., 1994). One of these mutations of *BRCA1* was a two base pair deletion in codon 23, termed 185delAG. It was detected in about 10% of cases of hereditary breast cancer, but varied depending on the proportion of individuals of Ashkenazi Jewish descent included in the population under study (Simard et al., 1994; Struewing et al., 1995; Tonin et al., 1995; Struewing et al., 1995a; Offit et al., 1996a). The mutation was found predominantly, but not exclusively, in individuals of Ashkenazi Jewish origin (Friedman et al., 1997). A Jewish woman with breast cancer before the age of 40 had about a 20% chance of harboring this single mutation (Offit et al., 1996b; Fitzgerald et al., 1996), which was also found in about a third of Ashkenazi families characterized by multiple cases of breast and ovarian cancer (Offit et al., 1996b). This same mutation was present in one out of a hundred Ashkenazi men and women in the general population (Struewing et al., 1995a).

It was estimated that the 185delAG mutation was transmitted from a common ancestor who lived some six centuries ago (Neuhausen et al., 1996b). The mutation was also observed in 29–45% of ovarian cancer cases in an Israeli population, and, surprisingly, in 3 of 650 (0.46%) unselected Iraqi Jews (Friedman et al., 1996; Levy-Lahad et

TABLE 4-3 Common Founder Mutations of *BRCA1* and *BRCA2*

Population	*BRCA1* Mutation	*BRCA2* Mutation	Reference
African-American	1832del5		Gao et al., 1997
	5296del4		
Ashkenazi Jewish	185delAG		Simard et al., 1994
	5382insC		
		6174delT	Neuhausen et al., 1996a
Britain	4184del4		Gayther et al., 1995
		6503delTT	Mazoyer et al.,1996
Finland		L2776X	Vehmanen et al., 1997
France	5149del4		Stoppa-Lyonnet et al., 1997
		9254del5	Serova-Sinilnokova et al.,
		A2951T	1997
Hungary	5282insC		Ramus et al., 1997b
Iceland		999del5	Thorlacius et al., 1996
Italy	1499insA		Montagna et al., 1996;
			de Benedetti et al., 1996
Netherlands	2804delAA		Peelan et al., 1997
Norway	1136insA		Andersen et al., 1996
Sweden	3166insTGAGA		Johannsson et al., 1996
	2595delA		
	1201del11		
	G563X		
		4486delG	Hakansson et al., 1997
Russia	5382insC		Gayther et al., 1997
	4153delA		

al., 1997). These latter results suggest independent origins for this mutation.

The second *BRCA1* mutation initially noted to demonstrate haplotype sharing in the initial study of Canadian families was the 5382insC mutation in codon 1756 (Simard et al., 1994). This mutation appears more commonly in Northern and Eastern Europeans, and may also be more common in Ashkenazi Jews. Another mutation, 188del11 was described in several individuals of Jewish background (Berman et al., 1996), but was not confirmed in larger series (Tonin et al., 1996).

A particular mutation of *BRCA2*, a single base pair deletion in codon 1982 of exon 11, 6174delT, was observed in about 8% of early onset (before age 42) breast cancer patients of Ashkenazi Jewish ancestry (Neuhausen et al., 1996a). Together, the 185delAG and 5382insC *BRCA1* mutations, and the 6174delT *BRCA2* mutation accounted for over a quarter of kindreds with at least two cases of breast cancer, one before the age of 50 years, and 90% of kindreds with two or more breast cancer cases and two or more ovarian cancer cases (Tonin et al., 1996) (Table 4-4). There also appeared to be an excess of pancreatic cancers in the Ashkenazi families with *BRCA2* mutations, and fallopian tube cancers were overrepresented in both the *BRCA2* and *BRCA1*-associated Jewish kindreds.

Table 4-4 Probability of Detection of *BRCA1* or *BRCA2* Founder Mutations in Ashkenazi Individuals

Family History	Number with Founder Mutation[a]	Percent
A. Families with Two Breast Cancers, One before Age 50:		
2 Breast cancers	12/48	25
3 Breast cancers	11/43	26
4+ Breast cancers	17/47	36
2+ Breast, 1 ovarian	35/54	65
2+ Breast, 2+ ovarian	25/28	89
B. Women with or without Family History of Breast or Ovarian Cancer:		
Unaffected, age <50		
Affected FDR or SDR	34/854	3.9
No family history	9/ 951	1
Unaffected, age >50		
Affected FDR or SDR	17/752	2
No family history	4/877	0.5
Affected, with FDR or SDR	20/161	12
Affected, no family history	7/141	5
Affected age <40	9/34	27
Affected age 40-49	11/109	10
Affected age 50-59	6/82	7
Affected age 60+	1/71	1.4

Sources: Part A based on 220 familes analyzed by Tonin P, Weber B, Offit K, et al. 1996. Frequency of recurrent *BRCA1* and *BRCA2* mutations in Ashkenazi Jewish breast cancer families. Nature Medicine 2:1179–83; Part B data from JP Struewing et al. 1997. The risk of cancer associated with specific mutations of BRCA1 and BRCA2 among Ashkenazi Jews. New Engl J Med 336:1401–8 and personal communication.
Note: "Affected" refers to breast cancer; FDR = first-degree relative; SDR = second-degree relative
[a]Founder mutations include 185delAG and 5382insC *BRCA1* mutations and 6174delT *BRCA2* mutation.

In Israeli cohorts, one of the three founder mutations was observed in 13 of 21 (62%) Ashkenazi women with ovarian cancer, 13 of 43 (30%) women with breast cancer before the age of 40 in one series (Abeliovich et al., 1997), and in 25 of 42 high-risk breast/ovarian families in another series (Levy-Lahad et al., 1997). The 6174delT *BRCA2* mutation was observed at about the same frequency (1%) in the Ashkenazi Jewish population as the 185delAG *BRCA1* mutation (Oddeux et al., 1996; Benjamin et al., 1996). The greater frequency of the 185delAG mutation in early-onset breast cancer cases (Offit et al., 1996a; Abeliovich et al., 1997; Levy-Lahad et al., 1997; Krainer et al., 1997) suggests that the risk for early-onset breast cancer was approximately three times greater for the *BRCA1* mutation (Oddoux et al., 1996). A population-based survey confirmed a twofold greater risk for breast cancer before age 40 in 185delAG heterozygotes, compared to 6174delT heterozygotes (Struewing et al., 1997). In this population-based study, family history information was self-reported, and genotyping of first-degree relatives was statistically inferred and not actually tested. Given these limitations, the lifetime penetrance for these mutations was comparable and was about 60% overall.

Including the 5382insC *BRCA1* mutation, about 1 in 40 Ashkenazi Jews harbored one of the common mutations of *BRCA1* or *BRCA2* (Oddeux et al., 1996; Benjamin et al., 1996; Struewing et al., 1997), a relatively high carrier frequency for a potentially lethal genetic disease. Given this high frequency, it is perhaps not surprising that a compound heterozygote for both *BRCA1* and *BRCA2* mutations was described (Ramus et al., 1997a). Another patient, with both the 6174delT *BRCA2* mutation and a 3888delAG *BRCA1* mutation, was described (Randall et al., 1997). The phenotype of both of these cases was severe, with both breast and ovarian cancer occurring at an early age.

Are there mutations of *BRCA1* or *BRCA2* in Ashkenazi Jews other than the founder mutations? This question is important for both practical as well as scientific reasons, because the cost of single mutation screening is considerably less than the cost of full sequencing. Ashkenazi individuals with private mutations have been observed (Robson and Offit, 1997a; Randall et al., 1997; Schubert et al., 1997). As evidence of this observation, 10% of Ashkenazi families with greater than two cases of breast cancer and two cases of ovarian cancer did not have one of the three founder *BRCA* mutations (Tonin et al., 1996). Similarly, 40% of families in a cancer genetics clinic in Israel did not segregate one of the three founder mutations (Levy-Lahad et al., 1997). These data should be provided to Jewish individuals considering "three-mutation" testing.

Despite the frequency of these mutations, the relative risk for breast cancer did not appear to be markedly increased in Jews compared to non-Jews. The relative risk of breast cancer was 1.1 in a study of over 6000 Jewish cases and 9000 non-Jewish controls (i.e., increased 10%). However, the relative risk was 3.8 in Jewish individuals with a history of a first-degree relative with breast cancer, compared to 1.6–1.7 for non-Jews with similar family histories (Egan et al., 1996). These figures suggest that the hereditary component of breast cancer may be greater in Jewish individuals.

Founder mutations in populations other than the Ashkenazim have also been observed. A specific mutation of *BRCA2,* 999del5, was identified in 40% of male breast cancer cases, 7.7% of female breast cancer patients, and 25% of female breast cancer cases before age 40 diagnosed in Iceland (Thorlacius et al., 1996; Thorlacius et al., 1997). Indeed, the carrier frequency for this mutation was estimated to be 0.6% in the entire Icelandic population. This same mutation was observed in Finland, and was attributed to a common Viking ancestor in the era 800–1050 A.D. (Vehmanen et al., 1997). In addition, a nonsense mutation in exon 18 of *BRCA2,* leu2776ter, was also a founder mutation in the Finnish population (Vehmanen et al., 1997).

The 1136insA *BRCA1* mutation was identified in Norwegian breast and ovarian cancer families (Andersen et al., 1996). In Sweden, at least 4 founder *BRCA1* mutations were documented: 3166insTGAGA, 2595delA, 1201del11 and gln563ter (Johannson et al., 1996), as well as a *BRCA2* founder mutation, 4486delG (Hakansson et al., 1997). In the Netherlands, the 2804delAA *BRCA1* mutation accounted for 24% of all mutations studied (Peelan et al., 1997).

In Russia, two mutations of *BRCA1*, 5382insC and 4153delA accounted for 86% of all mutations reported in ovarian (or breast/ovarian) cancer families (Gayther et al., 1997b). The 5382insC mutation was also observed frequently in Hungarian breast cancer families (Ramus et al., 1997b). These families shared the founder haplotype originally described by Neuhausen in 1996, and observed in Ashkenazi Jews and other Northern and Eastern European groups.

Searches for other founder mutations in North American families are underway. A polymorphism in the 3' UTR region of *BRCA1* has been observed in African Americans, and may be associated with a very modest increase in risk for breast cancer (Newman et al., 1996). Two recurrent mutations, 943ins10 and 1832del5, have been noted in unrelated African-American families (Arena et al., 1996; Gao et al., 1997). Analysis of African kindreds is also being performed.

Threshold for *BRCA* Testing

Several models have been proposed for predicting likelihood of detecting *BRCA* mutations given differing family histories (Shattuck-Eidens et al., 1995; Shattuck-Eidens et al., 1997; Couch et al., 1997). Table 4-5 compares two models to estimate the probabilities that families segregate *BRCA1* mutations. In general, the frequency of *BRCA1* mutations among families with breast cancer was lower than predicted by linkage studies. For example, for a family with two or more breast cancers, there was greater than a 10% probability of detection of a *BRCA1* mutation only if the average age of the women at the time they were affected by breast cancer was 39 or younger, or if one of the women was affected before age 35 (see Table 4-5). Both of these models emphasized the important role of (1) age of onset of breast cancers, and (2) a family or personal history of ovarian cancer. For example, there was a >50% probability of detecting a *BRCA1* mutation in a family with two individuals with both breast and ovarian cancer occurring at any age (Couch et al., 1997), or in a family in which one of the cases of breast and ovarian cancer occurred before the age of 50 (Shattuck-Eidens et al., 1997). Similarly, the probability for detecting a *BRCA1* mutation was also >50% when the proband had ovarian cancer before the age of 40 in the setting of a family history of breast and ovarian cancer in the same individual (Shattuck-Eidens et al., 1997). Interestingly, in one study, the number of cases in the family affected by breast cancer and the presence of bilateral breast cancer did not correlate with the probability of detecting a mutation in a breast cancer susceptibility gene (Couch et al., 1997). This result may have been due to the exclusion of some larger families participating in linkage studies, and the lack of *BRCA2* mutation analysis.

DNA Diagnosis

BRCA1 Because of its extremely large size (over 100,000 bases of genomic DNA with 22 coding and 2 noncoding exons), detection of mutations in *BRCA1* has remained a technical challenge. An update of mutations reported to date can be accessed through the Internet at

TABLE 4-5 Probability Thresholds for Detection of a *BRCA1* Mutation Using Two Models in All Affected Families and in Ashkenazi Jewish Families (parentheses)

Criterion	Probability of *BRCA1* Mutation Detection		
	>10%	>40%	>70%
Average age of breast cancer in families with breast cancer and no ovarian cancer	<39 (<55)	— (—)	— (—)
Age of breast cancer in proband with family history of breast cancer and no ovarian cancer	<35 (<54)	— (<30)	— (—)
Average age of breast cancer in family with breast and ovarian cancer in different individuals	<60 (all)	<40 (<55)	— (<40)
Age of breast cancer in proband with family history of breast and ovarian cancer in different individuals	<45 (<64)	— (<38)	— (—)
Average age of breast cancer in family with breast and ovarian cancer in a single member	all (all)	<50 (<60)	<35 (<50)
Age of breast cancer in proband with family history of breast and ovarian cancer in a single member	<50 (<69)	<30 (<45)	— (<30)

Sources: Data on average age of breast cancer in affected families taken from Table 3 in Couch FJ, De-Shano ML, Blackwood MA et al. *BRCA1* mutations in women attending clinics that evaluate the risk of breast cancer. New Engl J Med 1997; 336:1409–15; data on age of breast cancer in probands of affected families taken from Shattuck-Eidens D, Oliphant A, McClure M et al. *BRCA1* sequence analysis in women at high risk for susceptibility mutations. JAMA 1997 278:1242–50.

htpp://www.nhgri.nih.gov/Intramural_research/Lab_transfer/Bic

Numerous reports have summarized the spectrum of mutations catalogued to date (Shattuck-Eidens et al., 1995, 1997; Couch et al., 1996b). Over 100 mutations have been documented. The two most common mutations include the 185delAG and the 5382insC, located at opposite ends of the *BRCA1* gene. A third mutation, 4184del4 in codon 1355 was also seen recurrently in multiple series.

Of the *BRCA1* mutations identified, the large majority cause premature truncation of the peptide by frameshift or nonsense sequence changes (Figure 4-2). These truncation mutations have predominantly included deletions of up to 40 basepairs or insertions of up to a dozen basepairs, seen less frequently. By shifting the reading frame, these mutations cause a premature stop codon downstream. The nonsense mutations, which comprise about 10% of cases, result in stop codons at the site of the single base pair substitution. An additional 5–10% of cases are comprised of regulatory mutations outside of the coding regions that result in loss of expression of the mutant allele, or splice site mutations that cause abnormal translation of the gene.

A minority (about 5%) of *BRCA1* mutations reported are missense mutations that are known to be deleterious. More problematic for the clinician, however, are the

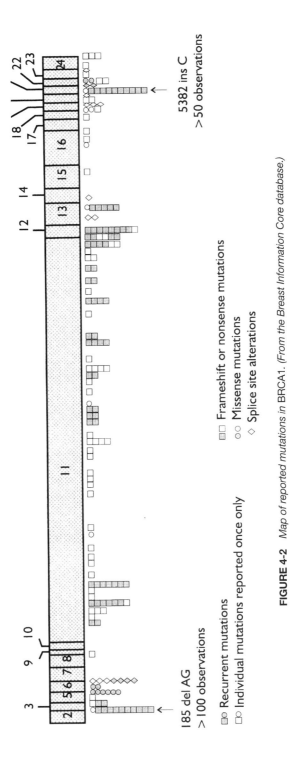

FIGURE 4-2 *Map of reported mutations in BRCA1. (From the Breast Information Core database.)*

larger number of missense mutations of unknown clinical significance. As explained in Chapter 3, missense mutations may pose serious diagnostic challenges. Of 798 samples analyzed by automated sequencing, 102 (13%) were clearly deleterious (including truncating mutations and deleterious missense mutations), 26 (3%) were neutral polymorphisms, and 38 (5%) were polymorphisms of unknown significance (Shattuck-Eidens et al., 1997). Put another way, of 166 mutations detected, 38 (23%) were of unknown significance. A list of recurrent deleterious mutations, neutral polymorphisms, and missense changes of unknown significance derived from this study are listed in Table 4-6.

A European series of 160 cases analyzed for *BRCA1* mutations revealed 38 truncating mutations and 15 missense mutations, of which 7 were of unknown significance (Stoppa-Lyonnet et al., 1997). A similar analysis of 77 cases for *BRCA2* mutations revealed 14 truncating mutations and 2 missense variants of unknown significance (Serova-Sinilnikova et al., 1997).

The report of a polymorphism of unknown significance poses special challenges for both clinician and family member. As discussed in Chapter 3, the clinician may need to test other members of the family to see if the mutation segregates with the cancers observed. If information from the literature or websites is not helpful, one may be left to infer whether the mutation lies in a region of the gene critical for its function. For example, *BRCA1* mutations in exons 2 through 5 are felt to be significant because they occur in a region that encodes a zinc finger RING motif that is felt to be critical to

TABLE 4-6   Most Common Recurrent Mutations in *BRCA1* Sequence Analysis of 798 Samples

Deleterious Mutations (seen twice or more)	Rare Polymorphisms	Variants of Unknown Significance (seen twice or more)
185delAG[a,c]	K38K	Y179C
5382insC[b]	T327T	F486L
4184del4	A622A	N550H
R1443X	R841W	K820E
G61G	G911G	R1347G[c]
917delTT	P938P	R1495M
K467X	P1238L	
Q563X	R1443G	
K679X	S1512I	
5085del19	Q1604Q	
	M1652I[c]	
	IVS8-17G → T	
	IVS12+31 delGT	

Source: Shattuck-Eidens D, Oliphant A, McClure M et al. *BRCA1* sequence analysis in women at high risk for susceptibility mutations. JAMA 1997 278:1242–1250.

[a]Also called 187delAG.

[b]Also called 5385insC.

[c]Most commonly recurring.

Case Example 4.3. A 30-year-old woman came for a second opinion after having obtained *BRCA1* mutation testing from a local health-care professional. She had a family history of maternal breast cancer at age 58. She was not told that testing would be most informative if it began with her mother and was not counseled about the possibility of ambiguous results. Her test revealed a missense mutation of *BRCA1* of "unknown significance." The patient reviewed a copy of her laboratory report provided to her and was confused about the results.

After consultation with a cancer geneticist, it was suggested that the parents come in for genetic counseling. They agreed to genetic testing. The same *BRCA1* sequence variation was found in the proband's father but not the mother. There was no cancer family history on the paternal side. The counselor informed the family that this most likely represents a normal polymorphism, although it was emphasized that this will need to be confirmed when it is observed in other "normal" individuals, or when a test is available to determine if this particular mutation has any affect on the function of the *BRCA1* protein.

Although the outcome of this evaluation was ultimately informative, individuals may experience distress and disappointment if pretest counseling does not address the possibility of ambiguous results. The high prevalence of *BRCA1* polymorphisms of unknown significance, discussed in the text, will be addressed by the availability of population-based statistics and the development of a "functional" assay (see text).

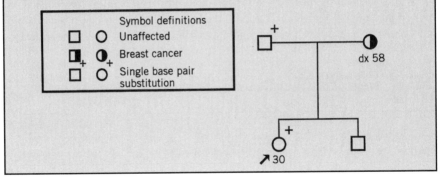

the DNA-binding function of the gene. As additional sequences of *BRCA1* are shown to be binding domains for other proteins, mutations in these regions will more likely be deleterious.

An example of the difficulties posed in the interpretation of the significance of *BRCA1* missense mutations is the ser1040asn mutation, which was initially reported to be associated with breast cancers in families by one set of authors (Friedman et al. 1994), but felt to be a common polymorphism by other authors (Castilla et al., 1994). An arg841trp missense mutation was associated with a moderate phenotype of late onset breast and ovarian cancer in one report (Barker et al., 1996), but was classified as a neutral polymorphism in another series (Shattuck-Eidens et al., 1997). A functional assay for *BRCA1* mutations allows assessment of the significance of rare missense mutations. An initial version of such a functional assay has been developed for mutations in the C terminal region of *BRCA1* (Humphrey et al., 1997). Until such tools are available in commercial laboratories, the counseling of families with missense mutations of unknown significance must be viewed as an ongoing and evolving challenge.

It is also possible that some seemingly "benign" polymorphisms of *BRCA1* and *BRCA2* will be shown to be of low penetrance, or to modify the penetrance of other mutations. Thus far, epidemiologic analysis has failed to demonstrate even a low breast cancer risk associated with three common *BRCA1* variants in the European population (Dunning et al., 1997). Further such studies will be necessary to exclude a lesser cancer risk associated with other polymorphisms.

BRCA2 *BRCA2* testing, previously performed by demonstrating linkage to chromosome 13q, can now be accomplished by direct sequencing. The gene is encoded by a transcript of 10–12 kb, corresponding to a known sequence of over 3418 amino acids. Like *BRCA1*, *BRCA2* was found to be a large gene, consisting of 27 exons distributed over 70 kb of genomic DNA. By coincidence, like *BRCA1*, *BRCA2* has a very large 11th exon (Figure 4-3). *BRCA2* was found to have only slight homology to *BRCA1*. Preliminary analysis of mutations of *BRCA2* did not show evidence of mutational hotspots (Wooster et al., 1995; Tavtigian et al., 1996). Like those of *BRCA1*, mutations of *BRCA2* appear to be distributed over the entire coding sequence and to be dominated by truncating mutations. One truncating mutation, 6503delTT, at the tail end of the *BRCA2* gene, involves a region that shows homology to the granin family of secreted proteins. Interestingly, this mutation did not appear to be deleterious, suggesting that the granin region was not critical to *BRCA2* function (Mazoyer et al., 1996).

Methods of Mutation Detection Direct detection of specific *BRCA1* or *BRCA2* mutations, by allele-specific-oligonucleotide (ASO), band shift on acrylamide gel electrophoresis, or similar techniques (see Chapter 7), can be performed on very small quantities of DNA, including DNA extracted from paraffin blocks. Because direct se-

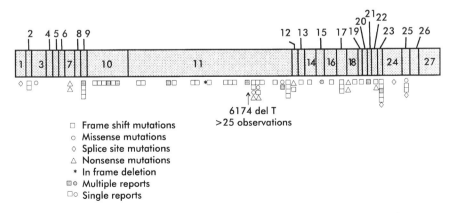

FIGURE 4-3 *Map of reported mutations in BRCA2. (From the Breast Information Core database.)*

quencing generally requires larger quantities of DNA of high purity, blood or tissue samples have been required. Similarly, analysis of regulatory mutations, utilizing cDNA (from RNA), and assays for truncated *BRCA1* proteins, are best performed on live lymphocytes from fresh blood or tissue samples. While each of these methods has been utilized in published reports, the relative sensitivities and specificities of these techniques have not been established (see Chapter 6).

OPTIONS FOR PREVENTION, EARLY DETECTION, AND TREATMENT

Options for the Unaffected Individual at Risk: Examination and Mammography

The three elements of breast surveillance are self-examination, clinician examination, and mammography. Self-examination is a skill that must be taught. Instructional booklets and tapes are available, and practice manikins with different sized lumps are also useful to make available to women to master examination techniques. Self-exams (and mammography) are best performed about a week after the menstrual cycle when the breasts are least lumpy. The evidence for the efficacy of physical examination is largely based on retrospective studies. The proportion of stage I tumors was 54% when detected by physician exam, 38% by self-exam, and 27% when detection was accidental. Tumors found during routine examination tended to be 6 mm smaller than those discovered accidentally (Greenwald et al., 1978).

There is widespread consensus that routine mammography reduces breast cancer mortality (Kopans, 1994a; Kerlikowske, 1995). Metanalyses have documented a 20–30% decrease in mortality for women age 50–74. Despite these statistics, a 1992 National Health Interview Survey indicated that only 35% of women over the age of 50 had a mammogram during the previous year. The controversy, at least in the United States, has concerned women younger than age 40–49, the ages of greatest risk for *BRCA1* gene carriers. This debate followed the publication of the Canadian National Breast Screening Study in 1992. This study surprisingly showed an increase, albeit statistically insignificant, in breast cancer deaths in a group of women age 40–49 randomly assigned to mammography. The considerable methodologic and technical shortcomings of this trial have been summarized elsewhere (Kopans, 1994a); however, the ensuing debate and metanalyses led to the modification of the official recommendations of the U.S. National Cancer Institute (NCI). In 1993, the NCI recommended that mammography decisions for women in their 40s should be individualized after a doctor–patient discussion. An NCI panel repeated this position in 1997, but later the same year the National Cancer Advisory Board and the American Cancer Society reaffirmed the importance of regular mammograms for women in their forties.

The reason for the contradictory "expert panel" recommendations in 1997 emerged from a review of the larger studies on which the recommendations were based. Metanalyses have shown that the 20–40% reductions in mortality from breast cancer in the age 40–49 age group lacked statistical significance, largely due to the limited number of women in the studies. A significant decrease for breast cancer mortality in this age

Case Example 4.4. A 34-year-old nurse was contemplating genetic testing because of a family history of breast and ovarian cancer. She decided to defer testing until after she completed childbearing. She was planning to attempt to initiate a pregnancy in the coming year. She was advised to have a baseline mammogram before pregnancy and before further discussion of testing options. She agreed and mammography revealed clustered microcalcifications. A "lumpectomy" revealed an intraductal carcinoma.

This case highlights that genetic testing should be provided in the context of preventive oncologic consultation. Baseline mammography should, as a routine, precede genetic testing.

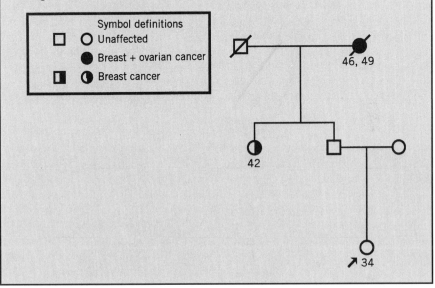

group did emerge, however, at 10–12 year follow-up. In addition, only three of the larger studies in the metanalyses utilized two-view mammography, and in these studies a decrease in mortality was noted (Feig, 1996a,b; Kerlikowske, 1995). More recent metanalyses have shown a significant 24% mortality reduction in the 40–49 year age group (Smart et al., 1995).

For women at high risk for breast cancer, the data are still evolving. A greater predictive value of mammography was documented in those with a family history of breast cancer compared to those without this history, and this advantage was documented in the 40–49 age group (Kerlikowske et al., 1993). However, a later study showed that the sensitivity of mammography in those 40–49 with a family history of breast cancer was significantly less than in those without a family history (Kerlikowske et al., 1996). Thus, the current data indicate a greater positive predictive value and a lesser sensitivity for screening mammography for young women with a family history of breast cancer. While the quantitative basis for these concepts will be more fully explored in Chapter 6, this means in general terms that for each mammogram performed, the probability that an abnormal result will turn out to be a tumor is higher for a young woman with a family history of breast cancer. However, for each tumor in such a woman, the chance that it will be missed by routine mammograms is also higher compared to a young woman without a family history of breast cancer. Given the fact that the risk of dying of breast cancer before age 50 is five times greater for women with a family history of breast cancer, a potential explanation emerges. Breast tumors in young women with a family history may be faster growing (hence missed more often). Preliminary data are consistent with greater indices of proliferation for *BRCA1*-associated tumors (Bignon et al., 1995; Jacquemier et al., 1995; Marcus et al., 1996; Eisinger et al., 1996; Lakhani et al., 1997). This argument would favor more frequent mammography screening in this group. Alternatively, it may simply be that mammography in the younger women has decreased sensitivity because of technical limitations due to the decreased fat in the breasts of younger women (Figure 4-4).

In view of these and other considerations, it seems prudent to initiate mammography at an early age for individuals at increased cancer risk. For *BRCA* gene carriers, the risk of breast cancer by age 40 is as high as 14–16% compared to less than 0.5% in the general population (Table 4-2). Because the earliest age of onset of breast cancer in

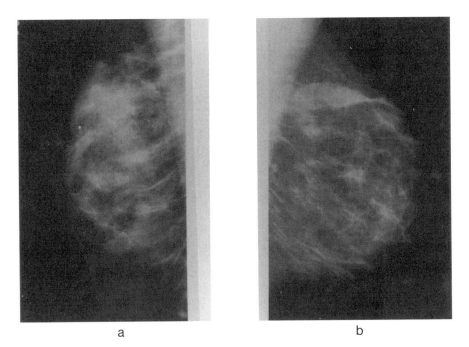

a   b

FIGURE 4-4 a. *Densely glandular breast with numerous pleomorphic microcalcifications that were found to be an intraductal carcinoma. The rounded white dot represents a metallic marker placed on the patient's skin. This pattern of breast density presents limitations to the radiologist's ability to diagnose a small mass; however, calcifications are still observable. b. Mildly glandular breast demonstrating a spiculated mass in the central portion of the breast. The density of this breast is more amenable to screening by mammography. (Cases courtesy of E. B. Sonnenblick, M.D.)*

hereditary syndromes is around 25, this is a reasonable time to begin mammography screening in the setting of a known mutation carrier. Because of the arguments about a faster growth rate in hereditary tumors, some investigators recommend twice yearly mammography for those at highest risk.

In the setting of lesser familial risks, guidelines must be individualized; one approach is to recommend mammography to begin 10 years before the earliest onset of breast cancer in the family (but not before age 25).

Patients will ask about the possibly deleterious effect of mammography. The amount of radiation from a modern mammogram is now substantially less than one rad (cGy), and can be compared to the amount of radiation from a cross-country airline flight. For the average woman, the risk of causing a cancer from radiation exposure due to mammography is negligible compared to its potential benefit. It has been estimated that for a woman who begins screening at age 35 and continues to age 75, the benefit is at least 25 times greater than the potential radiation risk (Mettler et al., 1996). A different set of recommendations may apply to women in families affected by ataxia telangiectasia, a rare recessive condition in which homozygotes have an increased sensitivity to ionizing radiation. As noted previously, the degree to which heterozygotes for mutations of the ataxia telangectasia gene (*ATM*) are sensitive to radiation remains to be established.

Digital mammography is a technique that utilizes a routine X-ray exposure to record the image of the breast in a computer and then displays it in an enhanced format. Although not yet in routine use, the technique offers promise to improve imaging of the breast and may be applied to women at hereditary risk (Schmidt and Nishikawa, 1994). Magnetic resonance imaging (MRI) of the breast offers the advantage of eliminating X-ray exposure and has been utilized to localize known lesions and to assist in preoperative planning of selected cases. Because of the need for multiple images and cost, MRI has not been utilized for screening, and considerable uncertainties remain regarding technique and interpretation of images (Heywang-Kobrunner, 1994; Adler and Wahl, 1995). However, MRI may have a role in assisting in the evaluation of the patient at highest hereditary risk who also has "dense" breasts on mammogram, or in the patient for whom radiation risks are a particular concern.

Options for the Unaffected Individual at Risk: Prophylactic Surgery

For women at the highest hereditary risk for breast cancer (>50% lifetime risk) it is appropriate to discuss the option of removing the healthy breasts as a preventative measure (prophylactic mastectomy). A survey of surgeons indicated that they would be willing to perform prophylactic mastectomy for women at risks ranging from 41% to 54%, depending on which type of surgeon was asked. Plastic surgeons were inclined to consider the procedure in lower risk groups, while gynecologists reserved discussion of the procedure unless risk was quite high. Of 741 surgeons surveyed, an average of 293 such surgeries were recommended during the year of the survey, with 101 actually performed (Houn et al., 1995). Although very little follow-up data on these patients had been reported, very high rates of patient satisfaction following these procedures was observed (Stefanek, 1995).

Case Example 4.5. A woman, age 27, came for counseling and testing with a striking family history of breast cancer. She decided that irrespective of the result of genetic testing, she would not undergo a preventive surgical procedure but would opt for increased surveillance.

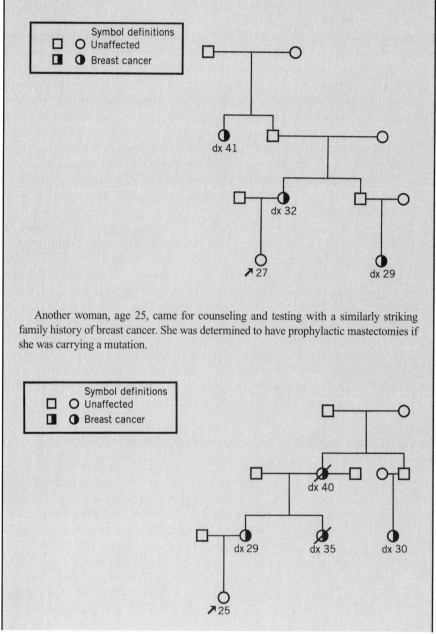

Another woman, age 25, came for counseling and testing with a similarly striking family history of breast cancer. She was determined to have prophylactic mastectomies if she was carrying a mutation.

The family histories differed with respect to the clinical outcome of the patients affected with breast cancer. For the 25-year-old woman who witnessed the unsuccessful struggle of many of her relatives, the decision to opt for the prophylactic surgical approach was without hesitation; for the 27-year-old woman whose family experienced a more favorable outcome, the diagnosis of breast cancer was viewed very differently.

Both women tested positive for *BRCA* mutations that cosegregated with the cancers in their families. The first woman elected breast and ovarian surveillance. The second woman decided to proceed with prophylactic mastectomy and consider oophorectomy after childbearing.

These cases illustrate the different contexts for decisions regarding prophylactic surgery.

In reviewing four large studies of prophylactic mastectomy, Ziegler and Kroll calculated that the proportion of patients who subsequently developed cancer ranged from .81% in a study of 1,500 women to 19% in a study of 285 women. These authors estimated the true risk in a subset of high risk patients from the largest study to be 1.18% (Ziegler and Kroll, 1991). However, the criteria for high risk in these studies varied, and the surgical techniques were not uniform. Many surgeons in these studies performed subcutaneous mastectomies. In this procedure the surgeon left behind a substantial amount of glandular tissue in the tail of the breast, beneath the nipple, and in the thick skin flaps that were created. The nipple-areolar complex, also left intact, represents another potential sanctuary site. It was estimated that 5% of the breast tissue remained after such procedures.

For these reasons, most surgeons now perform total mastectomy, in which all of the breast tissue is excised, along with the nipple-areolar complex and the pectoralis fascia underlying the breast. Following mastectomy, there are two options for reconstruction. The first utilizes subpectoral tissue expanders, which are gradually filled with saline to overstretch the skin, followed by an exchange operation in which implants are put into place. Silicon-containing implants, which have a more natural feel, are no longer utilized because of the controversy raised regarding a possibly increased frequency of autoimmune disease in these patients. (Although this association has not been confirmed by large studies, silicon-containing implants are reserved only for women seeking reconstruction after breast cancer surgery.) Saline implants are now routinely utilized in the prophylactic setting, but these devices gradually leak their contents, and up to 50% need to be replaced as early as 5 years from time of implantation. A third surgical procedure is necessary to build a nipple-areolar-complex by a combination of transplants of tissue from the vulva, earlobe, or toe, with darker pigmented skin from the upper thigh, or tattooing used to make the areolar complex.

The second type of reconstruction involves tissue transfer. In one of the most common procedures, a flap of abdominal skin, underlying fat, and blood supply from the rectus muscle is transplanted to the chest wall (Figure 4-5). The advantage of the transrectus abdominis myocutaneous flap (TRAM) procedure is that the abdominal fat is soft and simulates a natural breast. Reconstruction of the nipple-areolar complex is as described previously. No prosthesis is necessary, and the patient undergoes a surgical

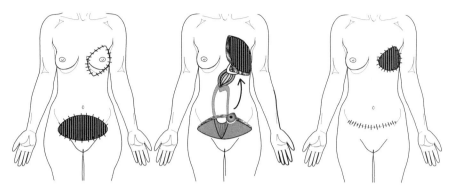

FIGURE 4-5 *The transrectus abdominis myocutaneous flap (TRAM) procedure of prophylactic mastectomy/reconstruction. A flap of abdominal skin, underlying fat, and blood supply from the rectus muscle are transplanted to the chest wall.*

"tummy tuck" in the process. A review of over 2000 cases of prophylactic mastectomy, including 203 cases suggestive of a dominant susceptibility syndrome, revealed fewer cases of breast cancer (10 overall) than would have been expected, suggesting that prophylactic mastectomy was "protective" (Hartmann et al., 1997). The downside is that this significant surgical procedure has a risk of graft failure as well as an increased risk of abdominal hernia (Elliott et al., 1992).

There are no firm indications for prophylactic mastectomy. In 1993, the Society of Surgical Oncology suggested that the following indications should be considered: (1) atypical hyperplasia of lobular or ductal origin, especially if present in multiple sites or in the contralateral breast; (2) family history of early onset or bilateral breast cancer in a first-degree relative; or (3) fibronodular breasts that are difficult to follow by exam or mammography in the setting of the diagnosis of atypia or a family history of the disease. With the advent of genetic cancer susceptibility testing, an emerging indication for discussion of these procedures is the detection of a deleterious mutation of *BRCA1* or *BRCA2*.

A concern of many, particularly those in nononcologic subspecialties, is that prophylactic mastectomy has not been proven to be effective in a population of women at highest genetic risk for breast cancer. The presence after mastectomy of even a single breast cancer cell with a *BRCA1* germline mutation could account for the chest wall recurrences that have been noted in some cases. A pathology study confirmed the presence of residual breast tissue after total mastectomy, particularly in the pectoralis major muscle and the lower skin flap (Temple et al., 1991).

The discussion of prophylactic mastectomy must be approached with special sensitivity. To simply recommend the procedure as medically indicated may absolve the clinician of perceived liabilities, but does little to empower individuals to make a difficult decision. It is helpful to emphasize that the choice for prophylactic surgery is a personal one, and no decision is wrong. Some individuals at the highest hereditary risk will start each day with fear about impending breast cancer, and may be overwhelmed by a perceived risk that will only be ameliorated if the organ-at-risk is removed. For others, the measure of life is quality not quantity. For them, the notion of removal of a healthy organ is not tenable. For the majority of individuals who are uncertain about these options, referral to a team of surgical subspecialists (including a plastic surgeon) can be enormously helpful. The purpose of this consultation is to discuss the potential surgical risks, as well as possible outcomes of the procedure, and to inspect photographs of actual cosmetic results. By demystifying the procedure, health professionals can assist the individual in a nondirective manner. The overall goal of the discussion of the option for prophylactic surgery is to provide education about the procedure, knowledge that it may not offer 100% protection, and support for the decision mutually achieved.

A formal evaluation by a mental health professional is recommended for all individuals scheduled to undergo prophylactic mastectomy. Even in the setting of a maximal cancer risk (by Mendelian analysis or DNA testing), prophylactic surgery will not be a prudent course if a breast cancer phobia is part of a spectrum of psychological issues that will not be addressed by surgery. Documentation of family history is also vital when a psychological evaluation raises concerns. A number of cases of Munchausen syndrome (fabrication of medical history and symptoms) have been documented in patients scheduled to undergo these procedures.

Medical and surgical options for *BRCA* heterozygotes are listed in Table 4-7. Options for prophylactic oophorectomy and ovarian cancer screening are also best included in the counseling regarding prophylactic mastectomy. These procedures are discussed in Chapter 5.

TABLE 4-7 Options for Cancer Prevention in *BRCA1* Mutation Carriers

Option	Interval
Breast self examination	Monthly (beginning at 18)
Clinician breast examination	Annual or semiannual beginning age 25
Mammography	Annually beginning age 25
Pelvic examination	Semiannually beginning age 25–35
Transvaginal ultrasound with color Doppler and CA 125	Biannually beginning age 25–35
Prostate cancer surveillance: rectal examination, and PSA	Annually beginning age 50
Flexible sigmoidoscopy (or colonoscopy)	Every 3–5 years beginning age 50
Prophylactic bilateral simple mastectomy (± reconstruction)	Discussed as an option
Prophylactic bilateral oophorectomy	Discussed as an option

Modified from: Cancer Genetic Studies Consortium, Ethical, Legal, and Social Implications Branch, National Center for Human Genome Research. Burke W, Daly M, Garber J et al. Recommendations for follow-up care of individuals with an inherited predisposition to cancer: *BRCA1* and *BRCA2*. JAMA 1997; 277:997–1003.

Options for the Unaffected Individual at Risk: Hormonal Factors

Much of what is known about the causative and protective effects of hormones and female cancers is derived from the widespread use of hormone replacement therapy (HRT) and oral contraceptives (OC) in this country over the past 30 years (Henderson, et. al., 1993). Although the slight increase in breast cancer risk in users of OCs remains controversial, the association of estrogen replacement therapy and breast and endometrial cancer risk is clearly recognized. The widespread use of unopposed estrogens as HRT starting in the 1960s led to an increase in the number of cases of endometrial cancer by the early 1970s. It also led to the observation that breast cancer risk was increased about 3% per year in postmenopausal HRT users. With the addition of progestins to the estrogen (typically 5–10 mg of medroxyprogesterone for 10–12 days per month), and the lowering of the estrogen dose, incidence and mortality from endometrial cancer declined 28% and 14% respectively from the early 1970s to the late 1980s. The effect of the addition of progestins on breast cancer risk were not as encouraging, with the same or slightly increased rates noted for breast cancer incidence and mortality during this same period.

In some clinical settings, for example, women at average or low hereditary risk for breast cancer, the beneficial effects of estrogen may offset the increased risk of breast cancer (Grady et al., 1992). The use of HRT has a significant effect on lowering risk for cardiovascular disease up to 50% and lowering risk of hip fracture 30–40%. In addition, there is evidence that estrogen use may decrease risk for Alzheimer's disease as well as colon cancer (see Part C of this chapter). The precise risks and benefits of HRT will be defined by the Women's Health Initiative, a randomized trial of HRT versus placebo. The results of this trial will be known by early in the next century. Until then, there remains the concern that women at genetically increased risk for breast cancer may be specially susceptible to the risks of estrogen. This view is supported by evidence for an increased risk of breast cancer among HRT users with a family history of the disease (Schurman et al., 1995; Stanford et al., 1995; Newcomb et al., 1995).

Limited data are available regarding the role of oral contraceptives (OC) in modifying breast cancer risk in the setting of a family history of the disease. There was no evidence from preliminary epidemiologic studies that the hormonal histories of women with a family history of breast cancer were different from other women (Brinton et al., 1982; Anderson, 1992). Indeed, such factors as late age of menarche, multiparity, and early age of first birth conferred little protection against breast cancer in women with a family history of the disease (Colditz et al., 1996; Parazzini et al., 1996). In contrast, greater numbers of births correlated with a lesser breast cancer risk in *BRCA1* carriers (Narod et al., 1995). In addition, studies of OC in both older (age 55–69) and younger (age 20–44) women revealed that women with a family history of breast cancer had a greater risk of breast cancer than women with no family history (Schuurman et al., 1995; Brinton et al., 1995). Sizes of the subsets were small, however, and results were of borderline statistical significance (Brinton et al., 1995).

There is preliminary evidence that long-term OC use may increase breast cancer risk in *BRCA1* heterozygotes (Ursin et al., 1997). In the absence of definitive data, there is a concern that for *BRCA1* and *BRCA2* heterozygotes, estrogens, even if opposed by progestins, may potentiate the growth of breast tumor cells that are more likely to appear in these individuals. As will be seen in the next part of this chapter, OCs remain the best studied means to prevent ovarian cancers. The risk–benefit ratio for OC use in *BRCA* heterozygotes has not been resolved. Pending larger clinical trials, the potential for increased breast cancer risk and decreased ovarian cancer risk should be considered in the counseling of *BRCA* heterozygotes.

Because of its antiestrogen properties, tamoxifen became a leading candidate for a hormonal chemopreventive agent in the 1980s (Jordan, 1990). A summary of data from randomized trials showed that tamoxifen lowered the risk of contralateral breast cancer by about 30–40% after an average of two years of treatment in affected patients (EBCTCG, 1992). In a trial in Scotland there was a beneficial effect on risk for mortality due to acute myocardial infarction, and other studies demonstrated slight increases in bone density of the lumbar spine in women on tamoxifen. These effects were presumably due to the paradoxical estrogen-like effects of long-term tamoxifen use. At the inception of the national tamoxifen prevention trial in the United States in 1992, and similar trials in Italy and the United Kingdom, there was the anticipation that an increased rate of endometrial cancers might be observed. When this increase was documented in 1994, the trial was modified to include ultrasound examinations to monitor endometrial thickness and allow biopsy of suspicious lesions. The trial was slow to accrue the necessary 16,000 participants necessary to provide the statistical power to detect the chemopreventive effect on breast cancer incidence. However, by 1996, the accrual at the 320 participating centers had improved. Eligibility for the trial, which was designed to include randomization between 20 mg/day of tamoxifen and placebo for 5 years, was calculated by the BDDP model described in Chapter 6. Enrollment of women at increased familial risk has offered the opportunity to document the preventive effects of tamoxifen in *BRCA1* heterozygotes. In addition to tamoxifen, novel anti-estrogens such as raloxifene may offer estrogen-like cardiovascular protection and effects on bone density, while decreasing breast cancer risk (Ziegler, 1996).

An alternative strategy for the hormonal chemoprevention of breast cancer is the use of oral contraceptives utilizing agonists of gonadotropin-releasing hormone (GnRHA), combined with a very low dose of estrogen and progesterone. This formulation would not give as great a breast cancer protection as GnRHA alone, but could cut breast cancer risk considerably. A pilot trial of leuprolide acetate (Lupron), with low doses of conjugated estrogen (Premarin) and medroxyprogesterone (Provera) has been undertaken (Spicer et al., 1993).

In addition to hormonal agents, a number of other compounds offer promise as chemoprevention agents (reviewed by Noguchi et al., 1996). Retinoids are analogues of vitamin A that induce and enhance cellular differentiation. A synthetic retinoid, N-(-4 hydroxyphenyl) retinamide (4-HPR), also called Fenretinade, was evaluated in a phase-III trial in patients with stage I/II breast cancer. Other agents under evaluation as chemopreventive drugs include selenium compounds, indole 3 carbinol, calcium glucarate, difluoromethylornithine (DFMO), and limonene, the major component of orange peel oil (Rose, 1994; Noguchi et al., 1996).

Diets with 20–25% of calories as fat, with equal proportions of polyunsaturated, saturated, and monounsaturated fat, have been proposed as "cancer preventive" and were included as part of adjuvant trials in patients. There is evidence that fish oils rich in n-3 polyunsaturated fatty acids protect against human breast cancer. Dietary modulation to decrease breast cancer risk remains an important research question (Noguchi et al., 1996).

Options for the Individual Already Affected by Breast or Ovarian Cancer: Tailoring of Treatments

The greatest amount of public attention has been focused on the importance of *BRCA1* and *BRCA2* mutations in unaffected women at risk for breast cancer. However, the most immediate clinical impact of breast cancer genetic testing will be for women with newly diagnosed breast cancer or women who are being followed in remission after a prior diagnosis. This group of individuals is large. The number of women with germline *BRCA1* or *BRCA2* mutations in these groups includes 10,000–20,000 women each year with newly diagnosed disease, and as many as 150,000 breast cancer survivors in remission after treatment of their localized disease. The extent to which these individuals are offered genetic testing depends on several factors. The family members of affected individuals will be a motivating factor in this testing, since these at-risk sisters and daughters (and also sons and brothers) will seek to know if a *BRCA1* or *BRCA2* mutation can be identified in their family.

Even in the absence of a striking family history, affected individuals may seek to undergo genetic testing so as to guide their own therapies. The prognostic importance of the detection of germline mutations is suggested by the observation that from 40–60% of mutation carriers already affected by breast cancer had secondary breast or ovarian cancers. For younger women with localized disease, a positive genetic test in this setting may be an important consideration in the choice to have, or not to have, breast conserving surgery. Based on current knowledge about the natural history of hereditary breast cancer, it may seem difficult to justify conservative approaches (e.g., lumpectomy and radiation therapy) in the setting of such a high risk for subsequent ipsilateral (or contralateral) disease. In counseling these individuals, however, it should be noted that some trials of patients with early stage disease have not detected an adverse affect of a positive family history. In a study of over 500 patients with stage I or II breast cancer, a history of 3 or more relatives with breast cancer decreased the risk for relapse after breast conserving surgery and radiation therapy (Peterson et al., 1994). Other studies have also suggested that breast cancer patients with family histories of the disease may have an improved survival (Ruder et al., 1988; Malone et al., (1996b). Recent functional studies of the *BRCA* genes have pointed to the potential for radiation sensitivity of the tumors in these patients, possibly providing an explanation for these clinical observations (Sharan et al., 1997; Kinzler and Vogelstein, 1997). However, in other series the presence of a family history of breast cancer has not correlated with improved outcome (Slattery et al., 1993; Israeli et al., 1994), leaving open the issue of the most prudent integration of *BRCA* testing into the management of these patients (Offit et al., 1996b).

Initial observations failed to demonstrate survival differences among prevalent cases of Jewish women with *BRCA* mutations, although a trend for decreased relapse-free survival was documented in incident cases with *BRCA* mutations (Robson et al., 1997b).These findings will require confirmation in large prospective trials.

In studies including patients with advanced as well as localized disease, retrospective analysis of survival and relapse based on *BRCA1*- and *BRCA2*-associated cases did not detect an adverse prognostic impact of *BRCA1*, but did find that *BRCA2*-associated cases had an increased relapse rate (Marcus et al., 1996). Retrospective review of *BRCA1*-associated ovarian cancers revealed a striking advantage in survival for these patients (Rubin et al., 1996). In these series the participants had to be alive in order to donate blood samples, and ascertainments were subject to bias of self-selection for testing. These considerations limit the utility of retrospective studies in guiding current therapeutic decisions. Prospective age-, stage-, and treatment-matched trials, incorporating direct detection of *BRCA1* and *BRCA2* germline mutations, as well as other known prognostic markers (e.g., estrogen receptor status, *HER2*/neu expression, etc.), will be necessary to define a uniform prognostic model. When these studies are complete, it is possible that *BRCA* germline testing will become part of the standard workup for young patients with breast cancer, or patients with significant family histories of disease.

Modeling the Benefits of Medical and Surgical Interventions in *BRCA* Heterozygotes

Attempts have been made to predict the benefits of surgical and medical interventions in carriers of *BRCA* mutations. Assuming a range 40–85% for penetrance (by age 70) for *BRCA* mutations, and assuming 85% and 50% cumulative reductions following prophylactic surgery for breast and ovarian cancer, respectively, a 30-year-old woman would gain 2.9 to 5.3 years of life following prophylactic mastectomy, and 0.3 to 1.7 years of life following prophylactic oophorectomy (Schrag et al., 1997). Importantly, the 30-year-old woman could delay oophorectomy 10 years with little loss of life expectancy. This model was highly sensitive to assumptions regarding penetrance and efficacy of interventions. Thus, prophylactic mastectomy resulted in 3, 4, and 5 additional years of life, assuming penetrance of 40%, 60%, and 85% respectively.

The model's assumptions regarding prophylactic oophorectomy were more conjectural. For example, the model assumed that younger women would receive hormone replacement therapy following oophorectomy, that oophorectomy resulted only in a 50% reduction in risk, and that the life expectancy gain for women following oophorectomy was based on the "more favorable" prognosis for *BRCA1* heterozygotes with ovarian cancer described in the study by Rubin et al., 1996 (Schrag et al., 1997). Another analysis assumed that oophorectomy would decrease ovarian cancer risk by 95% and mastectomy would decrease breast cancer risk by 98.8% (Grann et al., 1997). Based on these assumptions, oophorectomy and combined mastectomy/oophorectomy led to increases in survival of 2.6 and 6.5 years, respectively.

Future Options for Gene Therapy Based on Knowledge of *BRCA* Function

The development of more rational cancer treatments based on an understanding of the function of the *BRCA* genes remains a critical research challenge. Initial studies did not lead to a consistent model of the function of the *BRCA1* protein. The first such report suggested that *BRCA1* encoded a nuclear phosphoprotein, with abnormal cytoplasmic localization in tumors (Chen et al., 1995). Subsequent reports localized the protein product of the *BRCA1* protein to the cytoplasm (Scully et al., 1996) or in membrane vesicles (Jensen et al., 1996a). Homology of both *BRCA1* and *BRCA2* to the granin class of secreted proteins was suggested (Jensen et al., 1996a,b). These acidic calcium-binding proteins play a part in both intracellular and extracellular secretory pathways. The role of *BRCA* proteins as granins was not supported by lack of homology of murine *BRCA1* to a critical granin consensus sequence, or by the observation of a polymorphism of *BRCA2*, Lys3326ter, that results in loss of the putative granin domain, but which was not associated with increased risk for breast cancer (Mazoyer et al., 1996).

It was postulated that the *BRCA1* protein entered the nucleus from the cytoplasm and formed a complex with other proteins. At least 15 *BRCA1*-associated proteins were identified, including *BARD1* (breast cancer associated ring domain protein). Like *BRCA1*, *BARD1* had a ring finger domain (Wu et al., 1996). It was observed that both the *BRCA1* and *BRCA2* proteins bound *Rad51,* a homolog of a bacterial recombinase (Scully et al., 1997a; Sharan et al., 1997). These observations suggested that *BRCA1* and *BRCA2*, like the *ATM* gene product, played a fundamental role in the control of recombination that underlies the process of meiosis and mitosis in all human cells (Hawley and Friend, 1996). How these observations relate to the role of *BRCA1* as a transcription activator (Scully et al., 1997b), remains to be resolved. In addition, the role of *BRCA1* as a cell-cycle regulator was suggested by its ability to induce *p21* (Somasundaram et al., 1997), and the observation of a C-terminal *p53* binding motif (Koonin et al., 1996).

Mice deficient for both copies of the *BRCA1* gene died in utero at 7.5–13 days of gestation and showed abnormal neuroepithelial and mesodermal development (Gowen et al., 1996; Hakem et al., 1996). Similar experiments creating *BRCA2* "knockouts" revealed a similar phenotype (Suzuki et al., 1997). This suggested an important role for the *BRCA* genes, at least in mice, in embryogenesis. If the normal function for the *BRCA*-protein complex was as a transcriptional regulator of cell growth and division, then it might be possible to design cancer treatments that replace an abnormal *BRCA* protein in order to regain control of these processes.

Based on these principles, gene therapy was attempted in preliminary experiments. Initial studies demonstrated that retroviral transfer of a normal *BRCA1* gene inhibited the growth of breast and ovarian cell lines (Jensen et al., 1996b). Preliminary trials in humans have also been undertaken. In one of these trials, women with advanced ovarian cancer and *BRCA1* mutations were injected with normal copies of the *BRCA1* gene in a viral vector in an attempt to stem the growth of their tumors. In view of the caretaker function of the *BRCA* genes, in which *BRCA* mutations lead to mutations in other cancer-causing genes (Kinzler and Vogelstein, 1997), it seems less likely that injection of normal *BRCA* proteins will fully remedy the malignant phenotype. Nonetheless, as the function of *BRCA1* and *BRCA2* proteins are more fully resolved, other gene therapy trials will be undertaken.

REFERENCES: PART A

Abeliovich D, Kaduri L, Lerer I et al. 1997. The founder mutations 185delAG and 5382insC in *BRCA1* and 6174delT in *BRCA2* appear in 60% of ovarian cancer and 30% of early-onset breast cancer patients among Ashkenazi women. Amer J Hum Genet 60:505–14.

Adler DD, Wahl RL. 1995. New methods for imaging the breast: techniques, findings, and potential. Amer J Roentgenology 164:19–30.

Andersen TI, Borresen AL, Moller P. 1996. A common *BRCA1* mutation in Norwegian breast and ovarian cancer families? Am J Hum Genet 59:486–7.

Anderson DE. 1992. Familial versus sporadic breast cancer. Cancer 70:1740–6.

Anderson DE, Badzioch MD. 1993. Familial breast cancer risks: Effects of prostate and other cancers. Cancer 72:114–9.

Arena JF, Smith S, Plewinska M, Gayol L, Perera E, Murphy P, Lubs H. 1996. *BRCA1* mutations in African American women. Am J Hum Genet 59:169 (abstr).

Barker DF, Almeida ERA, Casey G et al. 1996. A strong candidate for a common *BRCA1* mutation with moderate phenotype. Genetic Epidemiology 13:595–604.

Berman DB, Wagner-Costalas J, Schultz DC, Lynch HT, Daly M, Godwin AK. 1996. Two distinct origins of a common *BRCA1* mutation in breast-ovarian cancer families: a genetic study of 15 185delAG-mutation kindreds. Am J Hum Genet 58:1166–76.

Bignon YJ, Fonck Y, Chassagne MC. 1995. Histoprognostic grade in tumours from families with hereditary predisposition to breast cancer. Lancet 346:258.

Boice JD Jr, Harvey EB, Blettner M et al. 1992. Cancer in the contralateral breast after radiotherapy for breast cancer. New Engl J Med 326:781–5.

Bowcock AM, Thai TH, Ou F et al. 1997. Rare germline BARD1 alterations in patients with breast, ovarian, and uterine cancer. Am J Hum Genet 61:241 (abstr).

Bradley A, Sharan SK. 1996. *BRCA1* protein products: secreted tumour suppressors. Nature Genet 13:268–9.

Breslow R, Kessler L. 1995. Stat bite: knowledge of breast cancer risk by age. J Natl Cancer Inst 87:1109.

Brinton LA, Hoover R, Fraumeni JF Jr. 1982. Interaction of familial and hormonal risk factors for breast cancer. J Natl Cancer Inst 69:817–22.

Brinton LA, Daling JR, Liff JM et al. 1995. Oral contraceptives and breast cancer risk among younger women. J Natl Cancer Inst 87:827–35.

Burke W, Daly M, Garber J et al. 1997. Recommendations for follow-up care of individuals with an inherited predisposition to cancer: *BRCA1* and *BRCA2*. JAMA 277:997–1003.

Cannon L, Bishop DT, Skolnick ML et al. 1982. Genetic epidemiology of prostate cancer in the Utah Mormon genealogy. Cancer Surv 1:1–12.

Cannon LA, Bishop DT, Skolnick MH. 1986. Segregation and linkage analysis of breast cancer in the Dutch and Utah families. Genet Epidem 1:43–8.

Cannon-Albright LA, Bishop DT, Goldgar C, Skolnick MH. 1991. Genetic predisposition to cancer. In Devita VT, Hellman S, Rosenberg SA (eds) Important Advances in Oncology. Philadelphia: J.B. Lippincott, 39–55.

Castilla LH, Couch FJ, Erdos MR et al. 1994. Mutations in the *BRCA1* gene in families with early onset breast and ovarian cancer. Nature Genet 8:387–91.

Chapman MS, Verma IM. 1996. Transcriptional activation by *BRCA1*. Nature Genet 382: 678–9.

Chen Y, Chen CF, Riley DJ et al. 1995. Aberrant subcellular localization of *BRCA1* in breast cancer. Science 270:789–91.

Claus EB, Risch N, Thompson WD. 1991. Genetic analysis of breast cancer in the Cancer and Steroid Hormone Study. Am J Hum Genet 48:232–42.

Claus EB, Risch N, Thompson WD, Carter D. 1993. Relationship between breast histopathology and family history of breast cancer. Cancer 71:147–53.

Colditz GA, Hankinson SE, Hunter DJ et al. 1995. The use of estrogens and progestins and the risk of breast cancer in postmenopausal women. New Engl J Med 332:1589–93.

Colditz GA, Rosner BA, Speizer FE. 1996. Risk factors for breast cancer according to family history of breast cancer. J Natl Cancer Inst 88:1003–4.

Couch FJ, Farid LM, DeShano ML et al. 1996a. *BRCA2* germline mutations in male breast cancer cases and breast cancer families. Nature Genet 13:123–5.

Couch FJ, Weber BL. 1996b. Mutations and polymorphisms in the familial early-onset breast cancer (*BRCA1*) gene. Human Mutation 8:8–18.

Couch FJ, DeShano ML, Blackwood MA et al. 1997. *BRCA1* mutations in women attending clinics that evaluate the risk of breast cancer. New Engl J Med 336:1409–15.

De Benedetti V, Radice P, Mondini P et al. 1996. Screening for mutations in exon 11 of the *BRCA* gene in 70 Italian breast and ovarian cancer patients by protein truncation test. Oncogene 13:1353–7.

de Waard F, Cornelis JP, Aoki K et al. 1977. Breast cancer incidence according to weight and height in two cities of the Netherlands and in Aichi Prefecture, Japan. Cancer 40:1269–75.

Deng G, Lu Y, Zlotnikov G, Thor AD, Smith HS. 1996. Loss of heterozygosity in normal tissue adjacent to breast carcinomas. Science 274:2057–9.

Dunning AM, Chiano M, Smith NR et al. 1997. Common *BRCA1* variants and susceptibility to breast and ovarian cancer in the general population. Hum Molec Genet 6:285–9.

Easton DF, Bishop DT, Ford D et al. 1993. Genetic linkage analysis in familial breast and ovarian cancer: results from 214 families. Am J Hum Genet 52:678–701.

Easton DF, Ford D, Bishop DT, Breast Cancer Linkage Consortium. 1995. Breast and ovarian cancer incidence in *BRCA1*-mutation carriers. Am J Hum Genet 56:265–71.

Easton DF.1997. Breast cancer genes—what are the real risks? Nature Genet 16:210–1.

EBCTCG. 1992. Systemic treatment of early breast cancer by hormonal, cytotoxic, or immune therapy. Lancet 339:71–85.

Egan KM, Newcomb PA, Longnecker MP et al. 1996. Jewish religion and risk of breast cancer. Lancet 347:1645–6.

Eisinger F, Stoppa Lyonnet D, Longy M et al. 1996. Germ line mutation at *BRCA1* affects the histoprognostic grade in hereditary breast cancer. Cancer Res 56:471–4.

Elliott LF, Eskenazi L, Beegle PH Jr et al. 1993. Immediate TRAM flap breast reconstruction: 128 consecutive cases. Plast Reconstr Surg 92:217–27.

Evans JS, Wennberg JE, McNeil BJ. 1986. The influence of diagnostic radiography on the incidence of breast cancer and leukemia. New Engl J Med 315:810–5.

Feig SA. 1996a. Methods to identify benefit from mammographic screening of women aged 40–49 years. Radiology 201:421–6.

Feig SA. 1996b. Strategies for improving sensitivity of screening mammography for women age 40–49 years. JAMA 276:73–4.

Feigelson HS, Coetzee GA, Kolonel LN, Ross RK, Henderson BE. 1997. A polymorphism in the CYP17 gene increases the risk of breast cancer. Cancer Res 57:1063–5.

Fitzgerald MG, MacDonald DJ, Krainer M et al. 1996. Germ-line *BRCA1* mutations in Jewish and non-Jewish women with early-onset breast cancer. New Engl J Med 334:186–8.

Fitzgerald MG, Bean JM, Hegde J et al., 1997. Heterozygous *ATM* mutations do not contribute to early onset of breast cancer. Nature Genet 15:307–310.

Ford D, Easton DF. 1995. The genetics of breast and ovarian cancer. Br J Cancer 72:805–12.

Ford D, Easton DF, Bishop DT, Narod SA, Goldgar DE, 1994. Breast Cancer Linkage Consortium. Risks of cancer in *BRCA1*-mutation carriers. Lancet 343:692–5.

Friedman E, Gak E, Theodur L et al. 1996. *BRCA1* 185delAG mutation in ovarian cancer patients and in Iraqi Jews in Israel. Am J Hum Genet 59:350 (abstr).

Friedman E, Bar-Sade RB, Gak E et al. 1997. The occurrence and origin of the 185delAG mutation in non-Ashkenazi Jews. Am J Hum Genet 61: 7571 (abstr).

Friedman LS, Ostermeyer EA, Szabo CI, Dowd P, Lynch ED, Rowell SE, King MC. 1994. Confirmation of *BRCA1* by analysis of germline mutations linked to breast and ovarian cancer in ten families. Nature Genet 8:399–404.

Friedman LS, Gayther SA, Kurosaki T et al. 1997. Mutation analysis of *BRCA1* and *BRCA2* in a male breast cancer population. Am J Hum Genet 60:313–9.

Gail MH, Brinton LA, Byar DP et al. 1989. Projecting individualized probabilities of developing breast cancer for white females who are being examined annually. J Natl Cancer Inst 81:1879–86.

Gao Q, Neuhausen S, Cummings S, Luce M, Olopade OI. 1997. Recurrent Germline *BRCA1* mutations in extended African American families with early onset breast cancer. Am J Hum Genet 60:1233–6.

Garcia-Foncillas J, Begier P, Martinez MJ et al. 1997. Variable penetrance of *BRCA1* mutations is associated with VNTR HRAS1 alleles. Proc Am Assoc Can Res 38:1122.

Gayther SA, Warren W, Mazoyer S et al. 1995. Germline mutations of the *BRCA1* gene in breast and ovarian cancer families provide evidence for a genotype-phenotype correlation. Nature Genet 11:428–33.

Gayther SA, Mangion J, Russell P et al. 1997a. Variation of risks of breast and ovarian cancer associated with different germline mutations of the *BRCA2* gene. Nature Genet 15:103–5.

Gayther SA, Harrington P, Russell P, Kharkevich G, Garkavtseva RF, Ponder BAJ. 1997b. Frequently occurring germ-line mutations of the *BRCA1* gene in ovarian cancer families from Russia. Am J Hum Genet 60:1239–42.

Goldgar DE, Fields P, Lewis CM et al. 1994. A large kindred with 17q-linked breast and ovarian cancer: genetic, phenotypic, and genealogical analysis. J Natl Cancer Inst 86: 200–9.

Gowen LC, Johnson BL, Latour AM et al. 1996. *BRCA1* deficiency results in early embryonic lethality characterized by neuroepithelial abnormalities. Nature Genet 12:191–4.

Grady D, Ernster V. 1991. Does postmenopausal hormone therapy cause breast cancer? Am J Epidemiology 134:1396–1406.

Grady D, Rubin SM, Petitti DB et al. 1992. Hormone therapy to prevent disease and prolong life in postmenopausal women. Ann Intern Med 117:1016–37.

Grann VR, Panageas K, Whang W. 1997. A decision analysis of prophylactic treatments in *BRCA1* gene positive patients. Proc Amer Soc Clin Oncol 16:532a (1918).

Greenwald P, Nasca PC, Lawrence CE et al. 1978. Estimated effect of breast self-examination and routine physician examinations on breast-cancer mortality. New Engl J Med 299: 271–3.

Haagensen CD, Bodian C, Haagensen DE. 1981. Lobular neoplasia (lobular carcinoma in situ) breast carcinoma: risk and detection. Philadelphia: WB Saunders.

Hakansson S, Johannsson O, Johansson U et al. 1997. Moderate frequency of *BRCA1* and *BRCA2* germ-line mutations in Scandinavian familial breast cancer. Am J Hum Genet 78:1068–1078.

Hakem R, de la Pompa JL, Sirard C et al. 1996. The tumor suppressor gene *BRCA1* is required for embryonic cellular proliferation in the mouse. Cell 85:1009–23.

Hartmann L, Jenkins R, Schaid D, Yanga P. 1997. Prophylactic mastectomy: preliminary retrospective cohort analysis. Proc Amer Assoc Can Res 38: 1123.

Hawley RS, Friend SH. 1996. Strange bedfellows in even stranger places: the role of ATM in meiotic cells, lymphocytes, tumors, and its functional links to p53. Genes and Development 10:2383–8.

Haywang-Kobrunner SH. 1994. Contrast enhanced magnetic resonance imaging of the breast. Invest Radiol 29:94–104.

Healy B. 1997. BRCA genes—bookmaking, fortunetelling, and medical care. New Engl J Med 336:1448–9.

Helzlsouer K. 1995. Epidemiology, prevention, and early detection of breast cancer. Current Opin in Oncol 7:489–94.

Henderson BE, Ross RK, Pike MC. 1993. Hormonal chemoprevention of cancer in women. Science 259:633–8.

Holt JT, Thompson ME, Szabo C, Robinson-Benion C, Arteaga CL, King MC, Jensen RA. 1996. Growth retardation and tumour inhibition by *BRCA1*. Nature Genet 12:298–302.

Houn F, Helzlsouer KJ, Friedman NB, Stefanek ME. 1995. The practice of prophylactic mastectomy: a survey of Maryland surgeons. Am J Public Health 85:801–5.

Humphrey JS, Salim A, Erdos MR, Collins FS, Brody LC, Klausner RD. 1997. Human *BRCA1* inhibits growth in yeast: potential use in diagnostic testing. Proc Natl Acad Sci 94:5820–5.

Israeli D, Tartter PI, Brower ST et al., 1994. The significance of family history for patients with carcinoma of the breast. J Amer Coll Surg 179:29–32.

Jacquemier J, Eisinger F, Birnbaum D, Sobol H. 1995. Histoprognostic grade in *BRCA1*-associated breast cancer. Lancet 345:1503.

Jensen RA, Thompson ME, Jetton TL et al. 1996a. *BRCA1* is secreted and exhibits properties of a granin. Nature Genet 12:303–8.

Jensen RA, Thompson ME, Jetton TL et al. 1996. *BRCA1* protein products: secreted tumour suppressors. Nature Genet 13:269–71.

Johannsson O, Ostermeyer EA, Hakansson S et al. 1996. Founding *BRCA1* mutations in hereditary breast and ovarian cancer in southern Sweden. Am J Hum Genet 58:441–50.

Johannsson OT, Idvall I, Anderson C, Borg A, Barkardottir RB, Egilsson V, Olsson H. 1997. Tumor biological features of *BRCA1*-induced breast and ovarian cancer. Eur J Cancer 33:362–71.

Jolly KW, Malkin D, Douglass EC, Brown TF, Sinclair AE, Look AT. 1994. Splice-site mutation of the p53 gene in a family with hereditary breast-ovarian cancer. Oncogene 9:97–102.

Jordan VC. 1990. Long-term adjuvant tamoxifen therapy for breast cancer: the prelude to prevention. Cancer Treat Rev 17:15–36.

Kerlikowske K, Grady D, Barclay J, Sickles EA, Eaton A, Ernster V. 1993. Positive predictive value of screening mammography by age and family history of breast cancer. JAMA 270:2444–50.

Kerlikowske K, Grady D, Rubin SM, Sandrock C, Ernster VL. 1995. Efficacy of screening mammography; a meta-analysis. JAMA 273:149–54.

Kerlikowske K, Grady D, Barclay J, Sickles EA, Ernster V. 1996. Effect of age, breast density, and family history on the sensitivity of first screening mammography. JAMA 276:33–38.

Kerlikowske K, Barclay J, Grady D, Sickles EA, Ernster V. 1997. Comparison of risk factors for ductal carcinoma *in situ* and invasive breast cancer. J Natl Cancer Inst 89:76–82.

King MC, Rowell S, Love SM. 1993. Inherited breast and ovarian cancer: what are the risks? What are the choices? JAMA 269:1975–80.

Kinzler KW, Vogelstein B. 1997. Gatekeepers and caretakers. Nature 386:761–2.

Koonin EV, Altshul SF, Bork P. 1996. *BRCA1* protein products: functional motifs. Nature Genet 13:266–8.

Kopans DB. 1994a. Breast cancer screening: women 40 to 49 years of age. In Devita VT, Hellman S, Rosenberg SA (eds) PPO Updates. Philadelphia: JB Lippincott, 9.

Kopans DB. 1994b. Accuracy of mammographic interpretation. New Eng J Med 331:1521–2.

Krainer M, Silva-Arrieta S, Fitzgerald MG et al. 1997. Differential contributions of *BRCA1* and *BRCA2* to early-onset breast cancer. New Engl J Med 336:1416–21.

Lagios MD, Rose MR, Margolin FR. 1980. Tubular carcinoma of the breast: association with multicentricity, bilaterality, and family history of mammary carcinoma. Am J Clin Path 73:25–30.

Lakhani SR, Sloane JP, Gusterson BA et al. 1997. The pathology of familial breast cancer: evidence for differences between breast cancers developing in carriers of *BRCA1* mutations, *BRCA2* mutations and sporadic cases. Lancet 349:1488–1510.

Langston AA, Malone KE, Thompson JD, Daling JR, Ostrander EA. 1996. *BRCA1* mutations in a population-based sample of young women with breast cancer. New Engl J Med 334; 137–42.

Levy-Lahad E, Catane R, Eisenberg S et al. 1997. Founder *BRCA1* and *BRCA2* mutations in Ashkenazi Jews in Israel: frequency and differential penetrance in ovarian cancer and in breast-ovarian cancer families. Am J Hum Genet 60:1059–1067.

Liaw D, Marsh D, Li J. 1997. Germline mutations of the PTEN gene in Cowden disease, an inherited breast and thyroid cancer syndrome. Nature Genet 16:64–7.

Lindblom A, Sandelin K, Iselius L, Dumanski J, White I, Nordenskjöld M, Larsson C. 1994. Predisposition for breast cancer in carriers of constitutional translocation 11q;22q. Am J Hum Genet 54:871–6.

LiVolsi VA, Kelsey JL, Fischer DB, Holford TR, Mostow ED, Goldenberg IS. 1982. Effect of age at first childbirth on risk of developing specific histologic subtype of breast cancer. Cancer 49:1937–40.

Lobaccaro JM, Lumbroso S, Belon C et al. 1993. Androgen receptor gene mutation in male breast cancer. Hum Mol Genet 11:1799–1802.

Longnecker MP, Newcomb PA, Mittendorf R et al. 1995. Risk of breast cancer in relation to lifetime alcohol consumption. J Natl Cancer Inst 87:923–9.

Lynch HT, Krush AJ. 1971. Carcinoma of the breast and ovary in three families. Surg Gynecol Obstet 133:644–8.

Lynch HT, Albano WA, Heieck JJ et al., 1984. Genetics, biomarkers, and control of breast cancer: a review. Cancer Genet Cytogenet 13:43–92.

MacMahon B. 1994. Pesticide residues and breast cancer? J Natl Cancer Inst 86:572–3.

MacMahon B, Cole P, Brown J. 1973. Etiology of human breast cancer: a review. J Natl Cancer Inst 50:21–42.

Malkin D, Li FP, Strong LC et al. 1990. Germ line p53 mutations in a familial syndrome of breast cancer, sarcomas, and other neoplasms. Science 250: 1233–8.

Malone KE, Thompson JE, Daling J, Ostrander EA. 1996a. *BRCA1* mutations in women with first degree family history of breast cancer identified from a population based case-control study. Amer J Hum Genet 59:13 (abstr).

Malone KE, Daling JR, Weiss NS et al.,1996b. Family history and survival of young women with invasive breast carcinoma. Cancer 78:1417–25.

Marcus JN, Watson P, Page DL, Lynch HT. 1994. Pathology and heredity of breast cancer in younger women. Monogr Natl Cancer Inst 16:23–34.

Marcus JN, Watson P, Page DL, Narod SA, Lenoir GM, Tonin P, Linder-Stephenson L, Salerno G, Conway TA, Lynch HT. 1996. Hereditary breast cancer: Pathobiology, prognosis, and *BRCA1* and *BRCA2* gene linkage. Cancer 77:697–709.

Marshall E. 1993. Breast cancer research, a special report: epidemiology. Science 259:618–21.

Mazoyer S, Dunning AM, Serova O et al. 1996. A polymorphic stop codon in *BRCA2*. Nature Genet 14:253–4.

McLemore ML, Whelan AJ, Mortimer JE. 1997. Is risk of breast cancer increased in individuals with Peutz-Jegher syndrome? Proc Amer Soc Clin Oncol 16:536a (1930).

Mettler FA, Upton AC, Kelsey CA, Ashby RN, Rosenberg RD, Linver MN, 1996. Benefits versus risks from mammography: a critical reassessment. Cancer 77:903–9.

Miki Y, Swensen J, Shattuck-Eidens D et al. 1994. A strong candidate for the breast and ovarian cancer susceptibility gene *BRCA1*. Science 266:66–71.

Miller BA, Feuer DJ, Hankey BF. 1993. Recent incidence trends for breast cancer in women and relevance of early detection: an update. CA Cancer J Clin 43:27–41.

Montagna M, Santacatterina M, Corneo B et al. 1996. Identification of seven new *BRCA1* germline mutations in Italian breast and breast/ovarian cancer families. Cancer Res 56:5466–9.

Narod S, Lynch H, Conway T, Watson P, Feunteun J, Lenoir G. 1993. Increasing incidence of breast cancer in a family with *BRCA1* mutation. Lancet 341:1101–2.

Narod SA, Goldgar D, Cannon-Albright L, Weber B, Moslehi R, Ives E, Lenoir G, Lynch H. 1995. Risk modifiers in carriers of *BRCA1* mutations. Int J Cancer 64:394–8.

Nelen MR, Padberg GW, Peeters EAJ et al. 1996. Localization of the gene for Cowden disease to chromosome 10q22-23. Nature Genet 13:114–6.

Neuhausen S, Gilewski T, Norton L et al. 1996a. Recurrent *BRCA2* 6174delT mutations in Ashkenazi Jewish women affected by breast cancer. Nature Genet 13:126–8.

Neuhausen SL, Mazoyer S, Friedman L et al. 1996b. Haplotype and phenotype analysis of six recurrent *BRCA1* mutations in 61 families: results of an international study. Am J Hum Genet 58:271–80.

Newcomb PA, Longnecker MP, Stover BE et al. 1995. Long-term hormone replacement therapy and risk of breast cancer in post-menopausal women. Amer J Epidemiol 142:788–95.

Newman B. 1996. The North Carolina Breast Cancer Study. 1996 June 26. Abstract presented at Second Plenary Meeting of Principal Investigators, NCI, Frederick, MD.

Noguchi M, Rose DP, Miyazaki I. 1996. Breast cancer chemoregulation: clinical trials and research. Oncology 53:175–81.

Oddoux C, Struewing JP, Clayton CM et al. 1996. The carrier frequency of the *BRCA2* 6174delT mutation among Ashkenazi Jewish individuals is approximately 1%. Nature Genet 14: 188–90.

Offit K. 1996a. *BRCA1*—A New Marker in the Management of Patients with Breast Cancer? Cancer 77:599–601.

Offit K, Gilewski T, Norton L et al. 1996b. Germline *BRCA1* 185delAG mutations in Jewish women with breast cancer. Lancet 347:1643–6.

Ozcelik H, Schmocker B, Di Nicola N et al. 1997. Germline *BRCA2* 6174delT mutations in Ashkenazi Jewish pancreatic cancer patients. Nature Genet 16:17–18.

Padberg GW, Schot JD, Vielvoye GJ, Bots GT, de Beer FC. 1991. Lhermitte-Duclos disease and Cowden disease: a single phakomatosis. Ann Neurol 29:517–23.

Parazzini F, La Vecchia C, Chatenoud L, Negri E, Franceschi S. 1996. Re: Risk factors for breast cancer according to family history of breast cancer (letter). J Natl Cancer Inst 88:1003–4.

Peelan T, van Vliet M, Petrij-Bosch A et al. 1997. A high proportion of novel mutations in *BRCA1* with strong founder effects among Dutch and Belgian hereditary breast and ovarian families. Am J Hum Genet 60:1041–9.

Peterson M, Fowble B, Solin LJ, Schultz DJ. 1994. Family history status as a prognostic factor for breast cancer patients treated with conservative surgery and radiation. Breast J 4(1):202–9.

Phelan CM, Rebbeck TR, Weber BL et al. 1996. Ovarian cancer risk in *BRCA1* carriers is modified by the *HRAS1* variable number of tandem repeat (VNTR) locus. Nature Genet 12:309–11.

Pike M, Bernstein L, Spicer D. 1993. Exogenous hormones and breast cancer risk. In Neiderhuber J (ed). Current Therapy in Oncology. St Louis: BC Decker.

Porter DE, Cohen BB, Wallace MR, Smyth E, Chetty U, Dixon JM, Steel CM, Carter DC. 1994. Breast cancer incidence, penetrance and survival in probable carriers of *BRCA1* gene mutation in families linked to *BRCA1* on chromosome 17q12-21. Br J Surg 81:1512–15.

Ramus SJ, Friedman LS, Gayther SA et al. 1997a. A breast/ovarian cancer patient with germline mutations in both *BRCA1* and *BRCA2* (letter). Nature Genet 15:14–15.

Ramus SJ, Kote-Jarai ZF, Friedman LS et al. 1997b. Analysis if *BRCA1* and *BRCA2* mutations in Hungarian families with breast or breast-ovarian cancer. Am J Hum Genet 60:1242–6.

Randall TC, Chiu HC, Bell KA, Rebane BA, Rubin SC, Boyd J. 1997. Germline mutations of the *BRCA1* and *BRCA2* genes in a breast and ovarian cancer patient: molecular genetics and clinical implications (submitted).

Rebbeck TR, Couch FJ, Kant J et al. 1996. Genetic heterogeneity in hereditary breast cancer: role of *BRCA1* and *BRCA2*. Am J Hum Genet 59:547–53.

Reichman ME, Judd JT, Loncope C et al. 1993. Effects of alcohol consumption on plasma and urinary hormone concentrations in premenopausal women. J Natl Cancer Inst 85:722–7.

Ries LAG, Hankey BF, Edwards BK eds. 1990. Cancer statistics review, 1973–1987. Bethesda MD: National Institutes of Health; National Institutes of Health publication 90-2789.

Roa BB, Boyed AA, Volcik K, Richards CS.1996. Ashkenazi Jewish population frequencies for common mutations in *BRCA1* and *BRCA2*. Nature Genet 14:185–7.

Robbins SL, Cotran RS. 1979. Patrologic Basis of Disease. Philadelphia: WB Saunders, pp 1305–33.

Robson ME, Gilewski T, Haas B et al. 1997b. BRCA-associated breast cancer in young Jewish women. Amer Soc Hum Genet (abstr., 1997).

Robson M, Offit K. 1997. A new *BRCA2* mutation in an Ashkenazi Jewish family with breast and ovarian cancer. Lancet 350:117–118.

Rose DF. 1994. Dietary fat and breast cancer: controversy and biologic plausibility. In: Weisberger EK (ed.): Diet and breast cancer. New York, Plenum Press, pp.1–10.

Rosen PP, Kosloff C, Lieberman PH, Adair F, Braun DW JR. 1978. Lobular carcinoma *in situ* of the breast: detailed analysis of 99 patients with average follow-up of 24 years. Am J Surg Pathol 2:225–51.

Rosen PP, Lesser ML, Senie RT, Kinne DW. 1982. Epidemiology of breast carcinoma III: relationship of family history to tumor type. Cancer 50:171–9.

Roy JA, Piccart MJ. 1995. Adjuvant systemic therapy for breast cancer. Current Opin in Oncol 7:517–22.

Rubin SC, Benjamin I, Behbakht K et al. 1996. Clinical and pathological features of ovarian cancer in women with germ-line mutations of *BRCA1*. New Engl J Med 335:1413–6.

Ruder AM, Moodie PF, Nelson NA et al. 1988. Does family history of breast cancer improve survival among patients with breast cancer? Am J Obstet Gynecol 158:963–8.

Schmidt RA, Nishikawa RM. 1994. Digital screening mammography. In: Devita VT, Hellman S, Rosenberg SA (eds), PPO Updates. Philadelphia: Lippincott, 8:1–16.

Schrag D, Kuntz KM, Garber JE, Weeks J. 1997. Impact of prophylactic mastectomy and oophorectomy on life expectancy of women with *BRCA1* or *BRCA2* gene mutations. New Engl J Med 336:1465–71.

Schrager CA, Schneider D, Gruener BA, Tsou HC, Peacocke M. 1997. Clinical and pathological features of breast disease in Cowden's syndrome: an underrecognized syndrome with an increased risk of breast cancer. Hum Path (in press).

Schubert E, Lee MK, Mefford HC et al. 1997. *BRCA2* in American families with four or more cases of breast or ovarian cancer: recurrent and novel mutations, variable expression, penetrance, and possibility of families whose cancer is not attributable to *BRCA1* or *BRCA2*. Am J Hum Genet 60:1031–40.

Schuurman AG, van den Brandt P, Goldbohm RA. 1995. Exogenous hormone use and the risk of postmenopausal breast cancer: Results from the Netherlands cohort study. Cancer Causes Control 6:416–24.

Scully R, Ganesan S, Brown M et al. 1996. Location of *BRCA1* in human breast and ovarian cancer cells (letter). Science 272: 123–6.

Scully R, Chen J, Plug A et al. 1997a. Association of *BRCA1* with Rad51 in mitotic and meiotic cells. Cell 88:265–75.

Scully R, Anderson SF, Chao DM et al. 1997b. *BRCA1* is a component of the RNA polymerase II holoenzyme. Proc Natl Acad Sci 94:5605–10.

Serova OM, Mazoyer S, Puget N et al. 1997. Mutations in *BRCA1* and *BRCA2* in breast cancer families: are there more breast cancer-susceptibility genes? Amer J Hum Genet 60:486–95.

Serova-Sinilnikova OM, Boutrand L, Stoppa-Lyonnet D et al. 1997. *BRCA2* mutations in hereditary breast and ovarian cancer in France. Am J Hum Genet 60:1236–9.

Sharan S, Morimatsu M, Albrecht U et al. 1997. Embryonic lethality and radiation hypersensitivity mediated by Rad51 in mice lacking Brca2. Nature 386:804–10.

Shattuck-Eidens D, McClure M, Simard J et al. 1995. A collaborative survey of 80 mutations in the *BRCA1* breast and ovarian cancer susceptibility gene. Implications for presymptomatic testing and screening. JAMA 273:535–41.

Shattuck-Eidens D, Oliphant A, McClure M et al. 1997. *BRCA1* sequence analysis in women at high risk for susceptibility mutations. JAMA 278:1242–50.

Sidransky D, Tokino T, Helzlsouer K et al. 1992. Inherited p53 mutations in breast cancer. Cancer Res 52:2984–6.

Simard J, Tonin P, Durocher F et al. 1994. Common origins of *BRCA1* mutations in Canadian breast and ovarian cancer families. Nature Genet 8:392–8.

Simpson J, Page DL. 1995. Pathology of preinvasive and excellent prognosis breast cancer. Current Opin in Oncol 7:501–5.

Slattery ML, Berry TD, Kerber RA. 1993. Is survival among women with breast cancer influenced by a family history of breast cancer? Epidem 4:543–8.

Smart CR, Hendrick RE, Rutledge JH III, Smith RA. 1995. Benefit of mammography screening in women ages 40–49 years: current evidence from randomized controlled trials. Cancer 75: 1619–26 (correction: Cancer 1995; 75:2788).

Society of Surgical Oncology Statement on Prophylactic Mastectomies. 1993. SSO Newsletter, 10.

Somasundaram K, Zhang H, Zeng Y et al. 1997. Arrest of the cell cycle by the tumour-suppressor *BRCA1* requires the CDK-inhibitor *p21*. Nature 389:185–188.

Spicer DV, Pike MC, Pike A et al. 1993. Pilot trial of a gonadotropin hormone agonist with replacement hormones as a prototype contraceptive to prevent breast cancer. Contraception 47:427–44.

Stanford JL, Weiss NS, Voigt LF et al. 1995. Combined estrogen and progestin hormone replacement therapy in relation to risk of breast cancer in middle aged women. JAMA 274:137–42.

Starink TM. 1984. Cowden's disease: analysis of fourteen new cases. Am Acad Dermatol 11:1127–41.

Stefanek ME. 1995. Bilateral prophylactic mastectomy: issues and concerns. Monogr Natl Cancer Inst 17:37–42.

Stoppa-Lyonnet D, Fricker JP, Essioux L et al. 1996. Segregation of two *BRCA1* mutations in a single family. Am J Hum Genet 59:479–81.

Stoppa-Lyonnet D, Laurent-Puig P, Essioux L et al. 1997. *BRCA1* sequence variations in 160 individuals referred to a breast/ovarian family cancer clinic. Am J Hum Genet 60:1021–30.

Struewing JP, Abeliovich D, Peretz T, et al. 1995a. The carrier frequency of the *BRCA1*

185delAG mutation is approximately 1% in Ashkenazi Jewish individuals. Nature Genet 11: 198–200.

Struewing JP, Brody LC, Erdos MR et al. 1995b. Detection of eight *BRCA1* mutations in 10 breast/ovarian cancer families, including 1 family with male breast cancer. Am J Hum Genet 57:1–7.

Struewing JP, Hartge P, Wacholder S et al. 1997. The risk of cancer associated with specific mutations of *BRCA1* and *BRCA2* among Ashkenazi Jews. New Eng J Med 336:1401–8.

Sturgeon SR, Schairer C, Gail M, McAdams M, Brinton LA, Hoover RN. 1995. Geographic variation in mortality from breast cancer among white women in the United States. J Natl Cancer Inst 87:1846–53.

Suzuki A, de la Pompe JL, Hakem R et al. 1997. *BRCA2* is required for embryonic cellular proliferation in the mouse. Genes and Devel 11:1242–52.

Swift M, Morrell D, Massey RB, Chase CL. 1991. Incidence of cancer in 161 families affected by ataxia telangiectasia. New Engl J Med 325:1831–6.

Tavtigian SV, Simard J, Rommens J et al. 1996. The complete *BRCA2* gene and mutations in chromosome 13q-linked kindreds. Nature Genet 12:333–7.

Temple WJ, Lindsay RL, Magi E, Urbanski SJ. 1991. Technical considerations for prophylactic mastectomy in patients at high risk for breast cancer. Am J Surg 161:413–5.

Thorlacius S, Olafsdottir S, Tryggvadottir L et al. 1996. A single *BRCA2* mutation in male and female breast cancer families from Iceland with varied cancer phenotypes. Nature Genet 13:117–21.

Thorlacius S, Sigurdsson S, Bjarnadottir H et al. 1997. Study of a single *BRCA2* mutation with high carrier frequency in a small population. Am J Hum Genet 60:1079–84.

Thune I, Brenn T, Lund E, Gaard M. 1997. Physical activity and the risk of breast cancer. New Engl J Med 336:1269–75.

Tirkkonen M, Johannsson O, Agnarsson BA et al. 1997. Distinct somatic genetic changes associated with tumor progression in carriers of *BRCA1* and *BRCA2* germ-line mutations. Cancer Res 57:1222–27.

Tonin F, Serova O, Lenoir G et al. 1995. *BRCA1* mutations in Ashkenazi Jewish women. Am J Hum Genet 57:189.

Tonin P, Weber B, Offit K et al. 1996. Frequency of recurrent *BRCA1* and *BRCA2* mutations in Ashkenazi Jewish breast cancer families. Nature Med 2:1179–83.

Trichopoulos D, MacMahon B, Cole P. 1972. Menopause and breast cancer risk. J Natl Cancer Inst 48:605–13.

Tulinius H, Egilsson V, Olafsdottir GH, Sigvaldsson H. 1992. Risk of prostate, ovarian and endometrial cancer among relatives of women with breast cancer. Br Med J 305:855–7.

Ursin G, Henderson BE, Haile RW et al. 1997. Does oral contraceptive use increase the risk of breast cancer in women with *BRCA1/BRCA2* mutations? Cancer Res 57:3678-81.

van de Vijver MJ, Peterse JL, Mooi WJ et al. 1988. Neu-protein overexpression in breast cancer: association with comedo-type ductal carcinoma *in situ* and limited prognostic value in stage II breast cancer. New Engl J Med 319:1239–45.

Vehmanen P, Friedman L, Eerola H et al. 1997. A low proportion of *BRCA2* mutations in Finnish breast cancer families. Am J Hum Genet 60:1050–8.

Vorechovsky I, Rasio D, Luo L et al. 1996. The *ATM* gene and susceptibility to breast cancer: analysis of 38 breast tumors reveals no evidence for mutation. Cancer Res 56:2726–32.

Whittemore AS, Gong G, Itnyre J. 1997. Prevalence and contribution of *BRCA1*/2 mutations in breast cancer and ovarian cancer: results from three U.S. population based case-control studies of ovarian cancer. Amer J Hum Genet 60:496–504.

Willet WC, Hunter DJ, Stampfer MJ et al. 1992. Dietary fat and fiber in relation to risk of breast cancer; an 8 year follow-up. JAMA 268: 2037–44.

Woods JE. 1986. Breast reconstruction: current state of the art. Mayo Clin Proc 61: 579–85.

Wooster R, Mangion J, Eeles R et al. 1992. A germline mutation in the androgen receptor gene in two brothers with breast cancer and Reifenstein syndrome. Nature Genet 2:132–4.

Wooster R, Neuhausen SL, Mangion J et al. 1994. Localization of a breast cancer susceptibility gene, *BRCA2*, to chromosome 13q12-13. Science 265:2088–90.

Wooster R, Bignell G, Lancaster J et al. 1995. Identification of the breast cancer susceptibility gene *BRCA2*. Nature 378:789–92.

Wu LC, Wang ZW, Tsan JT et al. 1996. Identification of a RING protein that can interact in vivo with the *BRCA1* gene product. Nature Genet 14:430–40.

Zigler J. 1996. Raloxifene, retinoids and lavender: "me too" tamoxifen alternatives under study. J Natl Cancer Inst. 88:1100–2.

Ziegler LD, Kroll SS. 1991. Primary breast cancer after prophylactic mastectomy. Am J Clin Oncol 14:451–4.

PART B: OVARIAN CANCER SYNDROMES

CLINICAL AND EPIDEMIOLOGIC FEATURES

Ovarian cancer is a relatively uncommon malignancy, but more than half of the 27,000 women diagnosed in 1997 will die of their disease. Like breast cancer, there is a steady increase in ovarian cancer incidence with age. Ovarian cancer before the age of 40 is relatively rare (0.2% probability), with the greatest increase in risk occurring between the ages of 50 and 60, peaking in the mid 70s. Overall, about 1 in 70 women (1.4%) will be diagnosed with ovarian cancer during the course of a lifetime.

A reduced risk of ovarian cancer is associated with factors that lead to decreased ovulation. These include pregnancy, lactation, and oral contraceptives. The protective effect of oral contraceptives is striking and little known by most physicians. There is a clear dose–response relationship, with a 40–50% reduction in risk in women who took oral contraceptives for 10–15 years (see Options for Prevention and Early Detection).

There are few known environmental or occupational risks for ovarian cancer (Daly, 1992; Runowicz, 1992). Dietary galactose, one of two sugars that constitute lactose found in milk, has been correlated with increased ovarian cancer risk, although associations with overall dietary fat have also been observed. An initial report of talc particles in ovarian tissues led to a study that implicated cosmetic talc, applied to the genital area, as a risk factor for ovarian cancer. Talc has subsequently been removed from most cosmetic products. In addition to these epidemiologic associations, risk for ovarian cancer is strongly associated with family history of the disease.

PATHOLOGY

About 90% of ovarian cancers is this country are of epithelial type, arising from the serosal mesothelial layer of the ovary. By far the most frequent subtypes of epithelial tumors are the serous cystadenocarcinomas, seen in more than 40% of cases. Mucinous cystadenocarcinomas, endometrial carcinomas, undifferentiated carcinomas, and clear cell carcinomas make up the remainder of epithelial tumors. In perhaps 10–15% of cases, epithelial tumors may be classified as of "borderline" malignancy, i.e., of low malignant potential, because of a lack of obvious invasion of the stroma in the biopsy specimen. These tumors progress and metastasize more slowly.

About 10% of ovarian tumors are derived from the gonadal stroma or germ cells. Of the former, the granulosa cell tumors are most common, and constitute a fortuitous finding when an epithelial tumor is suspected preoperatively. Granulosa cell tumors have a better prognosis than their epithelial counterparts. Germ cell tumors are diagnosed in younger women. These include dysgerminomas (which resemble seminomas in males), endodermal sinus tumors, and embryonal carcinomas. Although less common, the nonepithelial ovarian cancers are associated with a number of rare Mendelian conditions (see Appendix A). The diagnosis of any of these disorders should be accompanied by a careful family history and a search for associated congenital abnormalities.

HEREDITARY SYNDROMES

In 1950 Liber described ovarian cancer in a mother and five daughters. Through the next decades, familial ovarian cancer was documented in series of collected families. In 1989, a popular comedienne, Gilda Radner, died of ovarian cancer. Over 60 million Americans were told about familial ovarian cancer on prime time television programs in the first 6 months of 1990, and a registry of hundreds of families with ovarian cancer was compiled (Piver et al., 1993; Jashmi et al., 1995). Families with two or more cases of ovarian cancer among first- or second-degree relatives were entered into the registry. Of 143 families containing 508 ovarian cancers, a 2.5-fold excess risk for breast cancer, and a fivefold excess risk for uterine cancer were noted among female relatives of patients. For males a 4.5-fold increased risk for prostate cancer was noted. No increase in colon cancer risk was observed (Jashmi et al., 1995).

The findings of the Gilda Radner registry and other reports of familial ovarian cancer are largely consistent with three patterns of hereditary predisposition. These include (1) site-specific ovarian cancer; (2) hereditary breast-ovarian cancer; and (3) ovarian cancer as a component in hereditary nonpolyposis colon cancer (HNPCC), which includes colon, endometrial, and other tumor types.

Despite the documented risks in hereditary ovarian cancer families, large epidemiologic studies showed that familial clustering was not common. In the Cancer and Steroid Hormone Study (CASH), of 493 patients with ovarian cancer age 20-54, only 31 (7%) gave a history of a first-degree relative affected by ovarian cancer, and only 3 (0.6%) had more than one relative affected (Schildkraut et al., 1988). Other population-based studies confirmed this observation; while about 5% of patients with ovarian cancer had a family history of the disease, cases suggesting a highly penetrant dominant trait accounted for less than 1% of the total.

For the individuals with a single first-degree relative affected, however, the risk for ovarian cancer was increased three to four times over that of the risk in the general population. In selected families with multiple cases of ovarian cancer, the risk approached the 50% probability observed in dominant syndromes, and the age of onset appeared to be 10–15 years younger than the general population. The median age of onset of ovarian cancer in high risk individuals in 16 families studied at the National Cancer Institute was 47, with 17% of diagnoses made by the age of 40 (Amos et al., 1992). This statistic is of interest to individuals in hereditary breast–ovarian kindreds seeking to decide on an age to consider preventive or screening procedures. It also reveals that the majority of risk for ovarian cancer, even in a hereditary setting, occurred after childbearing.

Ovarian cancer is also a component in the hereditary nonpolyposis colon cancer syndrome (HNPCC) (see later in this chapter). In HNPCC families, the risk for ovarian cancers is increased up to fourfold.

BRCA1, BRCA2, and Ovarian Cancer

Of 374 cases of ovarian cancer identified at one center, 13 (3%) had germline *BRCA1* mutations (Stratton et al., 1997). A study of 145 families with at least one ovarian cancer and three or more cases of early onset breast cancer showed that 135 families were linked to *BRCA1* while the remaining 10 were linked to *BRCA2* (Narod et al., 1995b). Of families with two or more cases of ovarian cancer as well as multiple cases of breast cancer, 92% were linked to *BRCA1*. However, when 125 families with two or more cases of ovarian cancer were ascertained without regard to presence of breast cancer in the family, *BRCA1* mutations were noted in 37% and *BRCA2* mutations in 9%. Of families with 3 or more cases of ovarian cancer, mutations were detected in 61% of cases (Gayther et al., 1996). Thus, when direct mutation screening is performed in families with site-specific ovarian cancer, a significant proportion of cases may be due to genes other than *BRCA1* or *BRCA2*.

As presented in the prior section, there is a marked heterogeneity of risk of ovarian cancer in *BRCA1*-linked families. The lifetime risk for ovarian cancer in *BRCA1*-linked families varied from 10–80% (Easton et al., 1993, 1995; Narod et al., 1995a), and was 16% (confidence interval 4–30%) in a population based series (Struewing et al., 1997). Although some studies have suggested that ovarian cancer families less frequently demonstrated mutations in the 5′ end of the *BRCA1* gene (Gayther et al., 1995), there remain significant exceptions. For example, the kindred shown in Figure 4-6 would be termed a "site-specific ovarian cancer family," and yet it carried a 5382insC mutation, one of the most 5′ of the *BRCA1* mutations. This same mutation was the most common mutation observed in Russian ovarian cancer families described by these same authors, further weakening the correlation with site-specific breast cancer (Gayther et al., 1997).

As discussed earlier, the lifetime risk of ovarian cancer was 22% higher in *BRCA1*

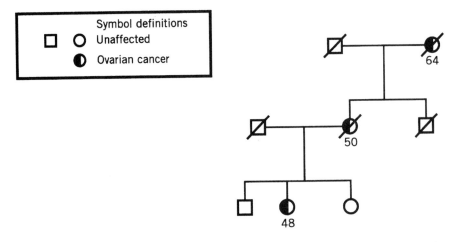

FIGURE 4-6 *A pedigree demonstrating site-specific ovarian cancer. This family was segregating* a BRCA1 *insertion mutation.*

heterozygotes with common alleles of the *HRAS1* variable number of tandem repeat polymorphism (Phelan et al., 1996). In addition to gene–gene interactions, environmental or hormonal factors may determine ovarian cancer risk in *BRCA1* heterozygotes. Parity, which is a protective factor for sporadic ovarian cancer, increased ovarian cancer risk in *BRCA1*-linked kindreds. The relative risk for multiparous women was 1.4; each birth conferred an additional 40% increase in risk for up to 5 births (Narod et al., 1995a). Interestingly, however, late age of last birth was protective, so that women whose last birth was after 30 were at nearly half the risk of those with last birth before 30. Women who had all their children after age 30 had the same risk as women who had no children (Narod et al., 1995a).

These results have potential counseling implications. Although the effect of the 5′ versus 3′ position of *BRCA1* mutation or the presence of *HRAS1* polymorphisms are of unclear clinical utility, the findings about age and risk factors for ovarian cancer in *BRCA1* heterozygotes can offer some guidance to women in their childbearing years. First, while parity does increase ovarian cancer risk in these women, late age of parity appeared to abrogate much of that risk. In addition, since the median age of ovarian cancer is after childbearing (age 48 in the series by Stratton et al., 1997), family planning can proceed with later discussion of possible risk-reducing surgical interventions when childbearing is completed. Because of the striking relationship between OC use and reduced ovarian cancer risk (see next section), prospective trials of oral contraceptives in younger women heterozygous for *BRCA1* mutations in ovarian cancer kindreds may offer a potential preventive option in this group.

The relationship between *BRCA2* mutations and ovarian cancer risk have not been as extensively analyzed. Somatic mutations of *BRCA2* were as rare as somatic mutations of *BRCA1* in ovarian cancers (Merajver et al., 1995; Takahashi et al., 1996)). The cases of *BRCA1* mutations observed in ovarian tumors were characterized by early onset or were observed in the setting of a family history of breast or ovarian cancer. Of two germline *BRCA2* mutations identified in 130 ovarian tumors analyzed, both were late-onset cases without significant family histories of cancer (Takahashi et al., 1996). Interestingly, in a large Israeli series, the median age of onset for ovarian cancer was significantly later in *BRCA2* carriers compared to *BRCA1* carriers (68 years versus 50 years) (Levy-Lahad et al., 1997).

When the histologic features of *BRCA1*-linked cases was analyzed, mucinous tumors appeared to be underrepresented. In the Gilda Radner registry, mucinous adenocarcinoma and cystadenoma were both underrepresented. Only 1.4% of the 439 familial ovarian cases were mucinous, compared to 12.7% expected (Piver et al., 1993).

A prolonged survival was reported in a study of ovarian cancer patients with germline mutations of *BRCA1*. Median survival for 43 ovarian cancer patients with *BRCA1* mutations was 77 months, compared to 29 months for matched controls (Rubin et al., 1996). However, these results were not confirmed in two studies totalling 82 ovarian cancer patients with germline *BRCA1* mutations (Johannsson et al., 1997; Brunet et al., 1997), suggesting that the original observation may have been due to an ascertainment bias (Brunet et al., 1997).

In addition to HNPCC, an increased risk for ovarian cancer is also associated with a number of rarer genetic syndromes, including hereditary basal cell nevus syndrome, Peutz-Jegher syndrome, and the gonadal dysgenesis syndromes (see Appendix A).

OPTIONS FOR PREVENTION AND EARLY DETECTION

Ovarian Screening

The standard recommendations for individuals at increased risk for ovarian cancer have included pelvic examination, ultrasound imaging, and serum tumor markers. Unfortunately, none of these strategies has been proved effective as a screening modality. This is particularly disturbing because most ovarian cancers present at an advanced stage of disease, highlighting the need for early diagnostic tests. The indications and limitations of ovarian screening remain controversial (Carlson et al., 1994; Kramer et al. 1993; NIH Consensus Conference, 1995.).

Pelvic examination is completely dependent on the skill of the examiner and the anatomy of the patient, and is difficult to evaluate in a clinical trial. CA125 is an antigenic determinant of a glycoprotein that is shed into the bloodstream by ovarian cancer cells. CA125 levels are increased in ovarian cancer, but also in endometriosis, uterine leiomyoma, pelvic inflammatory disease, early pregnancy, and benign cysts. The sensitivity, which reflects the false negative rate, of CA125 as a screening test in the general population is poor (see Chapter 6). Only about half of early stage ovarian cancers are accompanied by CA125 levels greater than 35 U/Ml. On the other hand, specificity, which reflects the false positive rate, is about 95% at a cutoff of 35U/L. The specificity may be slightly greater in postmenopausal women, because of the decreased likelihood of false positives.

Sonographic imaging of the ovaries is more sensitive when the transducer is

Case Example 4.6. A 29-year-old woman came for counseling regarding a family history of ovarian cancer. Her sister, mother, and grandmother were affected. Her sister was tested for mutations of *BRCA1* and *BRCA2*, but none were detected. The options for ovarian screening utilizing color Doppler transvaginal ultrasound and CA 125, as well as options for prophylactic oophorectomy were discussed. The patient's gynecologist had advised her to take oral contraceptives because of the evidence for their preventive role in ovarian cancer. Regular mammography and breast examinations were also recommended.

This case illustrates the range of options that should be addressed in families with site-specific ovarian cancer. It is believed that the majority of these families will have mutations in genes other than *BRCA1/2*.

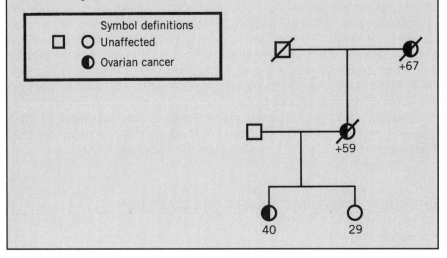

inserted into the vagina than when the transducer is located on the abdominal wall (Figure 4-7). In addition, the transvaginal approach is generally more convenient for the patient. A transabdominal approach requires a full bladder, while a transvaginal study is done when the bladder is emptied. Indices to assess abnormal findings of a cystic structure have been developed. These include measurements of ovarian volume, cyst wall thickness, and septal structure. In addition, a color flow Doppler examination can detect vessels with low resistance to flow, which are characteristic of tumors. In premenopausal women, examination should be performed during the first seven days of the menstrual cycle, so as to decrease the need to repeat the study after detection of a presumed functional cyst. Sensitivity of this technique has been estimated to be between 80% and 90%. The false positive rate of these examinations are their greatest shortcoming; a screening study of thousands of asymptomatic women resulted in a 10:1 ratio of benign to malignant lesions, with a yield of 4 malignant lesions found for every thousand women examined. Because of these false positives, the specificity of transvaginal ultrasound was estimated to be 94% (Carlson et al., 1994). A review of ultrasound screening of over 13,000 asymptomatic women indicated that 17 ovarian cancers were detected, 15 with stage I disease (reviewed by DePriest et al.,1997). All pa-

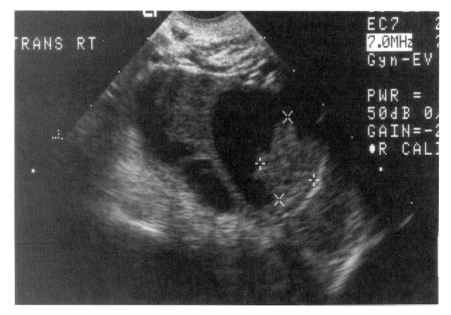

Figure 4-7 *Transvaginal ultrasound image of the ovaries. This ovarian cyst was observed during screening transvaginal ultrasound in a 36-year-old woman with a history of breast cancer at age 32. Within the ovary there was a cyst with a mural based soft tissue papillary excrescence, which proved to be an ovarian serous carcinoma.(Image courtesy of L. Hahn, M.D.)*

tients with ovarian cancers diagnosed in these reports were alive. A separate report of over 6470 women confirmed these results, with 6 cancers (5 stage I) detected. However, the major limitations of this approach were false positive results in 84 of the 90 women with suspicious findings on ultrasound examination (DePriest et al., 1997).

The specificity of ultrasound can be improved by the addition of CA125 screening. In fact, the two modalities are complementary. The sonogram will detect some of the CA125-negative ovarian masses, improving sensitivity, while the addition of CA125 to ultrasound decreases the false positive rate, improving specificity to 99.8% in one study.

In populations of women at increased familial risk for ovarian cancer, there is a marked improvement in the predictive value of the tests. Small trials have demonstrated the ability of ultrasound with Doppler and CA125 to find stage I ovarian cancers. For example, in a subset analysis of a study by Bourne et al. of 445 families with hereditary site-specific or multiple cancer syndromes, 21 had abnormal transvaginal doppler imaging, four of which proved to be ovarian cancer. Three of the four cases were stage Ia, one was stage III, with ages from 30–63 years (Bourne et al., 1993).

Based on similar data, the American College of Physicians recommended a combination of ultrasound and CA125 screening, preferably in a research setting, for women with a family history of ovarian cancer (American College of Physicians, 1994). A common recommendation is to screen twice yearly utilizing these modalities, starting at an early age (Lynch et al., 1982). The age to begin these evaluations is more difficult to assess. As mentioned, the median age for ovarian cancer in families with breast and ovarian cancer is in the late 40s. It seems prudent to begin ovarian screening at an early age. Some clinicians suggest the interval of ages 25–35; however, the earlier a woman's age at initiation of screening, the greater the risk for unnecessary biopsies.

Prophylactic Oophorectomy

Prophylactic removal of the ovaries is generally presented as an option to women with two first-degree relatives with ovarian cancer, in families linked to *BRCA1* or *BRCA2*, or women considering hysterectomy in the setting of a germline mutation associated with HNPCC. Newer techniques of laparoscopic surgery have made oophorectomy a one-day ambulatory experience with minimal morbidity. Unfortunately, prophylactic oophorectomy is not fail-safe. Cases of serous surface carcinoma, also called *papillary serous carcinoma,* have been reported in the literature. The tumor is indistinguishable from serous carcinoma of the ovary except that it spares the ovaries. In 1982, serous surface carcinoma was documented in 3 of 28 women (11%) who had prophylactic oophorectomies because of a family history of ovarian cancer. Subsequent case reports confirmed this observation. (Tobacman et al., 1982; Chen et al., 1985). Of 324 women from 100 families in the Gilda Radner registry, 6 cases (2%) occurred from 1 to 27 years post oophorectomy. An update of the original NCI series reported 8 cases of carcinomatosis in 44 oophorectomized women, with 460 person-years of follow-up. Although the confidence intervals in this study were wide, there was a trend for a decrease in ovarian cancer risk in the cohort post prophylactic oophorectomy, although their risk remained higher than population risks (Struewing et al., 1995).

One explanation for the failure of prophylactic oophorectomy is that the tumors arise from peritoneal tissues that have the same mesodermal origin as the germinal epithelium of the ovary. This explanation would limit the efficacy of the procedure in most patients at increased hereditary risk. However, another explanation for the origin of the peritoneal tumors is that micrometastases occurred prior to the prophylactic surgery. Preliminary evidence in support of this hypothesis stems from case reports in which microscopic ovarian cancers were retrospectively detected by careful dissection of the ovaries of high risk individuals after prophylactic surgery. In one case, the primary ovarian tumor was found by reexamination of ovaries prophylactically removed 3 years before the patient developed peritoneal carcinomatosis (Chen et al., 1985). In two additional cases, individuals heterozygous for *BRCA1* mutations were found to have small foci of cancer in ovaries that were prophylactically removed (Salazar et al., 1996).

As discussed in the previous section, decision-analysis models predicted very modest advantages (0.3 to 1.7 years of additional life gained) for the young *BRCA* heterozygote opting for prophylactic oophorectomy (Schrag et al., 1997). However, these models assumed a 50% failure rate for the surgical procedure, based the survival comparison on the "baseline" derived in the study by Rubin et al. (see Hereditary Syndromes above), and also assumed hormone replacement until menopause. The modification of any of these assumptions affects the benefit/risk ratio.

Hormonal Modulation

The major side effects of oophorectomy in young women include an increased risk of heart disease and osteoporosis associated with surgically induced menopause. Estrogen replacement therapy, if required in these circumstances, should utilize the lowest dose possible, due to the increased risk of breast cancer associated with estrogen replacement. Newer formulations of transdermal estrogen avoid the swings in blood levels after oral administration. The transdermal formulations do not require hepatic activation and give more stable blood levels of estradiol, simulating physiologic levels. At least in theory, in premenopausal women post oophorectomy, it should be possible to administer low doses of hormone, increasing breast cancer risk so as not to exceed the "baseline" risk associated with physiologic levels of estrogen.

Combination oral contraceptives (COC) contain an estrogen and high dose progestogen. Because COCs suppress ovulation, it was anticipated that the use of these agents would decrease ovarian cancer risk. This was because of the known protective effects of parity, and the "ovulation" hypothesis which suggests that ovarian cancer risk is related to the rapid turnover and repair by epithelial cells after each ovulation. A striking, time-dependent, protective effect of oral contraceptive use and ovarian cancer risk was demonstrated. Hormonal prevention has been suggested as a rational option for women at hereditary risk for ovarian cancer (Barber, 1993). Indeed, one metanalysis predicted that a 35-year-old woman who has one relative with ovarian cancer could virtually eliminate her increased risk for ovarian cancer by taking oral contraceptives for 10 or more years. A 35-year-old woman having two relatives with ovarian cancer could reduce her risk by half, to 3.7%, by following a similar course of oral contraceptives (Kerlikowske, 1992). There have not yet been longitudinal studies documenting a protective effect of oral contraceptives in the setting of hereditary ovarian or breast-ovarian cancer.

REFERENCES: PART B

American College of Physicians. 1994. Screening for ovarian cancer: recommendations and rationale. Ann Intern Med 121:141–2.

Amos CI, Shaw GL, Tucker MA, Hartge P. 1992. Age at onset for familial epithelial ovarian cancer. JAMA 268: 1896–9.

Barber HRK. 1993. Prophylaxis in ovarian cancer. Cancer 71:1529–33.

Bourne TH, Campbell S, Reynolds KM et al. 1993. Screening for early familial ovarian cancer with transvaginal ultrasonography and color blood flow imaging. Br Med Jour 306:1025–9.

Brunet JB, Narod SA, Tonin P, Foulkes WD. 1997. *BRCA1* mutations and survival in ovarian cancer (letter). New Engl J Med 336; 1256.

Carlson KJ, Skates SJ, Singer DE. 1994. Screening for ovarian cancer. Ann Intern Med 121:124–32.

Chen KT, Schooley JL, Flam MM. 1985. Peritoneal carcinomatosis after prophylactic oophorectomy in familial ovarian cancer syndrome. Obstet Gynecol 66:93–4 (suppl).

Daly M. 1992. The epidemiology of ovarian cancer. Hematol Oncol Clin N Amer 6(4): 729–38.

DePriest PD, Gallion HH, Pavlik EJ, Kryscio RJ, van Nagell JR. 1997. Transvaginal sonography as a screening method for the detection of early ovarian cancer. Gynecol Oncol 65:408–14.

Easton DF, Bishop DT, Ford D et al. 1993. Genetic linkage analysis in familial breast and ovarian cancer: results from 214 families. Am J Hum Genet 52:678–701.

Easton DF, Ford D, Bishop DJ, Breast Cancer Linkage Consortium. 1995. Breast and ovarian cancer in *BRCA1*-mutation carriers. Am J Hum Genet 56:265–71.

Gayther SA, Russell P, Harrington P et al. High frequency of germline *BRCA1* and *BRCA2* mutations in familial ovarian cancer. Am J Hum Genet 1996; 59: 173 (abstr).

Gayther SA, Warren W, Mazoyer S et al. 1995. Germline mutations of the *BRCA1* gene in breast and ovarian cancer families provide evidence for a genotype–phenotype correlation. Nature Genet 11:428–33.

Gayther SA, Mangion J, Russell P et al. 1997. Variation of risks of breast and ovarian cancer associated with different germline mutations of the *BRCA1* gene. Nature Genet 15:103–5.

Jashmi MF, Itnyre JH, Oakley-Girvan IA, Piver MS, Whittemore AS. 1995. Risks of cancer among members of families in the Gilda Radner familial ovarian cancer registry. Cancer 76:1416–21.

Johannsson O, Ranstam J, Borg A, Olsson H. 1997. *BRCA1* mutations and survival in ovarian cancer (letter). New Engl J Med 336:1255–6.

Kerlikowske K, Brown JS, Grady DG. 1992. Should women with familial ovarian cancer undergo prophylactic oophorectomy? Obstet Gynecol 80:700–7.

Kramer BS, Gohagan J, Prorok PC, Smart C. 1993. A National Cancer Institute sponsored screening trial for prostatic, lung, colorectal, and ovarian cancers. Cancer 71:589–93.

Levy-Lahad E, Catane R, Eisenberg S et al. 1997. Founder *BRCA1* and *BRCA2* mutations in Ashkenazi Jews in Israel: frequency and differential penetrance in ovarian cancer and in breast–ovarian cancer families. Am J Hum Genet 60:1059–67.

Lynch HT, Albano WA, Lynch JF, Lynch PM, Campbell A. 1982. Surveillance and management of patients at high genetic risk for ovarian carcinoma. Obstet Gynecol 59:589–96.

Merajver SD, Pham TM, Caduff RF et al. 1995. Somatic mutations in the *BRCA1* gene in sporadic ovarian tumours. Nature Genet 9:439–43.

Narod SA, Goldgar D, Cannon-Albright L, Weber B, Moslehi R, Ives E, Lenoir G, Lynch H. 1995a. Risk modifiers in carriers of *BRCA1* mutations. Int J Cancer 64: 394–8.

Narod SA, Ford D, Eyfjord J, et al. 1995b. Genetic heterogeneity of breast ovarian cancer revisited (letter). Am J Hum Genet 57:957–8.

NIH Consensus Conference. 1995. Ovarian Cancer: Screening, treatment, and follow-up. JAMA 273, 6:491–7.

Phelan CM, Rebbeck TR, Weber BL et al. 1996. Ovarian cancer risk in *BRCA1* carriers is modified by the *HRAS1* variable number of tandem repeat (VNTR) locus. Nature Genet 12: 309–11.

Piver MS, Baker TR, Jamshi MF et al. 1993. Familial ovarian cancer. A report of 658 families from the Gilda Radner Familial Ovarian Cancer Registry 1981–1991. Cancer 72:582–8.

Rubin SC, Benjamin I, Kehbakht K et al. 1996. Clinical and pathological features of ovarian cancer in women with germ-line mutations of *BRCA1*. New Engl J Med 335:1413–6.

Runowicz CD. 1992. Advances in the screening and treatment of ovarian cancer. Ca: Jour Clin 42(6):327–49.

Salazar H, Godwin A, Daly M et al. 1996. Microscopic benign and invasive malignant neoplasms and a cancer-prone phenotype in prophylactic oophorectomies. J Natl Cancer Inst 88:1810–20.

Schildkraut JM, Thompson WD. 1988. Familial ovarian cancer: a population based case-control study. Am J Epidem 128:456–66.

Schrag D, Kuntz KM, Garber JE, Weeks J. 1997. Impact of prophylactic mastectomy and oophorectomy on life expectancy of women with *BRCA1* or *BRCA2* gene mutations. New Engl J Med 336:1465–71.

Stratton JF, Gayther SA, Russell P et al. 1997. Contribution of *BRCA1* mutations to ovarian cancer. New Eng J Med 336:1125–30.

Struewing JP, Watson P, Easton DF, Ponder BAJ, Lynch HT, Tucker MA. 1995. Prophylactic oophorectomy in inherited breast/ovarian cancer families. Monogr Natl Cancer Inst 17:33–5.

Struewing JP, Hartge P, Wacholder S et al. 1997. The risk of cancer associated with specific mutations of *BRCA1* and *BRCA2* among Ashkenazi Jews. New Eng J Med 336:1401–8.

Takahashi H, Chiu HC, Bandera CA, et al. 1996. Mutations of the *BRCA2* gene in ovarian carcinomas. Cancer Res 56:2738–74.

Tobacman JK, Tucker MA, Kase R et al. Intra-abdominal carcinomatosis after prophylatic oophorectomy in ovarian cancer-prone families. Lancet 2:795–7.

PART C: COLON CANCER SYNDROMES

CLINICAL AND EPIDEMIOLOGIC FEATURES

Colon cancer is the third most common cancer in the United States, with about 150,000 cases occurring each year. It is the most common of the hereditary tumors affecting both men and women. In their lifetime 1 in 25 Americans will be affected with colon cancer. Other than genetic factors, risk factors for colon cancer include preexisting inflammatory bowel disease and diets high in fat and low in fiber.

Because it is known that polyps can progress to frank malignancy, it is assumed that most colon cancers take their origin from polyps. While the adenoma–colon cancer sequence has been documented, the true proportion of cancers that arise from polyps has not been measured directly. Histologic examinations of cancers, however, have shown traces of the residual polyp in some cases, and small tumors almost always bear these hallmarks of their origin.

As with breast cancer, there has been a trend for increased diagnosis of disease at the earliest most curable stages. Prognosis of colon cancer is dependent on the stage of the tumor at diagnosis. Whatever system of staging utilized, the survival of patients with the earliest stage lesions (e.g., Dukes A lesions confined to mucosa or submucosa) is 80%–100%. Disease that has spread past the muscularis mucosa (Dukes B disease) has only a 70% survival at 5 years. When the colon tumor has spread to regional lymph nodes (Dukes C disease) adjuvant chemotherapy is generally utilized along with surgery. Metastatic disease (Dukes D) is treated with palliative chemotherapy or radiotherapy.

Earlier detection of cancer is thought to explain the 10% decrease in mortality due to colon cancer among males (22% among females) noted from 1973 to 1990. Incidence rates actually increased during the early and mid 1980s, possibly reflecting the increase in diagnosis of early stage disease during this period (Chu et al., 1990).

PATHOLOGY

Polyps in the colon are outcroppings caused by tissue overgrowth. *Hyperplastic polyps* are areas of hyperplasia of the mucosa, of unknown cause. They may appear as slightly raised areas of mucosa or as polypoid lesions. They rarely, if ever, progress to malignancy. Adenomatous polyps appear redder and more granular than the surrounding mucosa, and may have stalks made of fibrous tissue that supports the glandular tissue in the head of the polyp. These polyps are also called *tubular adenomas* because of the branchlike tubules from the stalk embedded in the muscularis mucosa. Some adenomatous polyps are termed *villous* because of fingerlike projections of epithelial tissue extending from the stalk to the muscularis. The polyps may appear purplish in color and are softer in texture. They are also of greater clinical concern, because 40% of villous adenomas will progress to malignancy, compared to only 5% of tubular adenomas. An intermediate type of tubulo-villous adenoma is seen more often in older patients, or in larger lesions. It has an intermediate risk (about 20%) for malignant progression. Adenomatous polyps are the most common subtype, accounting for 50% of polyps less than 5 mm in size and 95% of polyps larger than 1 cm.

The time to progression from adenoma to cancer has been estimated to be about 5 years. This is based primarily on the difference in age frequencies of populations with these lesions; the median age for adenomatous polyps is around 58, while colon cancer incidence peaks in the early 60s. The doubling time of the colon tumors is quite slow, on the order of two years.

Almost all large bowel carcinomas are adenocarcinomas. Subtypes of mucinous adenocarcinoma and "signet ring" adenocarcinomas contain extracellular or intracellular mucin, respectively. Squamous or adenosquamous tumors are rarely seen, except at the anus.

HEREDITARY SYNDROMES

Highly penetrant dominant susceptibility syndromes account for about 5% of colon cancer. The most common syndrome is hereditary nonpolyposis colon cancer syndrome (HNPCC), with familial adenomatous polyposis (FAP) constituting a rarer familial syndrome. The extent to which HNPCC accounts for familial colon cancer remains to be established. Genetic epidemiologic analyses suggested the presence of a common susceptibility allele for both colon cancer and adenomatous polyps that accounted for at least 15% and possibly half of cases (Cannon-Albright et al., 1988; Houlston et al., 1992). A population-based ascertainment of over 1200 colon tumors confirmed that about 8% were due to highly penetrant genes (multiple cases in multiple generations), while 37% showed a less dramatic familial clustering, and 5% occurred at early age (<50 years). The remaining half of cases were "sporadic" (Ponz de Leon et al., 1996).

Epidemiologic analysis of a large follow-up study of individuals endoscopically evaluated for the presence of polyps revealed that the magnitude of increased risk for colon cancer in a first-degree relative of an individual with an adenomatous polyp diagnosed before age 60 (RR = 2.6) was similar to the risk for relatives of probands with colorectal cancer (Winawer et al., 1996). These empiric data are useful in counseling; however, they require an expanded family history that includes information on precancerous lesions (polyps).

HNPCC

"I will die of cancer of my female organs or bowels." This was the fear of the seamstress of the Michigan pathologist S. A. Warthin. She did indeed die of uterine cancer at an early age and in so doing followed the pattern of 17 members of her family over two generations (Warthin, 1925). Each succumbed to cancer of the bowel, uterus, stomach, or other organs, defining what was called "Warthin's Family G." Over the course of 50 years of study, this constellation of tumor types in a family became known as Lynch syndrome, or hereditary nonpolyposis colon cancer (HNPCC) (Marra and Boland, 1995). A statistical analysis of extracolonic tumors occurring in families with hereditary colon and uterine cancer revealed that four additional tumor sites had increased observed/expected (O/E) ratios: cancers of the stomach (O/E = 4.1), ovary (O/E = 3.5), small intestine (O/E = 25), ureter (O/E = 22), and kidney (mostly transitional cell tumors of renal pelvis and ureter) (O/E = 3.2) (Watson and Lynch, 1993).

Breast cancer was not statistically overrepresented in HNPCC families, and hence has not been considered a component tumor (Watson and Lynch, 1993). However, at least one report has documented the molecular hallmarks of HNPCC tumors in the breast cancer of a woman who was a member of an HNPCC kindred (Risinger et al., 1996).

Members of HNPCC families should be counseled regarding the 70%–75% risk of colon cancer by age 65. This risk is based largely on genetic epidemiologic studies (Bailey-Wilson et al., 1986; Scapoli et al. 1994). In a series of 41 HNPCC families studied by Vasen, the penetrance was 92% by age 60 (Vasen et al., 1994) (Figure 4-8). The median age at diagnosis for colon cancer was only 44–46 years in some series of hereditary cases (Vasen et al., 1994). Remarkably, the phenomenon of anticipation (Chapter 2) was observed in HNPCC families described initially by Warthin, and in a later series (Warthin, 1925; Menko et al., 1993; Vasen et al. 1994). The median age in three successive generations of 34 HNPCC families decreased from 45 to 32 to 28 years of age (Vasen et al., 1994). These results, however, could also be explained both by ascertainment bias as well as cohort effect (see case study). The penetrance of mutations associated with mutations of HNPCC genes has been derived based on a large number of HNPCC kindreds analyzed, but may be subject to the types of ascertainment bias present in all pedigree studies. As in the breast cancer penetrance estimates,

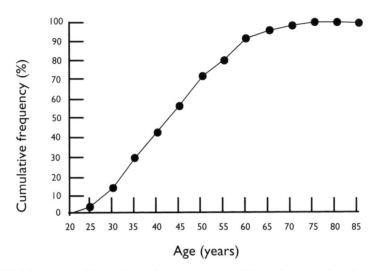

FIGURE 4-8 *Age specific penetrance for colon cancer in 41 hereditary nonpolyposis colon cancer families. The penetrance was 92% by age 60 (from Vasen et al., 1994, by permission).*

the risks of colon cancer for members of HNPCC families may be greater than the cancer risks for mutation carriers in the general population. In HNPCC families, synchronous cancers of the colon (several tumors presenting at the same time) were noted in 18% of cases, and metachronous tumors (multiple tumors at different times) were documented in up to 40%–50% at 10–15 year follow-up (Mecklin and Jarvinen, 1993). A 20%–30% risk of endometrial cancer by age 70 has been reported in these same pedigrees, with a median age of onset from the late forties to early fifties (Watson et al.,1994). This risk should be compared to the risk for endometrial cancer of 3% in the general population. The median age of onset for the associated ovarian cancers was around age 45.

At a 1991 meeting in Amsterdam, the International Collaborative Group on HNPCC defined the syndrome as (1) histologically verified colorectal cancer in three or more relatives, one of whom is a first-degree relative of the other two; (2) colorectal cancer involving at least two generations; and (3) one or more colorectal cancer cases diagnosed before 50 years of age. The most obvious limitation of the Amsterdam criteria, emphasized at the 1996 meetings of the International Collaborative Group on HNPCC was that it ignored the endometrial and extracolonic tumors. In a subsequent meeting, the Bethesda Criteria for HNPCC were defined to include the Amsterdam criteria, pedigrees with a colon cancer case before 40 years, and pedigrees with a higher incidence of tumors associated with HNPCC.

Although there do not appear to be defining histologic features of HNPCC tumors, mucinous types appear to be more common. Adenomas, like the cancers in HNPCC, appear more commonly on the right side. The adenomas appear as multiple lesions in about 20% of at-risk individuals. Less than 100 polyps are generally present in these cases (Marra, and Boland,1995). Tumors of HNPCC patients show a diploid genotype (Kouri et al., 1990), consistent with the improved survival of patients that is also noted (Sanikila et al., 1996).

A variant of HNPCC with multiple (50–100) small adenomas was described in six members of an HNPCC kindred (Lynch et al., 1988). This syndrome, termed *flat adenoma syndrome* in an earlier report (Muto et al., 1985), is now felt to be an attenuated form of familial adenomatous polyposis.

Muir-Torre Syndrome

Considered a variant of HNPCC, Muir-Torre syndrome was first described in 1967 in a proband with multiple sebaceous neoplasms, including keratoacanthomas, and neoplasms of the small and large bowel and larynx. The range of skin and internal malignancies was broad (Schwartz et al., 1989). Like HNPCC, tumors of the stomach, endometrium, kidney, and ovaries have been reported. In addition, cancers of the bladder, breast, larynx and other sites may be observed. These manifestations were rare, however, as the skin and colon cancers define the phenotype (Lynch et al., 1985). The skin lesions typically presented in the 40s. However, in some members of the kindreds described, the skin manifestations were absent altogether, with the phenotype more typical of HNPCC.

Familial Adenomatous Polyposis (FAP)

Originally described in the late nineteenth century (Lynch et al., 1997), FAP is a rare (1 in 7000–8000) syndrome characterized by a presentation with hundreds, or thousands, of colonic polyps in the late teens or early twenties and progression to colon cancer in virtually every case (Figure 4-9). A minimum of 100 polyps is generally necessary to make the diagnosis, whereas HNPCC families rarely have more than 50 polyps. The median number of polyps in one series of FAP patients was 842 (Debinski et al., 1996). There does appear to be a subset of attenuated FAP families in which the number of polyps may be significantly less than 100. One large Utah FAP kindred of over 4600 members was initially described by Burt and others. It has a highly variable number of polyps, with an average of 26 polyps per heterozygote (Burt and Samowitz 1988; Leppert et al., 1990). This phenotype may be related to the flat adenoma variant of HNPCC, which has been associated with mutations in the proximal portion of the *APC* gene (see section on *APC*).

In the absence of prophylactic colectomy, death from colon cancer will occur in virtually all of FAP cases by age 50, with 37% affected by colon cancer by age 37. There is a twofold greater risk for cancer in those with more than 1000 polyps, compared to FAP patients with less than 1000 polyps (Debinski et al., 1996). Upper GI malignancy may also occur in these patients and may be a cause of death after colectomy. There is a 10%–12% lifetime risk for duodenal cancer in FAP patients. Congenital hypertrophy of the retinal pigment epithelium (CHRPE) is a useful diagnostic marker for the syndrome. It consists of pigmented lesions in the retina that can be detected by fundoscopic examination (Figure 4-10).

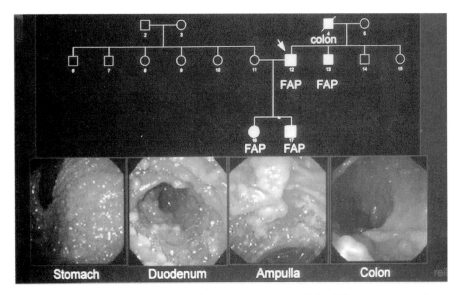

FIGURE 4-9 *Endoscopic appearance of upper intestinal polyps in familial adenomatous polyposis. The patient underwent subtotal colectomy; the retained portion of the sigmoid (right) demonstrated less diffuse polyposis. The patient and family members also had subcutaneous fibromas. (Courtesy of Dr. Hans Gerdes.)*

A variant form of FAP is Gardner's syndrome, in which the stigmata of FAP are accompanied by sebaceous cysts, lipomas, desmoid tumors, fibromas, facial bone osteomas, and impacted or supernumerary teeth.

Turcot's Syndrome

In 1949 Crail described a case of a 24-year-old man with medulloblastoma who subsequently was diagnosed with polyposis coli as well as papillary thyroid cancer. Ten years later, Turcot described two cases of familial polyposis in siblings, one of whom developed medulloblastoma and the other a glioblastoma. In 1988 a review of 50 similar cases revealed that the average age at presentation was 18 years, and virtually all had one of the two histologic types of brain tumor described by Crail and Turcot (Jarvis et al., 1988). There was extreme variability in the number of polyps, ranging from 1 to over 100, and also in the mode of inheritance. Some families showed a dominant pattern of inheritance, other families suggested a recessive pattern, and in still others there was no family history at all. Café au lait spots were described in several cases. In a series of 14 families, the age of onset of the polyposis ranged from 5 to 58, the age of medulloblastoma from 5 to 29 and the age of glioblastoma from 16 to 48 (Hamilton et al., 1995). Skin cysts and pigmented ocular-fundus lesions were also observed.

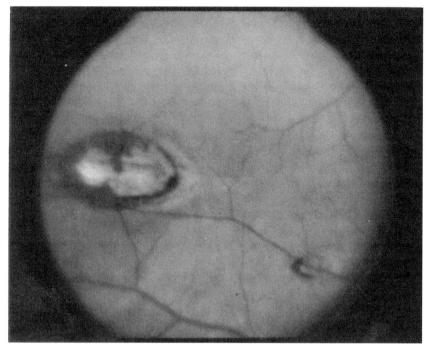

FIGURE 4-10 *Congenital hypertrophy of the retinal pigment epithelium in familial adenomatous polyposis. (Courtesy of Dr. M. H. Heinemann.)*

DNA DIAGNOSIS

APC

The biology and cloning of the *APC* gene for FAP and the *mutS* and *mutL* homologues associated with HNPCC were introduced in Chapter 3. Predictive testing for FAP has been hampered by the relatively large size of the gene and the wide spectrum of mutations observed (Mandl et al., 1994; Kinzler and Vogelstein, 1996). An analysis of 51 FAP families, using a variety of detection techniques revealed *APC* mutations in 42 (82%) of the families (Giardiello et al.,1997c). Based on data from hundreds of FAP kindreds in the world literature, 97% of the mutations in *APC* have been observed in the 5′ half of the gene, with a large number in a defined region within exon 15. Initial reports associated the location of a mutation in the *APC* gene with phenotypic features (Figure 4-11). Patients with mutations between codons 1250 and 1464 had profuse (>2000) polyps, compared to patients with other mutations (Nagase et al., 1992). Others were not able to find phenotypic correlations of exon 15 mutations (Paul et al., 1993). A preliminary genotype-phenotype correlation was noted between CHRPE and mutations in exons 9 through 15 (codons 463 to 1387), especially 3′ exon 9 mutations (Olschwang et al., 1993; Giardiello et al., 1997c). Truncating mutations in the region

APC Gene

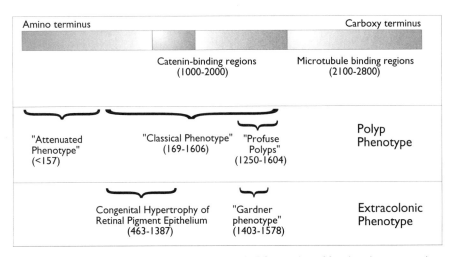

FIGURE 4-11   *Genotype-phenotype correlations of APC mutations. Mutations between codons 1250 and 1604 have been associated with profuse (>2000) polyps; retinal pigmentation has been associated with mutations in exons 9 through 15 (codons 463 to 1387). Truncating mutations in the region between codons 1403 and 1578 were associated with desmoid tumors and mandibular lesions of Gardner syndrome, but not with CHRPE. In an attenuated form of FAP, clustered mutations in the 5′ end of the APC gene were reported.*

between codons 1403 and 1578 were associated with the desmoid tumors and mandibular lesions of Gardner syndrome, but not with CHRPE (Davies et al., 1995).

In four families with the attenuated form of *APC* originally described by Burt et al., clustered mutations in the 5′ end of the *APC* gene, all within the first 4 exons, were reported (Spirio et al., 1993). The flat-adenoma subtype of HNPCC is also thought to be a form of attenuated FAP, since in the index family an *APC* mutation proximal to 5′ was described (Lynch et al., 1995; Spirio et al., 1993). Giardiello and colleagues compared the clinical features of seven FAP families with mutations proximal to codon 158 (5′ families) and seven families with mutations downstream of codon 158. A trend for lesser number of polyps, right-sided location, and increased survival was noted in the "5′ families" (Giardiello et al., 1997b). Recently, an even more attenuated form of FAP, characterized by familial desmoid tumor in the absence of the usual colonic or extracolonic features has been described (Eccles et al., 1996). In this syndrome, termed *hereditary desmoid disease,* mutations in the 3′ end of *APC* were observed, consistent with the trend for desmoid tumors noted in FAP patients with 3′ *APC* mutations (Eccles et al., 1996).

Up to a third of FAP cases may be due to new mutations of *APC.* The protein product of the *APC* gene was shown to associate with proteins (catenins) that bind to a cell surface molecule (cadherin), which is essential for cellular adhesion. These studies suggest that the *APC* protein may be a vital communications link between the cell surface and the microtubules necessary for cell division (Rubinfeld et al., 1993; Rubinfeld et al., 1996; Kinzler and Vogelstein, 1996). A mutation resulting in a T to A substitution at nucleotide 3920 creates a hypermutable region in the *APC* gene, resulting in a syndrome of familial colon cancer in individuals of Ashkenazi Jewish ancestry (Laken et al., 1997). This founder mutation, I1307K was detected in 6% of Ashkenazi Jews in the general population, and 7 of 25 Jewish individuals with a family history of colon cancer. Thus, in addition to the typical FAP phenotype, mutations of *APC* may be associated with a range of attenuated phenotypes of colon cancer susceptibility.

A variety of methodologies for detection of *APC* mutations have been proposed, including full sequencing and an *in vitro synthesized protein* (IVSP) assay (see Chapter 7). This later technique is commercially available for analysis of affected families. It will detect up to 90% of mutations and may be supplemented with allele-specific assays for the remaining 10% of cases (Powell et al., 1993). In a study of 105 Dutch FAP kindreds, denaturing gradient gel electrophoresis (DGGE) analysis (see Chapter 7) revealed mutations in 26% of families, protein truncation analysis of exon 5 picked up another 36%, and Southern blot identified an additional 2%, leaving 36% of families without *APC* mutations detected by these techniques (van der Luijt et al., 1997).

HNPCC

As predicted by linkage studies (Nystrom-Lahti et al., 1994), two genes on chromosomes 2p and 3p account for the majority of HNPCC kindreds. About 70% of HNPCC families were associated with mutations in one of the four known genes: *hMSH2*, *hMLH1*, *hPMS1* (post meiotic segregation 1), or *hPMS2* (Leach et al., 1993; Bronner et al., 1994; Nicolaides et al., 1994; Papadopolous et al., 1994; Liu et al., 1996). Of these, mutations of *hMSH2* and *hMLH1* are far more frequent than the others, accounting for about 30% each of families meeting Amsterdam criteria for HNPCC. The majority of mutations of *hMSH2* and *hMLH1* thus far reported have been inactivating insertions, deletions, alterations in premessenger RNA splicing signals, and nonsense mutations. However, some missense mutations have also been observed. The most common *hMSH2* mutation observed was an in-frame deletion of most of exon 5, from nucleotides 793-942. The remainder of *hMSH2* mutations have been scattered across the gene (Liu et al., 1996).

Mutations of the genes associated with HNPCC, as well as the genes *hGTBP* and *hMSH3*, result in the replication error repair (RER) phenotype in tumors. As introduced in Chapter 3, the RER phenotype is most commonly detected as microsatellite instability utilizing PCR screening of tumors with several microsatellite markers. The RER phenotype is present in about 80% of HNPCC-associated colon cancers (Aaltonen et al., 1993) and in about 15% of sporadic colon tumors (Thibodeau et al., 1993), as well as in other tumors associated with HNPCC (e.g., uterine, gastric cancers). The *RII* gene, which encodes the type II transforming growth factor receptor (TGF) β receptor, contains a 10 base pair adenine tract that is subject to mutation in RER positive adenomas and HNPCC tumors. Over 90% of RER positive sporadic and familial colon tumors showed *RII* mutations in this region (Parsons et al., 1995; Myeroff et al., 1995). The normal function of the family of TGF-β proteins is as an inhibitor of epithelial growth. Thus, mutations in these genes are consistent with the tumor suppressor model.

A novel method of detecting altered expression of the genes associated with HNPCC has been the development and commercial availability of monoclonal antibodies directed against the protein products of these genes (Leach et al., 1996). Immunohistochemical stains for these proteins are now available. Preliminary studies have shown decreased expression of hMSH2 and hMLH1 proteins in >90% of cases with germline mutations and RER posititivity, and also in most cases with RER positivity and no mutations. Decreased expression was not observed in cases without mutations or RER expression (Thibodeau et al., 1996). Decreased hMLH1 protein expression by immunohistochemical analysis was also identified in four RER-positive sporadic colon tumors without mutations in the coding sequence, but with evidence of DNA methylation of promotor regions (Kane et al., 1997). These findings suggest that immunohistochemical analysis of tumors for proteins expressed by HNPCC genes may be one method to identify some probands who may benefit from genetic counseling.

Mutations of *hMLH1* were shown to cluster in the Scandinavian families initially studied. More than half of *hMLH1* mutations in these early series clustered in a region encompassing exons 15 and 16 (Wijnen et al., 1996). Two founder mutations in *hMLH1* have been documented in Finland. One is a large deletion in exon 16 and flanking introns and the other is a single-base change at the splice acceptor site of exon 6. The common ancestors for these two mutations were born in the sixteenth and eighteenth centuries, respectively (Moisio et al., 1996). A recurring mutation at the splice donor site of exon 5 has been noted in about 12% of English HNPCC kindreds, although a common haplotype was not evident (Froggatt et al., 1995). In other kindreds, considerable heterogeneity was noted (Han et al., 1995; Kolodner et al. 1995). A codon 586 mutation in exon 16 was noted to be common in Korean HNPCC kindreds (Han et al., 1996).

Evidence for genotype–phenotype associations has been scanty. One *hMLH1* mutation, a deletion of codon 618 was observed in both a kindred with HNPCC and a kindred with Turcot's syndrome. The same *hMSH2* mutations have been observed in kindreds with typical HNPCC and a kindred with Muir-Torre syndrome (see following section). The clinical significance of the RER phenotype in HNPCC and related syndromes has been the subject of numerous studies. Of 181 colorectal tumors consecutively ascertained in one series, 24 demonstrated the RER phenotype. Of these, EBV-transformed lymphocytes were available for germline DNA analysis in 10 cases. Only one of these showed a mutation of an HNPCC gene. This tumor was from a 22-year-old with three relatives with colorectal or endometrial cancer. The tumor demonstrated homozygosity for the *hMLH1* mutation observed in the germline, consistent with the Knudson hypothesis. In seven colon cancer cell lines demonstrating the RER phenotype, only three had mutations in an HNPCC gene in the tumor samples. In at least one of these cases, the *hMLH1* mutation was not present in normal colon, suggesting that the mutation was somatic. In the tumor, there was no normal gene product detected, consistent with a somatic second hit to the other allele (Liu et al. 1995a). One explanation for the observation of the RER phenotype in the absence of mutations in the coding sequence of mismatch repair genes has been proposed. DNA methylation causing total inactivation of *hMLH1* expression has been documented in some RER positive tumors (Kane et al., 1997).

These findings suggest that the RER phenotype, observed in 15–20% of colorectal tumors, and 3–5% of sporadic adenomas, can be acquired as a somatic event in the absence of germline mutations. When RER-causing mutations do occur in the tumors, they may be due to other mechanisms than mutation of the known HNPCC genes. This would suggest that screening for the RER phenotype may not be an efficient way to identify those with germline HNPCC mutations. An exception to this rule may be in extremely early-onset cases (occurring before age 35). Of 189 cases of colorectal cancer occurring in patients not meeting Amsterdam criteria for HNPCC, the RER phenotype was observed in 37 (20)%, 18 of which were younger than age 35 (Liu et al., 1995b). Of these, 11 had no family history of colon or endometrial cancer. Of 12 cases on which EBV-transformed lymphocytes were available for analysis, a mutation of an HNPCC gene was observed in 5. Of note, in 4 of the cases, the mutation was identified in unaffected parents of the proband, suggesting a lesser penetrance, or shifted age-specific penetrance (Liu et al., 1995b).

Thus, in young patients (<35 years old), the detection of the RER phenotype is quite common (seen in 58%) and may be associated with detectable HNPCC gene mutations in about half of the cases with the RER phenotype. Regulatory mutations of the

Case Example 4.7. A 48-year-old woman was referred for *BRCA* testing because of a family history of gynecologic cancers, including malignancies of the ovary and uterus. In documenting the family history, the counselor uncovered a case of cancer of the gallbladder in a maternal relative. To confirm the diagnosis of hereditary nonpolyposis colon cancer, the family was enrolled in a protocol that provided genetic evaluation. Microsatellite instability was documented in the pathology sample of the mother's ovarian tumor. Sequencing of HNPCC-associated genes was expected to take several months. An immediate colonoscopy was recommended, as well as urine cytology and transvaginal ultrasound imaging of endometrial thickness and ovaries.

Colonoscopy revealed a villous adenoma with a small focus of adenocarcinoma.

This case illustrates the clinical diagnosis of HNPCC in the absence of a family history of a colonic neoplasm. Although the Amsterdam criteria of HNPCC do not include such kindreds, the phenotype of the syndrome is continuing to be defined by molecular markers.

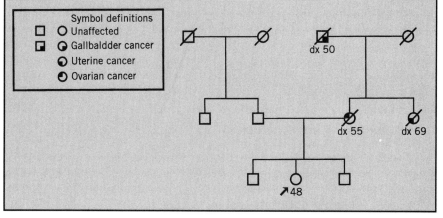

Symbol definitions
□ ○ Unaffected
▣ ◔ Gallbaldder cancer
◑ Uterine cancer
◗ Ovarian cancer

dx 50
dx 55
dx 69
↗48

HNPCC genes, methylation at promotor regions, or mutations in other genes, for example, DNA polymerase, or somatic mutations may be explanations for the RER positive early-onset cases without identifiable germline mutations in known HNPCC genes. The observation of variable expressivity—or altered age-specific penetrance—in the small number of kindreds identified to date, has important implications for counseling. This may best be explained to families as evidence for the possibly ameliorating role of dietary or other modifications, although this hypothesis has not been proved.

A case report has documented a germline *hMLH1* mutation and somatic loss of wild-type *hMLH1* expression in the tumor of a woman with both colon and breast cancer in an HNPCC kindred (Risinger et al., 1996). While breast cancers have not been statistically overrepresented in HNPCC kindreds, these findings, and the observation of breast cancer in a *MLH1* compound heterozygote, provide evidence that breast cancer should be added to the spectrum of extracolonic HNPCC manifestations (Risinger et al., 1996; Hackman et al., 1997).

Commercial laboratories offer a variety of techniques for identification of mutations of HNPCC genes. In addition to sequencing of coding regions of the genes, which is costly and time consuming, techniques of lower sensitivity and less cost are available. About 50%–70% of mutations in the "HNPCC genes" identified by sequencing can also be detected by an in vitro synthesized protein assay (IVSP) for truncated protein products (Liu et al., 1996). This assay will not detect regulatory mutations or large deletions or insertions. It will be very sensitive for nonsense and frameshift mutations that cause premature truncation of the protein (see Chapter 7). IVSP screening of 12 consecutive families meeting criteria for HNPCC revealed a truncated *hMSH2* or *hMLH1* protein in half of the cases (Luce et al., 1995).

In addition to IVSP, analysis of the replication error repair (RER) phenotype is available for frozen and paraffin embedded tumor specimens. A possibly cost-effective means to work-up families would include limiting RER testing to colon tumors from individuals with a family history of colon cancer, patients with a personal history of another HNPCC-associated tumor, or patients with early-onset colorectal cancer. These individuals would undergo RER analysis, and those with evidence of microsatellite instability would be offered sequencing analysis for HNPCC mutations. This approach is based on the data presented thus far in this chapter, which suggest that germline mutations of HNPCC-associated genes are detected in those with RER positive tumors in the setting of a family history of the disease, in those with metachronous HNPCC tumors, or in patients with early-onset colorectal cancer. This analysis assumes that the yield for finding HNPCC-associated gene mutations will be low in families without any of the clinical features of HNPCC, an observation that is being tested in population-based series.

Turcot's and Muir-Torre Syndromes

In 1995, the autopsy slides of one of the two cases in Turcot's original description were reanalyzed. Both the rectal adenomas and the glioblastoma multiforme showed evidence of errors in DNA repair characteristic of HNPCC. An additional three tumors from three other Turcot's syndrome families showed microsatellite instability. All of the brain tumors were glioblastomas. Two of these families, one of which met Amsterdam criteria for HNPCC, demonstrated germline mutations of *HPMS2* or *hMLH1*. The third case did not show germline mutations of any of the HNPCC genes or *APC*. Nine of 10 remaining cases showed germline mutations of *APC*. In this group, medulloblastoma predominated (Hamilton et al., 1995).

Two kindreds with Muir-Torre syndrome have been associated with mutations of the *hMSH2* gene. In addition, microsatellite instability has been documented in both the cutaneous and internal neoplasms of the syndrome. There does not appear to be an association of the phenotype with a specific *hMSH2* mutation; the exon 5 in-frame deletion observed in one Muir-Torre kindred has also been observed in 3 HNPCC kindreds without features of the Muir-Torre phenotype (Honchel et al., 1994; Liu et al., 1996). In addition, an exon 12 deletion was identified in another large kindred with Muir-Torre syndrome (Bapat et al., 1996)

Case Example 4.8. A 20-year-old man was referred because of a suspicion of the diagnosis of neurofibromatosis. He had three café au lait spots on his abdomen and thorax. He had no evidence of Lisch nodules, axillary freckling, or other signs of NF1. His brother died of a glioblastoma at early age, and there was a history of another brain tumor in a paternal uncle. DNA from the father was sent for analysis of mutations in the *APC*, *hMSH2*, and *hMLH1* genes. In the meantime, a colonoscopy was performed and 11 hyperplastic or adenomatous polyps were discovered in the descending and sigmoid colon and removed.

As noted in the text, Turcot's syndrome is a rare condition characterized by polyposis and CNS tumors. Some consider Turcot's syndrome to be a variant of hereditary nonpolyposis colon cancer syndrome (HNPCC). The phenotype is variable, and genetic heterogeneity also complicates the molecular diagnosis. In this kindred, the presence of the glioblastoma suggests that an HNPCC-associated mutation will be found.

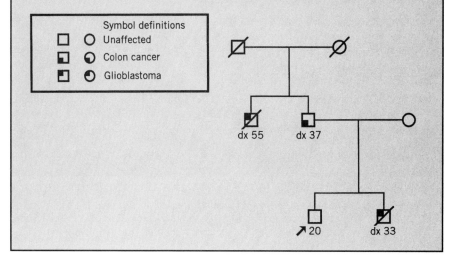

OPTIONS FOR PREVENTION AND EARLY DETECTION

Surveillance and Early Detection

HNPCC   In 1973, Shinya and colleagues introduced the procedure of colonoscopic polypectomy and set a new standard for the management of these lesions. Improvements in fiberoptics and other technical innovations have greatly impacted on the safety and efficacy of endoscopy. Identification, biopsy, or snare removal of polyps can now be accomplished with complications due to bleeding or perforation in the range of 1%. Upper endoscopy also provides a sensitive means to detect gastric neoplasms in kindreds with this extra-colonic feature of HNPCC (Figure 4-12).

There is now good evidence to believe that this procedure can prevent colon cancers. Of 1418 patients randomly assigned to various intervals of colonoscopic follow-up in the National Polyp Study, asymptomatic colon cancers (malignant polyps) were found in five patients, compared to 20–40 colon cancers expected from various control series (Winawer et al., 1993b). These results provided evidence that colonoscopy actually decreased the incidence of cancers in this population and supported the model of the adenoma–colon cancer sequence. Thus, the most commonly recommended option for HNPCC family members is screening colonoscopy at frequent intervals, ranging from 1 to 3 years, with annual screening being the most conservative recommendation.

Preliminary data support the efficacy of colonoscopy in reducing colorectal cancer in HNPCC families. A 7.4% difference in colorectal cancer incidence was observed in 133 members of HNPCC kindreds undergoing 3-year colonoscopy or barium enema, compared to 118 HNPCC controls without screening. The groups were not random-

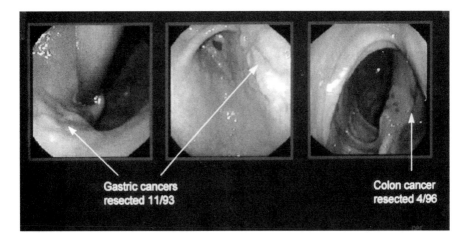

Gastric cancers
resected 11/93

Colon cancer
resected 4/96

FIGURE 4-12   *Endoscopic appearance of synchronous antral (left) and proximal gastric (center) tumors prior to gastrectomy in a 65-year-old woman. The patient subsequently had a partial colectomy for a colonic adenocarcinoma and was later found to have a T2 colorectal tumor (right) by endoscopic surveillance. The family history was consistent with hereditary nonpolyposis colorectal cancer (HNPCC). (Courtesy of Dr. Hans Gerdes.)*

ized, however. In comparison to the general population where 41 to 119 polypectomies were necessary to find one carcinoma (Winawer et al., 1993a, 1993b), only 2.8 polypectomies were needed in HNPCC kindreds to find one tumor (Jarvinen et al., 1995). Despite the presumptive beneficial effect of polypectomy in the HNPCC group, four cancers emerged during the screening interval, suggesting that more frequent surveillance may be prudent (Jarvinen et al., 1995). Indeed, polyp recurrences have anecdotally been noted within a year of colonoscopy, confirming the rationale for frequent surveillance (Vasen et al., 1995). Lynch has reported one case of a woman with two recurrent colon tumors diagnosed endoscopically just 5 months after a normal colonoscopy (Lynch et al., 1997). There remains the concern that polyps in HNPCC may behave differently, and *de novo* cancers may be more frequent. Clinical trials will be needed to prove the efficacy of colonoscopic surveillance in HNPCC heterozygotes.

A suggested age to begin colonoscopy screening in the unaffected mutation-carrier is 20–25, based on data regarding the frequency of the mutation in early-onset cases. Even in kindreds demonstrating anticipation, in which ages of onset appear to be younger with successive generations, the earliest onset of colorectal cancer was age 25 (Menko et al., 1993). (There are, however, anecdotal reports of colon cancer at even younger ages in rare HNPCC kindreds.) Since sigmoidoscopy will not detect right-sided lesions, it is rarely recommended in the setting of hereditary cancer risk. Barium enema remains a diagnostic option for individuals for whom invasive procedures are contraindicated.

Based on the very high rate of synchronous and metachronous colon cancers in HNPCC kindreds, subtotal colectomy has been recommended at the first diagnosis of colon cancer in a member of an HNPCC family (Lynch et al., 1997). This counseling discussion should include reference to the observation by Mecklin et al. (1993) of second (metachronous) colon cancers in 15 of 37 patients followed for 7 years after segmental colon resection. A difficult counseling scenario occurs when the mutation carrier already has had a partial colectomy. In these circumstances surgical options may be influenced by a number of considerations, including the status of the primary cancer, the amount of bowel remaining, the patient's age, and other medical concerns. Some oncologists feel, too, that subtotal colectomy should be offered at the time of first detection of a polyp in a member of an HNPCC kindred. This view is supported by the observations that some polyps in HNPCC patients can be flat and plaquelike, hence more easily missed by colonoscopy. In addition, there is evidence that adenomas in HNPCC kindreds may grow more rapidly or be more aggressive. DNA diagnosis of polyp tissue is unlikely to inform this decision; even in the setting of HNPCC, only 50–60% of polyps demonstrated the RER phenotype. Germline DNA analysis for specific mutations remains the most accurate approach in these instances.

The issues of prophylactic colectomy in HNPCC are complex, because the penetrance (risk for colorectal cancer) in mutation carriers is around 70%. In addition, there remains a 12% risk of rectal cancer generally occurring four to six years after prophylactic colectomy (Rodriguez-Bigas et al., 1997). Mortality from this surgical procedure has been about one percent (Herrera, 1991). Despite these risks, it was calculated that prophylactic colectomy at age 30 in an HNPCC patient would increase life

Case Example 4.9. A 55-year-old woman was referred after presenting with melena and a colonoscopy revealing a malignant polyp in the transverse colon. Five years earlier, she was diagnosed with a Dukes B lesion of the right colon, and ten years earlier she had a villous adenoma removed. Interval colonoscopies were negative. Her family history was significant for uterine and colon cancer. Genetic testing was not available in this patient's managed care plan. Nonetheless, a diagnosis of hereditary nonpolyposis colon cancer was evident.

After extensive counseling, a subtotal colectomy and hysterectomy/oophorectomy were recommended. She elected to return to her local physician, who decided to perform a segmental resection of the transverse colon.

This case illustrates the special challenges of counseling kindreds with hereditary nonpolyposis colon cancer syndrome. Decisions to elect major surgery require a coordinated educational effort that should include health care providers as well as patients.

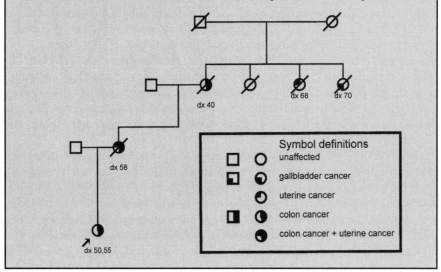

expectancy up to a year or more (Vasen, 1996). Nonetheless, prophylactic colectomy in HNPCC gene carriers remains a controversial recommendation (reviewed by Rodriguez-Bigas, 1996).

The posttest preventive oncology counseling following documentation of a mutation in one of the HNPCC-associated genes must cover a range of options. Virtually all of the data and options for preventive management have been extrapolated from the pre-DNA diagnosis era and are based on presumed rather than proven benefit. Recommendations for members of families with Muir-Torre syndrome are identical to those for HNPCC. The options for surveillance of HNPCC kindreds are listed in Table 4-8.

It has been recommended that women in HNPCC kindreds be screened for uterine cancer, at least with pelvic exams beginning annually at age 18. One potential method of screening for endometrial cancer is transvaginal ultrasound. The ovaries and kidneys, also organs at risk, can be visualized during the ultrasound examination. In one study of 140 symptomatic postmenopausal women, endometrial thickness of 4 or 2

TABLE 4-8   Options for Surveillance or Prevention in Carriers of HNPCC-Associated Mutations

Option	Interval
Colonoscopy	Every 1–3 years beginning at age 20–25
Colectomy	When cancer diagnosed (recommended by some at time of diagnosis of polyp)
Pelvic examination	Annually beginning at age 25–35
Mammography	Annually beginning at age 40[a]
Transvaginal ultrasound (with color Doppler)	Annually beginning at age 25–35
Transabdominal hysterectomy and bilateral salpingo-oophorectomy	Discuss as an option

Source: Cancer Genetics Consortium of the Ethical, Legal, and Social Implications Branch of the National Center for Human Genome Research. From Burke W, Petersen G, Lynch P et al. Recommendations for follow-up care of individuals with an inherited predisposition to cancer. I. Hereditary nonpolyposis colon cancer. JAMA 1997; 277:915–919.

[a] Not in Cancer Genetics Consortium recommendations.

mm yielded sensitivities of 98.2% and 82%, respectively (Van den Bosch et al., 1995). Blind biopsy with the Pipelle endometrial sampler missed most cases of endometrial polyps and myomas but diagnosed all cases of endometrial cancer. Additional studies in asymptomatic, premenopausal women are needed to support this approach to screening women at risk for HNPCC-associated endometrial cancer.

For women who have tested positive for a mutation in one of the HNPCC-associated genes, prophylactic hysterectomy and bilateral salpingo-oophorectomy remains a viable option to consider after childbearing, or around age 35–40. As noted above, the age for highest incidence of endometrial and ovarian cancer is around 45. Although breast cancer risk in HNPCC is controversial, several early onset cases have been reported in HNPCC kindreds, with preliminary molecular evidence supporting this association (Risinger et al., 1996; Hackman et al., 1997). For this reason, mammographic screening at an earlier age may increase the positive predictive value in these kindreds.

The genetic heterogeneity of Turcot's syndrome has obvious implications for the preventive management of these families. The demonstration of multiple polyps in the setting of a family history of a brain tumor should lead to endoscopic surveillance starting at an early age and *APC* testing of the offspring of the affected individual. Patients with a history of a brain tumor in the setting of multiple cases of colon cancer (or replication error repair defects in their tumors) merit colonoscopic surveillance for HNPCC, including screening for endometrial cancer and the other extracolonic manifestations of HNPCC as described above.

Familial Adenomatous Polyposis   The identification of an *APC* mutation, confirming the clinical diagnosis of FAP, is usually followed by discussion of prophylactic colectomy as the treatment of choice for adolescents with this condition. As indicated in Table 4-8, the discussion of surgery is planned after detection of polyps by endoscopy. Even in heterozygotes for *APC* mutations, colectomy is generally not performed on a polyp-free colon (Petersen et al., 1996). In addition, because current testing may still miss up to 20% of *APC* mutations, patients should be counseled about the possibility of false negative tests. Because of this, it has been suggested that a less intensive sigmoidoscopy schedule be maintained in children who "test negative" for *APC* mutations (Petersen et al., 1996) (Table 4-9). In the setting of a child who tests negative for a mutation known to segregate in the family, screening can revert to that of the general population.

Surgical options for mutant gene carriers include ileorectal anastomosis with frequent surveillance of the rectum, or total colectomy with creation of an ileal pouch. Surgery is generally performed in the late teens or at age 21. At-risk relatives for whom genetic testing is not available should receive diagnostic sigmoidoscopies by age 11 and continuing through the early teen years. In most cases the diagnosis is made by the age of 30; if no polyps are found by age 40, the risk is less than 1%. Following the documentation of adenomatous polyps, annual colonoscopic surveillance should be performed until prophylactic surgery is undertaken. Management of FAP patients requires prompt diagnosis and intervention; reviews of large series have revealed a substantial risk of mortality for members of affected kindreds (Arvanitis et al., 1990).

Reduction in the number of polyps in patients with FAP has been demonstrated after treatment with the nonsteroidal anti-inflammatory agent sulindac (Giardiello et al., 1993). This treatment is still considered investigational. Polyp number decreased in FAP patients taking vitamin C, alpha tocopherol, and a wheat fiber supplement (De Cosse et al., 1989). Aspirin and acarbose are being tested in a European study to prevent or reverse polyp development. Significantly, regression of rectal polyps has been noted after ileorectal anastomosis, suggesting possible environmental modulators of the phenotype. As noted, careful surveillance of the upper GI tract is recommended every 3 years in FAP patients postcolectomy.

Because of its potential impact on clinical care, *APC* testing meets the ethical requirements to allow testing of children (see Chapter 10). Petersen and Brensinger have

TABLE 4-9   Options for Surveillance for Familial Adenomatous Polyposis

APC *Mutation Identified*

Annual flexible sigmoidoscopy beginning age 10–11
Counseling for prophylactic colectomy in teen years, when polyps detected by endoscopy
Surveillance for extracolonic neoplasms, particularly upper gastrointestinal tract adenomatous
   polyps

No APC *Mutation Identified*

Flexible sigmoidoscopy at ages 18, 25, 35
Conventional colon cancer screening (e.g., colonoscopy every 3–5 years starting at age 50)

Source: After Petersen GM and Brensinger JD. Genetic testing and counseling in familial adenomatous polyposis. Oncology 1996; 10:90–94.

Case Example 4.10. A 41-year-old male underwent prophylactic colectomy at age 32 because of a history of childhood familial polyposis. He and his wife requested genetic counseling. They were planning on starting a family. He wanted to confirm his diagnosis of familial adenomatous polyposis with a blood test. If the test was positive the couple was interested in using this information for prenatal diagnosis during her planned pregnancy.

An in vitro synthesized protein assay was performed and a truncated *APC* protein product was found. A nonsense mutation was confirmed by sequencing. After receiving the result, and after further discussion, the couple had second thoughts about using the results to terminate a pregnancy. While considering this information, the proband was referred to a gastroenterologist for upper endoscopy as part of follow-up surveillance for FAP patients post-colectomy.

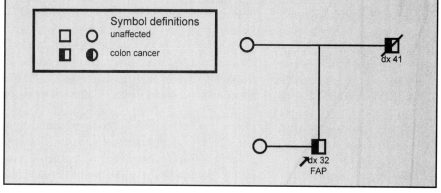

described counseling two brothers, age 7 and 14 about whether they wanted gene testing for FAP, which was recently diagnosed in their 10-year-old sister (Petersen and Brensinger, 1996). Both decided to be tested, and both tested negative, decreasing the need for invasive screening. Availability of age-appropriate educational materials and close involvement of a team of professionals with the parents and at-risk family members were recommended for genetic counseling of FAP kindreds. Unfortunately, an initial survey of oncologists, geneticists, and other medical specialists revealed that genetic counseling was provided in less than a quarter of cases (Giardiello et al., 1997a).

Familial Colon Cancer

In 1992 the American Society of Colon and Rectal Surgeons revised their guidelines for colon cancer screening of first-degree relatives of patients with colorectal cancer (American Society of Colon and Rectal Surgeons Standards Task Force, 1992). Recommended were yearly fecal occult blood testing beginning at age 35, combined with colonoscopy or contrast barium enema plus flexible sigmoidoscopy every 3 to 5 years beginning at age 40, or colonoscopy or double contrast barium enema every 5 years beginning at age 35 to 40 for individuals with one or more first-degree relatives with colon cancer before age 55. Similar recommendations may be appropriate for Ashkenazim with *APC*-associated familial colon cancer (Laken et al., 1997).

Chemoprevention and Diet

Another option to discuss with individuals at increased risk for colon cancer is chemoprevention and dietary modification. Three epidemiologic studies support the role of aspirin as a means to reduce colon cancer risk, and seven epidemiologic studies have shown that hormone replacement therapy in women has the same effect. In the largest of the aspirin studies, involving over 600,000 adults, mortality from colon cancer was decreased 40% with regular use of aspirin more than 15 times per month for a year (Peleg, 1994). A hypothesis emerging from these studies is that the aspirin use may have caused bleeding from early cancers, allowing their diagnosis and decreasing mortality. An NCI-sponsored chemoprevention trial is exploring the role of 325 mg of enteric-coated aspirin in patients surgically treated for early-stage colon cancer.

Some studies have supported the observation of a decreased rate of colon cancer associated with postmenopausal hormone replacement (Potter, 1995). In one study of nearly 700 cases and 1600 control subjects, use of oral, injectable, or transdermal noncontraceptive hormones, including estrogens and/or progestins for 3 months or more was associated with a 30% to 46% decrease in colon cancer incidence. In the setting of HNPCC, the long-term effects of estrogen are uncertain, especially in view of the increased risk for endometrial cancer. This latter risk should, in theory, be ameliorated by the progestin component.

The association of colon cancer risk and diet has been established by numerous epidemiologic studies (Vargas and Alberts, 1992). In a large prospective study of nurses, the risk for women who consumed red meat daily, compared to once per month, was 2.5 times greater. More than 30 studies have pointed to an inverse relationship between dietary fiber and colon cancer risk. Fiber may come from many sources, including vegetables, cellulose, rice, wheat, cereals, and whole grain breads. Laboratory studies indicate that high bran diets may protect against colon cancer by "diluting carcinogens" by increasing fecal bulk, and by direct effects on gut mucosa, gut pH, bile acids, and bacterial flora. Current NCI recommendations are for consumption of 20 to 30 grams of fiber per day, compared to the U.S. average of 11 to 13 grams per day. Given the average of 2–3 grams of fiber in a single serving of most fruits and vegetables, and 1–2 grams in servings of whole grain breads (or bagels), it is generally necessary to have one fiber-dense meal (cereal or beans) to reach this goal. The effects of these modulations in the setting of an hereditary colon cancer risk are not clear.

Evidence from laboratory studies indicates that dietary calcium in excess of 1250 mg per day may decrease the proliferation rates in the colon in patients with adenomas. These observations have stimulated interest in calcium as a potential chemoprevention agent. Other colon cancer chemoprevention agents under investigation include: DFMO, Cox-2 inhibitors, sulindac sulfone, oltipraz and ursodiol (Kelloff et al., 1996).

REFERENCES: PART C

Aaltonen LA, Peltomaki P, Leach FS et al. 1993. Clues to the pathogenesis of familial colorectal cancer. Science 260:812–6.

American Society of Colon and Rectal Surgeons Standards Task Force. 1992. Practice parameters for the detection of colorectal neoplasms. Dis Colon Rectum 35:391–4.

Arvanitis ML, Jagelman DG, Fazio VW, Lavery IC, McGannon E. 1990. Mortality in patients with familial adenomatous polyposis. Dis Colon Rectum 33:639–42.

Bailey-Wilson JE, Elston RC, Schuelke GS et al. 1986. Segregation analysis of hereditary non-polyposis colorectal cancer. Genet Epidemiol 3:27–38.

Bapat B, Xia L, Madlensky L et al. 1996. The genetic basis of Muir-Torre syndrome includes the *hMLH1* locus. Am J Hum Genet 59:736–39.

Bronner CE, Baker SM, Morrison PT et al. 1994. Mutation in the DNA mismatch repair gene homologue *hMLH1* is associated with hereditary non-polyposis colon cancer. Nature 368:258–61.

Burke W, Petersen G, Lynch P et al. 1997. Recommendations for follow-up care of individuals with an inherited predisposition to cancer. I. Hereditary nonpolyposis colon cancer. JAMA 277:915–9.

Burt R, Samowitz W. 1988. The hereditary polyp and the hereditary polyposis syndromes. Gastroenterol Clin N Amer 17:657–78.

Cannon-Albright LA, Skolnick MH, Bishop DT, Lee RG, Burt RW. 1988. Common inheritance of susceptibility to colonic adenomatous polyps and associated colorectal cancers. New Engl J Med 319:533–7.

Chu KC, Tarone RE, Chow WH et al. 1994. Temporal patterns in colorectal cancer incidence, survival, and mortality from 1950 through 1990. J Natl Cancer Inst 86:997–1006.

Davies D, Armstrong JG, Thakker N et al. 1995. Severe Gardner syndrome in families with mutations restricted to a specific region of the *APC* gene. Am J Hum Genet 57:1151–8.

Debinski HS, Love S, Spigelman AD, Phillips RK. 1996. Colorectal polyp counts and cancer risk in familial adenomatous polyposis. Gastroenterol 110:1028–30.

DeCosse JJ, Miller HH, Lesser ML. 1989. Effect of wheat fiber and vitamins C and E on rectal polyps in patients with familial adenomatous polyposis. J Natl Cancer Inst 81:1290–7.

Eccles DM, van der Luijt R, Breukel C et al. 1996. Hereditary desmoid disease due to a frameshift mutation at codon 1924 of the *APC* gene. Am J Hum Genet 59:1193–1201.

Froggatt NJ, Joyce JA, Davies R, Evans GD, Ponder BAJ, Barton DE, Maher ER. 1995. A frequent *hMSH2* mutation in hereditary nonpolyposis colon cancer syndrome. Lancet 345: 727.

Giardiello FM, Hamilton SR, Krush AJ et al. 1993. Treatment of colonic and rectal adenomas with sulindac in familial adenomatous polyposis. New Engl J Med 328:1313–6.

Giardiello FM, Brensinger JD, Petersen GM et al. 1997a. The use and interpretation of commercial *APC* gene testing for familial adenomatous polyposis. New Engl J Med 336:823–7.

Giardiello FM, Brensinger JD, Luce MC et al., 1997b. Phenotypic expression of disease in families that have mutations in the 5′ region of the adenomatous polyposis coli gene. Ann Intern Med 126:514–9.

Giardiello FM, Petersen GM, Piantadosis et al. 1997c. APC gene mutations and extra-intestinal phenotype of familial adenomatous polyposis. Gut 40:521–5.

Hackman P, Tannergärd P. Osei-Mensa S et al. 1997. A human compound heterozygote for two *MLH1* missense mutations. Nature Genet 17:135–6.

Hamilton SR, Liu B, Parsons RE et al. 1995. The molecular basis of Turcot's syndrome. New Engl J Med 332:839–47.

Han HJ, Maruyama M, Baba S, Park JG, Nakamura Y. 1995. Genomic structure of human mismatch repair gene, *hMLH1*, and its mutation analysis in patients with hereditary non-polyposis colorectal cancer (HNPCC). Hum Mol Genet 4:237–42.

Han HJ, Yuan Y, Ku JL et al. 1996. Germline mutations of *hMLH1* and *hMSH2* genes in Korean hereditary nonpolyposis colorectal cancer. J Natl Cancer Inst 88:1317–8.

Herrera L. 1991. The article reviewed. In: Jagelman DG (Ed) Extracolonic Manifestations of FAP. Oncology 5:31–3.

Honchel R, Halling KC, Schaid DJ, Pittelkow M, Thibodeau SN. 1994. Microsatellite instability in Muir-Torre syndrome. Cancer Res 54:1159–63.

Houlston RS, Collins A, Slack J, Morton ME. 1992. Dominant genes for colorectal cancer are not rare. Ann Human Genet 56:99–103.

Jarvinen HJ, Mecklin JP, Sistonen P. 1995. Screening reduces colorectal cancer rate in families with hereditary nonpolyposis colorectal cancer. Gastroenterol 108:1405–11.

Jarvis L, Bathurst N, Mohan D, Beckly D. 1988. Turcot's Syndrome. Dis Colon Rectum 31:907–14.

Kane MF, Loda M, Gaida GM et al. 1997. Methylation of the *hMLH1* promotor correlates with lack of expression of *hMLH1* in sporadic colon tumors and mismatch repair defective human tumor cell lines. Cancer Res 57:808–11.

Kelloff GJ, Hawk ET, Crowell JA, et al. 1996. Strategies for identification and clinical evaluation of promising chemopreventive agents. Oncology 10:1471–80.

Kinzler KW, Vogelstein B. 1996. Lessons from hereditary colorectal cancer. Cell 87:159–70.

Kolodner RD, Hall NR, Lipford J et al. 1995. Structure of the human *MLH1* locus and analysis of a large hereditary nonpolyposis colorectal carcinoma kindred for *MLH1* mutations. Cancer Res 55:242–8.

Kouri M, Laasonen A, Mecklin JP, Jarvinen H, Franssila K, Pyrhonen S. 1990. Diploid predominance in hereditary non-polyposis colorectal carcinoma evaluated by flow cytometry. Cancer 65:1825–9.

Laken SJ, Petersen G, Gruber S et al. 1997. An *APC* mutation associated with familial colorectal cancer in Ashkenazi Jews. Nature Genet 17:79–83.

Leach FS, Nicholaides NC, Papadappoulos N et al. 1993. Mutations of the MutS homolog in hereditary non-polyposis colorectal cancer. Cell 75:1215–25.

Leach FS, Polyak K, Burrell M et al. 1996. Expression of the human mismatch repair gene *HMSH2* in normal and neoplastic tissues. Cancer Res 56:235–40.

Leppert M, Burt R, Hughes JP et al. 1990. Genetic analysis of an inherited predisposition to colon cancer in a family with variable number of adenomatous polyps. New Engl J Med 322:904–8.

Levin B, Murphy GP. 1992. Revision in American Cancer Society recommendations for the early detection of colorectal cancer. CA Cancer J Clin 42:296–9.

Liu B, Parsons RE, Hamilton SR et al. 1994. *hMSH2* Mutations in hereditary nonpolyposis colorectal cancer kindreds. Cancer Research 54:4590–4.

Liu B, Nicolaides NC, Markowitz S et al. 1995a. Mismatch repair gene defects in sporadic colorectal cancers with microsatellite instability. Nature Genet 9:48–55.

Liu B, Farrington SM, Petersen GM et al. 1995b Genetic instability occurs in the majority of young patients with colorectal cancer. Nature Medicine 1:348–52.

Liu B, Parsons R, Papadopoulos N et al. 1996. Analysis of mismatch repair genes in hereditary non-polyposis colorectal cancer patients. Nature Medicine 2:169–74.

Luce MC, Marra G, Chauhan DP et al. 1995. In vitro transcription/ translation assay for the screening of *hMLH1* and *hMSH2* mutations in familial colon cancer. Gastroenterol 109: 1368–74.

Lynch HT, Fusaro RM, Roberts L, Voorhees GJ, Lynch JF. 1985. Muir-Torre syndrome in several members of a family with a variant of the cancer family syndrome. Br J Dermatol 113:295–301.

Lynch HT, Smyrk T, Lanspa SJ, Marcus JN, Kriegler M, Lynch JF, Appelman HD. 1988. Flat adenomas in a colon cancer-prone kindred. J Natl Cancer Inst 80:278–82.

Lynch HT, Smyrk T, McGinn T et al. 1995. Attenuated familial adenomatous polyposis (AFAP): a phenotypically and genotypically distinctive variant of FAP. Cancer 76:2427–33.

Lynch HT, Smyrk T, Lynch J. 1997. An update of HNPCC (Lynch syndrome). Cancer Genet Cytogenet 93:84–99.

Mandl M, Paffenholz R, Friedl W, Caspari R, Sengteller M, Propping P. 1994. Frequency of common and novel inactivating *APC* mutations in 202 families with familial adenomatous polyposis. Hum Mol Gen 3:181–4.

Marra G, Boland CR. 1995. Hereditary nonpolyposis colorectal cancer: the syndrome, the genes, and historical perspectives. J Natl Cancer Instit 87:1114–25.

Mecklin JP, Jarvinen H. 1993. Treatment and follow-up strategies in hereditary nonpolyposis colorectal carcinoma. Dis Col Rect 36:927–9.

Menko FH, Meerman GJ, Sampson JR. 1993. Variable age of onset in hereditary nonpolyposis colorectal cancer: clinical implications. Gastroenterol 104:946–7.

Moisio AL, Sistonen P, Weissenbach J, de la Chapelle A, Peltomaki P. 1996. Age and origin of two common *MLH1* mutations predisposing to hereditary colon cancer. Am J Hum Genet 59:1243–51.

Muto T, Kamiya J, Sawada T et al. 1985. Small "flat adenoma" of the large bowel with special reference to its clinicopathologic features. Dis Colon Rectum 28:847–51.

Myeroff LL, Parsons R, Kim S-J et al. 1995. A transforming growth factor β receptor type II gene mutation common in colon and gastric but rare in endometrial cancers with microsatellite instability. Cancer Res 55:5545–7.

Nagase H, Miyoshi Y, Horii A et al. 1992 Correlation between the location of germ-line mutations in the *APC* gene and the number of colorectal polyps in familial adenomatous polyposis patients. Cancer Res 52:4055–7.

Nicolaides NC, Papadopoulos N, Liu B, Wei YF et al. 1994. Mutations of two PMS homologues in hereditary nonpolyposis colon cancer. Nature 371:75–80.

Nyström-Lahti M, Parsons R, Sistonen P et al. 1994. Mismatch repair genes on chromosomes 2p and 3p account for a major share of hereditary nonpolyposis colorectal cancer families evaluable by linkage. Am J Hum Genet 55:659–65.

Olschwang S, Tiret A, Laurent-Puig P, Muleris M, Parc R, Thomas G. 1993. Restriction of ocular fundus lesions to a specific subgroup of *APC* mutations in adenomatous polyposis coli patients. Cell 75:959–68.

Papadopoulous N, Nicolaides NC, Wei YF et al. 1994. Mutation of a mutL homolog is associated with hereditary colon cancer. Science 263:1625–9.

Parsons R, Myeroff LL, Liu B, Wilson JK, Markowitz SD, Kinzler KW, Vogelstein B. 1995. Microsatellite instability and mutations of the transforming growth factor β type II receptor gene in colorectal cancer. Cancer Res 55:5548–50.

Paul P, Letteboer T, Gelbert L et al. 1993. Identical *APC* exon 15 mutations result in a variable phenotype in familial adenomatous polyposis. Hum Mol Genet 2:925–31.

Peleg II, Mailbach HT, Brown SH et al. 1994. Aspirin and nonsteroidal anti-inflammatory drug use and the risk of subsequent colorectal cancer. Arch Intern Med 154:394–9.

Petersen GM, Brensinger JD. 1996. Genetic testing and counseling in familial adenomatous polyposis. Oncology 10:89–94.

Ponz de Leon M, Benatti P, Roncucci L. 1996. Inheritance and susceptibility to tumors of the large bowel: a new classification of colorectal malignancies. Eur J Cancer 32A:2206–11.

Potter JD. 1995. Hormones and colon cancer. J Natl Cancer Inst 87:1039–40.

Potter JD, Slattery ML, Bostick RM et al. 1993. Colon cancer: a review of the epidemiology. Epidem Rev 15:499–545.

Powell SM, Petersen GM, Krush AJ, Booker S, Jen J, Giardiello FM, Hamilton SR, Vogelstein B, Kinzler KW. 1993. Molecular diagnosis of familial adenomatous polyposis. N Engl J Med 329:1982–7.

Risinger JI, Barrett JC, Watson P, Lynch HT, Boyd J. 1996. Molecular genetic evidence of the occurrence of breast cancer as an integral tumor in patients with the hereditary nonpolyposis colorectal carcinoma syndrome. Cancer 77:1836–43.

Rodriguez-Bigas MA. 1996. Prophylactic colectomy for gene carriers in hereditary non-polyposis colorectal cancer. Cancer 78:199–201.

Rodriguez-Bigas MA, Vasen HFA, Mecklin JP et al. 1997. Rectal cancer risk in hereditary nonpolyposis colorectal cancer. Ann Surg 225:202–7.

Rubinfeld B, Souza B, Albert I et al. 1993. Association of the *APC* gene product with β-catenin. Science 262:1731–4.

Rubinfeld B, Albert I, Porfiri E et al. 1996. Binding of GSK3–beta to the *APC*-beta-catenin complex and regulation of complex assembly. Science 262:1023–5.

Sanikila R, Aaltonen LA, Jarvinen H, Mecklin JP. 1996. Better survival rates in patients with *MLH1*–associated hereditary colorectal cancer. Gastroenterol 110:682–7.

Scapoli C, Ponz de Leon M, Sassatelli R et al. 1994. Genetic epidemiology of hereditary nonpolyposis colorectal cancer syndromes in Modena, Italy: results of a complex segregation analysis. Ann Hum Genet 58:275–95.

Schwartz RA, Goldberg DJ, Mahmood F, DeJager RL, Lambert WC, Najem AZ, Cohen PJ. 1989. The Muir-Torre syndrome: a disease of sebaceous and colonic neoplasms. Dermatologica 178:23–8.

Spirio L, Olschwang S, Groden J et al. 1993. Alleles of the *APC* gene: an attenuated form of familial polyposis. Cell 75:951–7.

Thibodeau SN, Bren G, Schaid D. 1993. Microsatellite instability in cancer of the proximal colon. Science 260:816–9.

Thibodeau SN, Tester DJ, Moslein G et al. 1996. Sequence analysis and protein expression of *hMSH2* and *hMLH1* in sporadic and inherited colon cancer. Second plenary meeting of Principal Investigators, June 26, Frederick, MD.

Van den Bosch T, Vandendael A, Van Schoubroeck D et al. 1995. Combining vaginal ultrasonography and office endometrial sampling in the diagnosis of endometrial disease in postmenopausal women. Obstet Gynecol 85:349–52.

Van der Luijt RB, Khan PM, Vasen HF. 1997. Molecular analysis of the APC gene in 105 Dutch kindreds with familial adenomatous polyposis: 67 germline mutations identified by DGGE, PTT, and Southern analysis. Hum Mut 9:7–16.

Vargas PA, Alberts DS. 1992. Primary prevention of colorectal cancer through dietary modification. Cancer Suppl 70:1229–35.

Vasen HF, Offerhaus GJ, den Hartog Jager FC et al. 1990. The tumor spectrum in hereditary non-polyposis colorectal cancer: A study of 24 kindreds in the Netherlands. Int J Cancer 46:31–4.

Vasen HF, Nagengast FM, Meera Kahn P. 1995. Interval cancers in hereditary non-polyposis colorectal cancer (Lynch syndrome). Lancet 345:1183–4.

Vasen HF, Taal BG, Griffioen G et al. 1994. Clinical heterogeneity of familial colorectal cancer and its influence on screening protocols. Gut 35:1262–6.

Vasen HFA Wijnen JT, Menko FH et al. 1996. Colorectal cancer risk in families with hereditary nonpolyposis colorectal cancer diagnosed by mutation analysis. Gastroenterology 110: 1020–7.

Warthin AS. 1925. The further study of a cancer family. J Cancer Res 9:279–86.

Watson P, Lynch HT. 1993. Extracolonic cancer in hereditary nonpolyposis colorectal cancer. Cancer 71:677–85.

Watson P, Vasen HF, Mecklin JP, Jarvinen H, Lynch HT. 1994. The risk of endometrial cancer in hereditary non-polyposis colorectal cancer. Amer J Med 96:516–20.

Wijnen J, M Khan PM, Vasen H, et al. 1996. Majority of *hMLH1* mutations responsible for hereditary nonpolyposis colorectal cancer cluster at the exonic region 15–16. Am J Hum Genet 58:300–7.

Winawer SJ, Zauber AG, O'Brien MJ et al. 1993a. Randomized comparison of surveillance intervals after colonoscopic removal of newly diagnosed adenomatous polyps. New Eng J Med 328:901–6.

Winawer SJ, Zauber AG, Ho MN et al. 1993b. Prevention of colorectal cancer by colonoscopic polypectomy. New Eng J Med 329:1977–81.

Winawer SJ, Zauber AG, Gerdes H, et al. 1996. Risk of colorectal cancer in the families of patients with adenomatous polyps. New Engl J Med 334:82–7.

PART D: PROSTATE CANCER SYNDROMES

CLINICAL AND EPIDEMIOLOGIC FEATURES

The statistics of prostate cancer are both alarming and paradoxical. The incidence of the disease in men is extraordinarily high, rivalling breast cancer in women. However, the prostate cancer mortality rate is not in proportion with the incidence rate, and its incidence rate is not in proportion with the true rate of the disease as estimated by autopsy series. Almost a quarter of a million men will be diagnosed with prostate cancer each year, but only about 40,000 deaths are due to the disease (Bales and Gerber, 1995).

The average man has about a 10% lifetime risk of developing clinically evident prostate cancer, with a 3% chance of dying due to the disease (Garnick, 1993). The proportion of individuals harboring undetected disease is probably higher for prostate cancer than any other known human tumor; from autopsy series 30–40% of men older than 50 had occult prostate cancer (Dhom, 1983). Looked at another way, of the 27 million men over 50 years of age in the United States, 8 million have occult prostate cancer, but only 86,000 have clinically detectable disease.

Prostate cancer affects primarily older men. The proportion of prostate cancers diagnosed in men older than 64 years of age is 83%; the median age of onset is 73. Because of the pattern of increased risk with age and the increasing proportion of elderly in the population, prostate cancer will pose an even greater public health concern in the twenty-first century (Potosky et al., 1995). The incidence is already rising at a rate of 1% per year in the Western world.

Surprisingly little is known about the causes of prostate cancer. For unknown reasons, the incidence of prostate cancer among African-Americans is the highest in the world. The risk in this group is 50% higher than in Caucasians. Like breast cancer, prostate cancer is less common in Asia and the third world. Unlike other cancers, there is no link between prostate cancer and smoking or any other known environmental exposure, including the radiation exposure resulting from the atomic explosions over Japan in 1945. Conflicting studies have been published seeking to associate prostate cancer risk with prior vasectomy, or coexistent benign prostatic hypertrophy. A large epidemiologic analysis of 51,000 males found that individuals who ate 89 grams of fat a day had twice the rate of advanced-stage prostate cancer than individuals who ate 53 grams of fat. However, there was no clear association between low fat and the overall incidence of disease, suggesting that dietary factors (perhaps linked to testosterone production or metabolism) may mediate spread of the disease, but not its occurrence. (Giovannucci et al., 1993; Pienta and Esper, 1993). With the exception of age and race, the only clearly defined risk factor for prostate cancer is a family history of the disease.

Early studies of familial aggregation of prostate cancer showed a relative risk ranging from 2 to 5 in first-degree relatives of those affected. In studies utilizing the unique database of the state of Utah (see Chapter 2), brothers of probands with prostate cancer diagnosed before the age of 62 had a relative risk of 4. Cases of prostate cancer in Utah were related to one another to a greater extent than a matched control population. As shown in Table 2–5, prostate cancer actually displayed a higher familial aggregation than breast cancer or colon cancer. In a series of studies by Carter et al. of over 600 men referred for surgery at a teaching hospital in Baltimore, the risk of prostate cancer was twofold, fivefold, and elevenfold higher in individuals with one, two, or three first-degree relatives affected, respectively. Of the total group, 15% had a father or brother affected by prostate cancer and an additional 5% had a second degree relative affected. The cumulative risk for prostate cancer for first-degree relatives of probands affected before the age of 53 was a striking 40%. These authors concluded that the identification of a family history of prostate cancer could serve as an important marker for individuals who could benefit the most from screening measures (Steinberg et al., 1990; Carter et al., 1992; Carter et al., 1993).

In a series of 6,390 men surveyed in another study, a family history of prostate cancer was observed in 658 (10.3%). The relative risk of detecting prostate cancer was elevated in those with a brother affected (RR = 2.6), but was not significantly elevated in those with an affected father (Narod et al., 1995).

PATHOLOGY

Most prostate cancers originate from the peripheral acinar ducts and are classified as adenocarcinomas. The Gleason scoring system is widely utilized to describe tumor grade. It ranges from grades 1 through 5, from well-differentiated to poorly-differentiated lesions. A modification of the Gleason system includes a primary and secondary score, which are added to give a total, which ranges from 2 to 10. Thus, a tumor with a mixture of well-differentiated and poorly differentiated cancers would be scored as, for example, a 2 + 4, or a 6/10. Gleason score has been shown to be a good predictor of lymph node involvement by tumor. Despite these observations, the enigma of prostate cancer pathology is its phenotypic heterogeneity. Tumors can range from occult disease to a clinically evident and often aggressive presentation. The elucidation of prognostic genetic markers for early stage prostate cancer remains a translational research need.

Less common forms of prostate neoplasms include periurethral duct tumors, adenoid cystic carcinoma, endometrioid tumors, choriocarcinoma, sarcoma, and lymphoma.

HEREDITARY SYNDROMES

Familial clustering of cases of prostate cancer is well established and may be due to a variety of inherited syndromes, including both dominant as well as recessive forms. One genetic epidemiologic analysis was performed on a large number of families with relatively early-onset prostate cancer (median age 59 years versus the population mean of 73). The data in this study were best explained by the existence of a single prostate cancer susceptibility gene. In fact, the estimated frequency of this gene (q = .003) was identical to that calculated by Claus et al. (see part A of this chapter) for a breast cancer susceptibility gene. This gene frequency means that about 1 in 170 individuals has an inherited genetic mutation which, in males, confers a susceptibility to prostate cancer.

The penetrance for this dominant syndrome of prostate cancer susceptibility was quite high, estimated to be 88% by age 85. The syndrome was estimated to account for 43% of prostate cancers diagnosed before age 56, and 9% by age 85 (Carter et al., 1992). While it was estimated that only 2% of prostate cancer in the general population was diagnosed before age 56, this proportion has been increasing with the introduction of newer screening modalities (Potosky et al., 1995). Perhaps 5–10% of cases are now diagnosed at this earlier age, underscoring the potential importance of an autosomal dominant hereditary syndrome. The clinical features, stage, histology, and PSA at diagnosis were comparable in hereditary and nonhereditary cases (Carter et al., 1993).

While a number of candidate genes, including the androgen receptor, were excluded based on linkage analysis of the Utah families, a number of other loci, including one at 10q24-26 remained (Cannon et al., 1982; Cannon-Albright and Eeles, 1995). A tumor suppressor gene, *PTEN* (also called *MMAC1*) at 10q23 was identified in a significant proportion of advanced prostate cancers, as well as other tumor types (Li et al., 1997; Steck et al., 1997). High grade and advanced stage disease were more common in 33 HPC1-linked kindreds (Grönberg et al., 1997). Analysis of 91 kindreds containing 600 individuals affected by prostate cancer revealed linkage to a locus on chromosome 1q24-q25. Individuals linked to this gene, called *HPC1*, demonstrated an 88% lifetime probability of developing prostate cancer, with an average age of disease of 66 years (Smith et al., 1996).

As with breast/ovarian cancer genetic counseling during the period immediately preceding the identification of *BRCA1*, counseling of prostate cancer kindreds requires an understanding of the statistical limitations of counseling small size families based on linked markers (Chapter 6). Genetic heterogeneity remains an important issue, since some studies have not confirmed 1q-linkage in hereditary prostate cancer kindreds (Gibbs et al., 1997). With the identification of *HPC1*, direct testing can replace the more cumbersome linkage analysis.

The data cited above were derived from a highly selected populations. Not all studies were consistent with the dominant model for a prostate cancer susceptibility locus. Two other population-based series were more suggestive of a recessive mechanism because risk of disease was greater in sibs than in children of those affected (Narod et al., 1995; Woolf, 1960). These and other findings suggested a heterogeneity of genetic mechanisms of susceptibility, including a multigenic etiology. Candidate susceptibility alleles for the majority of prostate cancers have included the genes encoding receptors for two steroid hormones that influence cell division within the gland. A case-control study of 57 prostate cancer cases and 169 controls revealed that individuals carrying polymorphisms in the genes encoding the androgen receptor (*AR*) and vitamin D receptors (*VDR*) were at increased risk for prostate cancer. Individuals with an *AR* CAG allele with fewer than 20 repeats, and individuals with a long *VDR* poly-A allele receptor had odds ratios of 2.1 and 4.6 respectively (Ingles et al., 1997). An earlier study associated a Taq I polymorphism in the *VDR* gene with a threefold increase in prostate cancer risk (Taylor et al., 1996). The small size, unclear biological mechanism, and possible confounders in these studies have been emphasized (Feldman, 1997).

In some families, prostate cancer may be associated with already known cancer predisposition syndromes. For example, prostate cancer was noted in excess in *BRCA1*-linked families, with a relative risk among carriers of approximately 3. This observation is supported by prior epidemiologic studies that observed twice the risk of breast cancer in individuals with a family history of prostate cancer. An analysis of 49 patients with prostate cancer at early age (<53), or in the setting of a family history of breast or prostate cancer, revealed one individual with a 185delAG mutation. An additional five cases had rare *BRCA1* sequence variants of unclear significance, suggesting the importance of further studies in this area (Langston et al., 1996). Prostate cancer may also be a component in the extended definition of the Li-Fraumeni syndrome, associated with germline mutations of the *p53* oncogene. Prostate cancer is not thought to be a component of the hereditary nonpolyposis colorectal cancer syndromes, or the *p16* associated melanoma susceptibility syndromes.

A number of rarer Mendelian syndromes have also been shown to include cases of prostate cancer (see Appendix A).

OPTIONS FOR PREVENTION AND EARLY DETECTION

The *New York Times* called it a "dilemma," and *Newsweek* described doctors "wrangling over the benefits" of screening and treatment for early-stage prostate cancer. Given the epidemiologic statistics previously summarized, it is perhaps not surprising that there is such controversy about screening for early-stage prostate cancer. It is difficult to imagine the rational use of even a perfect screening test for a disease that will be the cause of death in only a small fraction of the individuals affected. The screening tests in use today are far from perfect.

Although only about a third of prostate cancers are diagnosed at a stage when they are contained, the prognosis for this group is excellent. Curative treatment options include radical prostatectomy as well as radiation therapy. This has led to the routine inclusion of digital rectal examination (DRE) in clinical practice and use of other means to detect early prostate cancers. Starting in the late 1980s, newer serum markers of prostate cancer became commercially available. Prostate-specific antigen (PSA) is a protease produced by the prostate epithelium. The normal concentration for this enzyme in the serum is 0–4 ng/ml. It may be elevated in benign prostatic hypertrophy and prostatitis, as well as in prostate cancer. Values greater than 10 ng/ml are more likely to be associated with cancer. Values in the range of 4–10 are indeterminate. Transrectal ultrasound is commonly performed in the setting of an increased PSA, with transrectal needle biopsy of any suspicious area guided by ultrasound or DRE.

About a quarter of patients with localized prostate cancer will have normal PSAs, which translates to a sensitivity of only 75%. Specificity, the proportion of unaffected individuals with a negative test (see Chapter 6), is 92% if the cutoff for the upper normal range is set at 10, but falls significantly when the range is set at 5. The sensitivity is impacted by the fact that most patients with benign prostatic hypertrophy (BPH) will have PSA values in the 5–10 range. Methods to improve the accuracy of the PSA have included derivation of a PSA density, in which the volume of the prostate gland is taken into account, and adjustment of normal values according to the age of the individual. There is little question, based on large studies, that a combination of PSA and DRE can diagnose early prostate cancers. However, the positive predictive value (see Chapter 6) when these tests are abnormal is only 15–21% (Coley et al.,1997). In addition, a controversy relates to the need and costs of offering radical prostatectomy (or radiation therapy) to men whose tumors may be at an indolent stage (Kramer et al., 1993; Johansson et al., 1992; Krahn et al., 1994).

Decision analysis concluded that screening would vastly increase morbidity (due to complications of surgery) and lead to enormous costs (Krahn et al., 1994). A large prospective trial, sponsored by the National Cancer Institute, will randomize 148,000 individuals age 60–74 to observation versus screening for cancers of the prostate, lung, colon, and ovary. The prostate component of the study will measure the impact of DRE and PSA screening on disease-specific mortality. Unfortunately, the age range where prostate screening is likely to be most beneficial is 50 to 65, and hereditary prostate cancer is also manifest at these earlier ages. Pending the outcome of these trials, however, current recommendations by the American Cancer Society and a number of professional societies include DRE and PSA screening offered to men between the ages of 50 and 70 (Littrup et al., 1993). The FDA has approved the PSA test for this purpose.

In the setting of a family history, much of the controversy surrounding screening for prostate cancer seems to diminish. Individuals at increased familial risk stand to benefit the most from early detection. The positive predictive value of the PSA is significantly improved when the baseline risk and occurrence (prevalence) of the disease in the target population is high (see Chapter 6). Of 95 men with a family history of prostate cancer, a normal DRE, and a PSA > 3.0, the positive predictive value was 27%, compared to 12% for those without a family history of the disease (Narod et al., 1995). Interestingly in this study, a high false positive rate for DRE was noted in those with a family history of the disease, possibly due to a link between benign hyperplasia and a family history of prostate cancer (Narod et al., 1995). For these reasons, and because of the younger age of onset of familial prostate cancer, it seems prudent to initiate PSA and DRE annually at the age of 40 for high-risk individuals. There may be negative biopsies if DRE is relied upon exclusively, with PSA determinations particularly useful in this higher-risk subset. In addition, the documentation of disease in one family member improves risk estimates for other family members.

A study of 34 individuals at increased risk for prostate cancer by virtue of a family

---

Case Example 4.11. A 43-year-old male sought a second opinion for an elevated prostate-specific antigen of 8 ng/ml. Review of his family history revealed two maternal uncles with prostate cancer diagnosed at early age. Because of the family history, transrectal ultrasound was recommended. A hyperechoic lesion was detected, and multiple transrectal biopsies revealed a Gleason 4 adenocarcinoma.

This case illustrates the emerging awareness of hereditary susceptibilities to prostate cancer, in this circumstance being transmitted through the maternal lineage. A prostate cancer susceptibility gene (*HPC1*) linked to chromosome 1q has been identified (see text). While equivocal PSAs in the 5–10 ng/ml will be managed differently in many settings, when there is a family history of disease, a complete evaluation, including digital examination, ultrasound, and directed biopsy, is warranted.

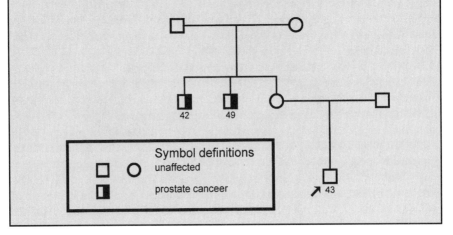

history (two brothers affected in each kindred) provided intensive screening to participating individuals. Screening included measurement of PSA, DRE, transrectal ultrasound (TRUS), and systematic as well as directed core biopsies. Eight cancers were detected. Unfortunately, five were stage C and three stage B (McWhorter et al., 1992). These data support the use of intensive screening in at-risk relatives of kindreds affected by multiple cases of prostate cancer, although the advanced stage of disease in the majority of cases in this series was discouraging. While such an approach remains investigational, it may constitute one option to offer individuals who test positive for mutations in prostate cancer susceptibility genes.

Future options for those at hereditary risk for prostate cancer include hormonal chemoprevention with antiandrogens, and, possibly, prophylactic prostatectomy. One such chemoprevention trial is a randomized placebo-controlled trial piloting finasteride (Proscar), a 5-alpha reductase inhibitor used to treat patients with symptomatic benign prostatic hypertrophy. Like the tamoxifen breast cancer chemoprevention trial, eligibility for the finasteride trial includes a positive family history for the disease (Donodeo, 1993). It has enrolled 18,000 healthy men older than 55, and includes PSA levels as well as digital examinations, with a randomization to finasteride for a 7-year duration.

REFERENCES: PART D

Bales GT, Gerber GS. 1995. Screening for the early detection of carcinoma of the prostate. PPO Updates 9, 6:1–9.

Cannon LA, Bishop DT, Skolnick M et al. 1982. Genetic epidemiology of prostate cancer in the Utah Mormon Genealogy. Cancer Surv 1:47–69.

Cannon-Albright L, Eeles R. 1995. Progress in prostate cancer. Nature Genet 9:336–8.

Carter BS, Beaty TH, Steinberg GD, Childs B, Walsh PC. 1992. Mendelian inheritance of familial prostate cancer. Proc Natl Acad Sci 89:3367–71.

Carter BS, Bova GS, Beaty TH, Steinberg GD, Childs B, Isaacs WB, Walsh PC. 1993. Hereditary prostate cancer: Epidemiologic and clinical features. J Urol 150:797–802.

Coley CM, Barry MJ, Flemming C, Mulley AG. 1997. Early detection of prostate cancer. Ann Intern Med 126:394–406.

Dhom G. 1983. Epidemiologic aspects of latent and clinically manifest carcinoma of the prostate. J Cancer Res Clin Oncol 106:210–8.

Donodeo F. 1993. Prevention trial for prostate cancer piques public interest. J Natl Cancer Inst 85:1801–2.

Feldman D. 1997. Androgen and vitamin D receptor gene polymorphisms: the long and short of prostate cancer risk. J Natl Cancer Inst 89:109–11.

Garnick MB. 1993. Prostate cancer: screening, diagnosis, and management. Ann Intern Med 118:804–18.

Gibbs M, McIdoe RA, Stanford JL et al. 1997. Linkage analysis of the HPC1 region in high risk prostate cancer families. Am J Hum Genet 61:71 (abstr).

Giovannucci E, Rimm EB, Colditz GA et al. 1993. A prospective study of dietary fat and risk of prostate cancer. J Natl Cancer Inst 85:1571–9.

Grönberg H, Isaacs SD, Smith JR et al. 1997. Characteristics of prostate cancer in families potentially linked to the hereditary prostate cancer 1 (HPC1) locus. JAMA 278:1251-5.

Ingles SA, Ross RK, Yu MC, Irvine RA, La Pera G, Haile RW, Coetzee GA. 1997. Association of prostate cancer risk with genetic polymorphisms in vitamin D receptor and androgen receptor. J Natl Cancer Inst 89:166–70.

Johansson JE, Adami HO, Andersson SO, Bergström R, Holmberg L, Krusemo UB. 1992. High 10-year survival rate in patients with early, untreated prostatic cancer. JAMA 267:2191–6.

Krahn MD, Mahoney JE, Eckman MH et al. 1994. Screening for prostate cancer: A decision analytic view. JAMA 272:773–80.

Kramer BS, Brown ML, Prorok PC, Potosky AL, Gohagan JK. 1993. Prostate cancer screening: What we know and what we need to know. Ann Intern Med 119:914–23.

Langston AA, Stanford JL, Wicklund KG, Thompson JD, Blazej RG, Ostrander EA. 1996. Germ-line *BRCA1* mutations in selected men with prostate cancer. Am J Hum Genet 58:881–4.

Li J, Yen C, Liaw D et al. 1997. PTEN, a putative protein tyrosine phosphatase gene mutated in human brain, breast, and prostate cancer. Science 275:1943–7.

Littrup PJ, Goodman AC, Mettlin CJ. 1993. The benefit and cost of prostate cancer early detection. CA Cancer J Clin 43:134–49.

McWhorter WP, Hernandez AD, Meikle AW et al. 1992. A screening study of prostate cancer in high risk families. J Urol 148:826–8.

Narod S, Dupont A, Cusan L, Diamond P, Gomez JL, Suburu R, Labrie F. 1995. The impact of family history on early detection of prostate cancer (letter). Nature Medicine 1:99–101.

Pienta KJ, Esper PS. 1993. Risk factors for prostate cancer Ann Intern Med 118:793–803.

Potosky AL, Miller BA, Albertsen PC, Kramer BS. 1995. The role of increasing detection in the rising incidence of prostate cancer. JAMA 273:548–52.

Smith JR, Freije D, Carpten JD et al. 1996. Major susceptibility locus for prostate cancer on chromosome 1 suggested by a genome-wide search. Science 274:1371–4.

Steck PA, Pershouse MA, Jasser SA et al. 1997. Identification of a candidate tumour suppressor gene, MMAC1, at chromosome 10q23.3 that is mutated in multiple advanced cancers. Nature Genet 15:356–62.

Steinberg GD, Carter BS, Beaty TH, Childs B, Walsh PC. 1990. Family history and the risk of prostate cancer. Prostate 17:337–47.

Taylor JA, Hirvonen A, Watson M, Pittman G, Mohler JL, Bell DA. 1996. Association of prostate cancer with vitamin D receptor gene polymorphism. Cancer Res 56:4108–10.

Woolf CM. 1960. An investigation of familial aspects of carcinoma of the prostate. Cancer 13:739–44.

5

Other Cancer Predisposition Syndromes

PART A: LI-FRAUMENI SYNDROME AND p53-*RELATED SUSCEPTIBILITIES*

CLINICAL AND PATHOLOGIC FEATURES

The association of the component tumors of the Li-Fraumeni syndrome resulted from painstaking epidemiologic inquiry. A report by Bottomley in 1971 described a family characterized by multiple cases of breast cancer and sarcoma. Based on a review of 280 medical records of patients with childhood rhabdomyosarcoma and 418 death certificates, Frederick E. Li and Joseph F. Fraumeni, Jr. identified five families with multiple cases of sarcoma and other tumors (Li and Fraumeni, 1969). Most frequently, soft tissue sarcomas and breast cancers were associated. Other tumors included osteosarcoma, leukemia, brain tumors, adrenal cortical tumors, and cancers of the lung, pancreas, and skin. Individuals were frequently affected by multiple primaries (Birch, 1994; Malkin, 1993).

Subsequent segregation analysis was consistent with a dominant mode of inheritance, with a probability of a component tumor reaching 50% by age 30 (compared to 1% in the general population) and 90% by age 70 (Lustbader et al., 1992). A follow-up of the original cohort of patients confirmed six of the initially reported tumors, but excluded cancers of the pancreas, lung, and skin from the list of component tumors. Subsequent series of families analyzed by Strong and colleagues showed an excess of prostate, cervical, and skin (melanoma) cancers in addition to sarcomas and breast cancer (Strong et al., 1992). The sarcomas, brain tumors, and leukemias in the Li-Fraumeni syndrome generally were diagnosed in childhood, although a small proportion presented later in life. The breast cancers usually occurred between the ages of 15 and

157

44 years. The adrenocortical tumors, both benign and malignant, were seen only in the pediatric patients, in contrast to the other malignancies, which were seen predominantly in adults. A recent review of 475 tumors in 91 families with the genetic hallmark of Li-Fraumeni syndrome (see following section) confirmed organ-specific differences in the mean age of the component tumors, which are summarized in Table 5-1.

Because of the variability of penetrance of *p53* mutations with age, it is possible, and has been observed, that a child may present with Li-Fraumeni syndrome before a component tumor is diagnosed in a parent.

GENETIC DIAGNOSIS AND OPTIONS FOR PREVENTION AND EARLY DETECTION

The association of germline mutations of *p53* was based on testing of a candidate gene (Malkin et al., 1990). Of the five families initially analyzed, affected members in each showed germline missense mutations within a highly conserved region of the protein. Approximately half of Li-Fraumeni kindreds had germline mutations in the coding region of the *p53* gene. These mutations were detected by single strand conformation analysis (see Chapter 7) followed by full sequencing. The *p53* mutations were generally located between exons 5 and 8. Most were missense mutations, although some nonsense mutations were also observed. A review of the 40 published constitutional *p53* mutations by Birch revealed a clustering within exon 7. However, this clustering may have been due to the focus of these studies on the conserved regions of the gene (Birch, 1994). A more recent review of 91 germline *p53* mutations revealed an identi-

TABLE 5-1   Mean Age at Diagnosis for Component Tumors in Li-Fraumeni Families

Tumor	Mean age (years)
Adrenal tumors	4.9
Bone sarcoma	14.6
Soft tissue sarcoma	15.5
Brain tumors	25.0
Hematologic malignancy	25.4
Breast cancer	36.5
Gynecologic malignancy	43.1
Lung cancer	46.5
Gastrointestinal tumors	47.3

Source: Data from Kleihues P, Schauble B, zur Hausen A, Esteve J, Ohgaki H. Tumors associated with *p53* germline mutations; a synopsis of 91 families. Amer J Pathol 1997; 150:1–13.

Note: Other rare (1% or less) component tumors include carcinomas of the prostate, pancreas, bladder, hepatocellular carcinoma, hepatoblastoma, Wilms' tumor, skin cancer, neuroblastoma, nasopharyngeal carcinoma, teratoma, ureteral cancers, testicular cancers, laryngeal carcinoma.

cal distribution of germline compared to sporadic cases (Figure 5-1). Most mutations occurred in exons 5 to 8, with clusters seen at codon 248 (14%) and codon 273 (10%) (Kleihues et al., 1997).

A detailed analysis of 15 Li-Fraumeni families revealed six mutations between exons 5 and 8, one nonsense mutation in exon 6, and one splicing mutation in intron 4. In three families a mutation of *p53* was observed in cell lines derived from the patient, but in one of these cases the same mutation could not be detected in the primary (blood) specimen. This finding suggests that the *p53* mutation was acquired as a result of cell culture. In four families no *p53* mutation was observed (Frebourg et al., 1995). In another series, no *p53* mutations were found in one "classic" and two Li-Fraumeni-like families (Evans et al. 1997).

In a screening study of 196 patients with malignant sarcoma, 8 (4%) had germline *p53* mutations. In all of the 8 cases there was a family history suggestive of Li-Fraumeni syndrome (Toguchida et al., 1992). A slightly greater proportion of children with rhabdomyosarcoma (3/33) had germline *p53* mutations (Diller et al., 1995). In contrast, fully half of children with sporadic adrenocortical carcinoma, a component tumor of Li-Fraumeni syndrome, had *p53* mutations (Wagner et al., 1994). Of 59 patients who had survived second cancers, 4 (7%) had germline mutations of *p53*. In these cases there was no family history suggestive of Li-Fraumeni syndrome; the tumors observed included lymphoma, colon and gastric cancer, and neuroblastoma (Malkin et al., 1992). In three large studies, 429 breast tumors were examined for *p53* mutations. A total of four germline mutations were found, all with family histories of cancers suggestive of variants of the Li-Fraumeni syndrome (Sidransky et al., 1992; Prosser et al. 1992; Borreson et al. 1992). In the series by Sidransky et al., the index case subsequently developed a melanotic spindle cell sarcoma of the mediastinum at age 35.

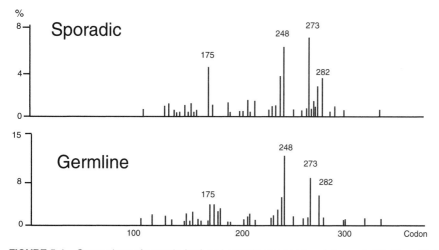

FIGURE 5-1 *Comparison of somatic (top) and germline (bottom) mutations of p53. (From Kleihues P, Schauble B, zur Hausen A, Esteve J, Ohgaki H. Tumors associated with p53 germline mutations; a synopsis of 91 families. Amer J Pathol 1997; 150:9.*

An assay for the detection of *p53* mutations based on its function as a transcriptional activator (see Chapter 7) has been described (Frebourg et al., 1992). In this assay the presence of an inactivating mutation was scored by its ability to interfere with the transcriptional function of *p53*. The endpoint of the clinical assay was a transformant's ability to grow on nutrient-deprived medium, resulting in different color colonies for wild-type and mutant *p53*. To date, this assay has been applied to tumor samples and cell lines, as well as lymphocytes from patients in a number of Li-Fraumeni families (Frebourg et al., 1995). There was a good correlation of results with direct sequencing in published reports, and the technique is offered commercially. This assay appears to be superbly sensitive for the missense mutations of *p53* that are seen in Li-Fraumeni syndrome. However these functional assays will not detect large deletions or mutant alleles that are poorly expressed due to promotor or splicing defects.

Unfortunately, with the exception of breast cancer, there are no proven means to screen for the component tumors of Li-Fraumeni syndrome. There is no evidence of

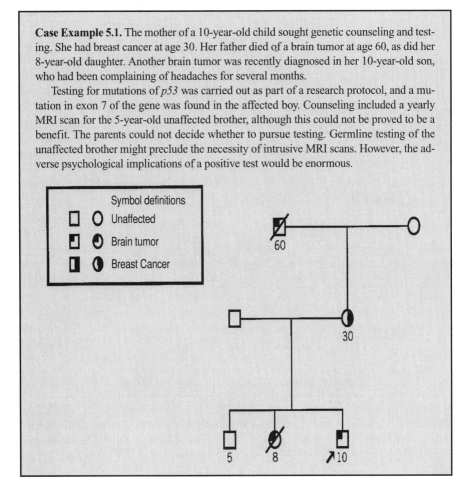

Case Example 5.1. The mother of a 10-year-old child sought genetic counseling and testing. She had breast cancer at age 30. Her father died of a brain tumor at age 60, as did her 8-year-old daughter. Another brain tumor was recently diagnosed in her 10-year-old son, who had been complaining of headaches for several months.

Testing for mutations of *p53* was carried out as part of a research protocol, and a mutation in exon 7 of the gene was found in the affected boy. Counseling included a yearly MRI scan for the 5-year-old unaffected brother, although this could not be proved to be a benefit. The parents could not decide whether to pursue testing. Germline testing of the unaffected brother might preclude the necessity of intrusive MRI scans. However, the adverse psychological implications of a positive test would be enormous.

Symbol definitions
□ ○ Unaffected
◧ ◑ Brain tumor
◪ ◑ Breast Cancer

mutational clustering associated with specific tumor types (Kleihues et al., 1997). If such clustering could be documented, there could be a theoretical benefit in the early diagnosis of the secondary tumors. In contrast to the pediatric acute leukemias, however, the other component tumors of this syndrome (sarcoma, brain tumors) have less effective therapies. Thus, of the human cancer predisposition syndromes, predictive testing for Li-Fraumeni syndrome perhaps most closely resembles that for Huntington disease. In many cases, at-risk individuals may elect not to undergo testing. As one mother wrote in the *Li-Fraumeni Newsletter* (published at the Dana Farber Cancer Center):

> I have twice been diagnosed with cancer, at ages 26 and 32 . . . I had lost my parents, two brothers, grandparents, and an aunt to cancer. I was still in treatment for lymphoma when my daughter suffered a malignant brain tumor. At this time we . . . heard of the *p53* gene. I now have a 5-month daughter, and in spite of our history, I will not have her tested. I see more problems from knowing than good. (*Li-Fraumeni Newsletter,* 1992)

Although germline *p53* testing is now commercially available, the decision to embark on this path is not one to be taken lightly (Li et al., 1992). The availability of DNA testing makes possible the molecular confirmation of the diagnosis, and raises the opportunity for predictive testing for other family members. However, the extraordinary medical, ethical, and legal implications of a positive test result and the enormous, sustained psychological support required must be taken into account before the test is considered.

REFERENCES: PART A

Birch JM. 1994. Li-Fraumeni syndrome. Eur J Cancer 30A (13):1935–41.

Borresen AL, Andersen TI, Garber J et al. 1992. Screening for germ line *p53* mutations in breast cancer patients. Cancer Res 52:3234–6.

Bottomley RH, Trainer AL, Condit PT. 1971. Chromosome studies in a "cancer family." Cancer 28:519–28.

Diller L, Sexsmith E, Gottleib A, Li FP, Malkin D. 1995. Germline *p53* mutations are frequently detected in young children with rhabdomyosarcoma. J Clin Invest 95:1606–11.

Evans S, Mims B, Foster C, Amos C, Strong L, Lozano G. 1997. Lack of p53 germline mutations in Li-Fraumeni families. Proc Amer Assoc Cam Res 38:1126.

Frebourg T, Barbier N, Kassel J, Ng Y-S, Romero P, Friend SH. 1992. A functional screen for germ line *p53* mutations based on transcriptional activation. Cancer Res 52:6976–8.

Frebourg T, Barbier N, Yan Y-x, Garber JE, Dreyfus M, Fraumeni JF Jr, Li FP, Friend SH. 1995. Germ-line *p53* mutations in 15 families with Li-Fraumeni syndrome. Am J Hum Genet 56:608–15.

Kleihues P, Schauble B, zur Hausen A, Esteve J, Ohgaki H. 1997. Tumors associated with *p53* germline mutations; a synopsis of 91 families. Amer J Pathol 150:1–13.

Li FP, Fraumeni JF Jr. 1969. Soft-tissue sarcomas, breast cancer, and other neoplasms. A familial syndrome? Ann Intern Med 71:747–52.

Li FP, Garber JE, Friend SH et al. 1992. Recommendations on predictive testing for germ line *p53* mutations among cancer-prone individuals. J Natl Cancer Inst 84:1156–60.

Li-Fraumeni Syndrome Newsletter 1992. 2(2):3.

Lustbader ED, Williams WR, Bondy ML et al. 1992. Segregation analysis of cancer families of childhood soft-tissue-sarcoma patients. Am J Hum Genet 51:344–56.

Malkin D, Li FP, Strong LC, Fraumeni JF Jr, Nelson CE, Kim DH, Kassel J, Gryka MA, Bischoff FZ, Tainsky MA, Friend SH. 1990. Germline *p53* mutations in a familial syndrome of breast cancer, sarcomas, and other neoplasms. Science 250:1233–8.

Malkin D, Jolly KW, Barbier N et al. 1992. Germline mutations of the *p53* tumor-suppressor gene in children and young adults with second malignant neoplasms. New Engl J Med 326:1309–15.

Malkin D. 1993. The Li-Fraumeni syndrome. PPO Updates 7, 7:1–14.

Prosser J, Porter D, Coles C et al. 1992. Constitutional *p53* mutation in a non-Li-Fraumeni cancer family. Br J Cancer 65:527–8.

Sidransky D, Tokino T, Helzlsouer K, et al. 1992. Inherited *p53* gene mutations in breast cancer. Cancer Res 52:2984–6.

Strong LC, Williams WR, Tainsky MA. 1992. The Li-Fraumeni syndrome: from clinical epidemiology to molecular genetics. Am J Epidemiol 135:190–9.

Toguchida J, Yamaguchi T, Dayton SH et al. 1992. Prevalence and spectrum of germline mutations of the *p53* gene among patients with sarcoma. New Engl J Med 326:1301–8.

Wagner J, Portwine C, Rabin K, Leclerc JM, Narod SA, Malkin D. 1994. High frequency of germline *p53* mutations in childhood adrenocortical cancer. J Natl Cancer Inst 86:1707–10.

PART B: MELANOMA SYNDROMES

CLINICAL AND EPIDEMIOLOGIC FEATURES

There are over 30,000 new cases of cutaneous malignant melanoma each year and about 7000 melanoma-related deaths (Parker et al., 1996). Since 1973, the incidence of melanoma has been increasing about 4% per year, a faster rate of rise than any other cancer in the United States. In fact, analysis of the Connecticut tumor registry data reveals that the melanoma rate has been increasing for at least 60 years, doubling every 10–12 years since 1934. A white child in the United States has about a 1% chance of developing melanoma, while in some areas of the country, the risk for fair-skinned individuals is 1 in 60. The median age of onset for sporadic melanomas is in the early 50s, although about one-fifth of cases occur before the age of 40 (Koh, 1991; NIH Consensus Statement, 1992; Balch et al., 1993). The 48% increase in melanoma deaths in males, documented between 1973 and 1992, represents the highest sex-specific increase for any human cancer (CDC, 1995)

Exposure to sunlight is the principal risk factor for melanoma. The incidence of the disease is greatest among fair-skinned peoples living nearest to the equator. However, unlike other forms of skin cancer, long-term sun exposure does not appear to be a factor, because those working outdoors (farmers, field laborers) are not at particularly increased risk. Instead, there are important constitutional factors that underlie the sensitivity to sun-induced melanoma, such as a tendency to sunburn. Known risk factors for melanoma are: white skin that does not tan easily, an early blistering sunburn as a child, blond or red hair, and the presence of multiple dysplastic nevi (MacKie et al., 1989). Limitation of sun exposure during childhood appears to be particularly important, because 80% of lifetime sun exposure occurs before the age of 18 (Stern et al., 1986).

Dysplastic nevi occur most commonly in sun-exposed areas. These are irregularly shaped lesions, with pigmentation of varying shades of brown. In some, the nevi arise in unusual places, including the palms, soles, scalp, or buttocks. They may become more frequent during pregnancy. The lesions have the potential to progress to malignant melanomas. Epidemiologic studies have shown that individuals with multiple dysplastic nevi have an increased risk for malignant melanoma, with a 7% lifetime risk cited by Tucker. In studies by MacKie and others, the relative risk increased several hundredfold when there was both a history of melanoma in another family member as well as documentation of dysplastic nevi in the proband (Tucker, 1988; Tucker et al., 1993; MacKie et al., 1989).

Unfortunately, the histologic and clinical recognition of dysplastic nevi may vary widely.This histologic uncertainty has led to differing estimates of the prevalence of dysplastic nevi in the general population (ranging from 1% to over 50%). Because of these discrepancies, an NIH consensus conference in 1992 suggested avoiding the term altogether (NIH Consensus Conference, 1992).

PATHOLOGY

Melanomas appear as irregularly shaped lesions with varying pigmentation (Figure 5-2). Melanomas come in four varieties: superficial spreading melanoma, nodular melanoma, acral lentiginous melanoma, and lentigo maligna melanoma. Superficial spreading melanomas are the most common subtype, often presenting on the trunk or limbs. Nodular melanomas appear as dark pigmented nodular lesions, although they may be without pigment in 5% of cases. They are more aggressive than superficial spreading melanomas. Acral lentiginous melanomas are diagnosed as dark specks on palms, soles, or mucous membranes. They are uncommon in whites, but more common in dark-skinned individuals. Lentigo maligna melanomas are commonly found on the faces of older patients, as large spots with darker speckles. They less frequently metastasize (Balch et al., 1993).

In each melanoma, the malignant cell is the pigmented dendritic cell within epithelial regions. The appearance of melanoma cells varies depending on whether the tumor grows horizontally or vertically. A spindle-shaped appearance is more common in the vertical phase, while an irregularly shaped cell with hyperchromatic nuclei distributed along the dermal-epidermal junction is more common in the horizontal phase. Prognosis for the patient is directly related to the depth of invasion of the tumor, with a depth greater than four millimeters chosen by many authors as the cut-off for poorest prognosis. Other adverse prognostic factors include ulceration, anatomic site of the primary, and gender.

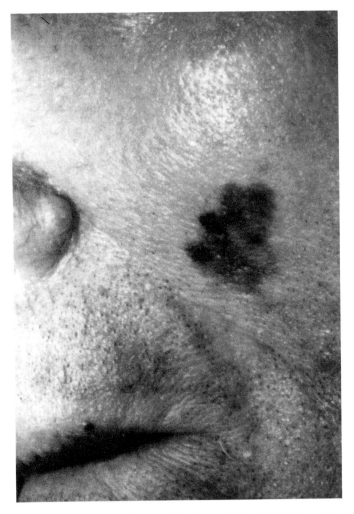

FIGURE 5-2 *Malignant melanoma. The type of melanoma illustrated, lentigo maligna, common-ly presents on the faces of older patients and infrequently metastasizes. These lesions demon-strate the irregular border and variation in pigmentation characteristic of other melanomas. (Cour-tesy of Dr. Patricia Myskowski.)*

HEREDITARY SYNDROMES

Of individuals with melanoma, 10–15% have a family history of the disease. In these families, the median age of onset is in the mid-40s, and multiple primaries are more common than the sporadic cases. Risk for melanoma is increased in kindreds with al-binism, Li-Fraumeni syndrome, and xeroderma pigmentosum (Appendix A).

In the late 1970s and early 1980s, several authors described a hereditary syndrome of susceptibility to melanoma in which family members had precursor lesions (Reimer

1978; Lynch et al., 1983; Greene et al., 1985; Tucker et al., 1988). The familial syndrome was termed *familial atypical mole malignant melanoma syndrome* (FAMMM), *B-K mole syndrome,* or *hereditary dysplastic nevus syndrome* (DNS). The median age of onset in these families was in the 30s, and the number of dysplastic nevi was highly variable. Analysis of 23 melanoma-prone kindreds revealed a lifetime risk of melanoma approaching 50% in individuals with dysplastic nevi who were part of affected families (Tucker et al., 1993). Although a review of eight epidemiological studies confirmed the approximately twofold increased risk of melanoma in individuals with a first-degree relative with the disease, this review was not able to confirm any association between familial risk and the number of dysplastic nevi (Ford et al., 1995). Attempts at genetic epidemiologic analyses of families with this syndrome were complicated by an overdiagnosis of dysplastic nevi in spouses and family members. In an attempt to avoid these diagnostic problems, Goldgar et al. derived a phenotype incorporating both number and size of nevi. This study confirmed that a major gene was responsible for some, but not all, variability in the density of nevi in families (Goldgar et al., 1991).

Linkage studies in melanoma/DNS kindreds were performed with differing findings. Initial studies reported linkage to markers on chromosome 1p, with lod scores ranging from 1.56 to 3 (Bale et al., 1989; Goldstein et al., 1993). In contrast to these results, analysis of 10 Utah kindreds and one Texas family showed evidence of strong linkage to a locus at 9p12–22 (Cannon-Albright et al., 1992). A 65% penetrance by age 80 was predicted for gene carriers (Cannon-Albright et al., 1994). The conflicting linkage results suggested genetic heterogeneity for hereditary melanoma.

Candidate gene investigations identified *CDKN2* as a likely candidate for the melanoma predisposing gene (also called *MLM*) (Kamb et al., 1994). Subsequent molecular studies have documented germline mutations of the gene *CDKN2*, in most, but not all, 9p21-linked families. *CDKN2* normally generates a protein product, p16^{INK4}, that is an inhibitor of the cyclin D1-dependent kinase 4 complex (see Chapter 3). Of 8 mutations described in one series, 6 were missense, 1 nonsense, and 1 splice donor site. Among 9 9p-linked families with lod scores greater than 0.5, 2 showed germline missense mutations. However, of 33 individuals in these 9 families who had dysplastic nevi, only 10 carried the *CDKN2* mutation, compared to 33 mutation carriers among 36 with melanomas (Hussussian et al., 1994). These findings suggest that there may be other genetic susceptibilities to account for the dysplastic nevi in these families.

Founder mutations for *CDKN2* have been demonstrated in Italian and Dutch kindreds. The gly93trp mutation was observed in 8 of 16 Italian families studied (Ghiorzo et al., 1996). A remarkably high proportion of Dutch melanoma-prone families studied showed *CDKN2* mutations. Of 15 Dutch melanoma kindreds putatively linked to 9p, 13 showed an identical 19 base pair deletion (218del19) in exon 2. Haplotype sharing among these families confirmed their common ancestry. Interestingly, two family members one of whom was unaffected, were homozygous for the deletion (Gruis et al., 1995). The risk-modifying effects of the gene encoding the melanocyte-stimulating hormone receptor, a determinant of skin and hair color, was demonstrated in a subset of Dutch families (Frants et al., 1996).

Recently, germline mutations of *CDK4* have also been observed in melanoma-prone kindreds (Zuo et al., 1996). The p15 protein is an additional inhibitor of CDK4 and CDK6. The gene encoding p15, termed *CDKN2B* was proposed as another candidate melanoma-susceptibility locus. No germline mutations in *CDKN2B* were detected in 100 Swedish melanoma kindreds (Platz et al., 1997). Thus, at least three genes (*CDKN2*, *CDK4*, a 1p-linked gene, and probably others) contribute to the genetic heterogeneity of hereditary melanoma syndromes (Goldstein and Tucker, 1997).

A number of associations between familial melanoma and other cancer types have been reported. A syndrome of melanoma and pancreatic cancer, originally described by Lynch, has been associated with germline mutations of *CDKN2*. In 10 kindreds with germline mutations of this gene, 4 had at least one family member with pancreatic cancer, compared to none in 9 melanoma-prone kindreds without these mutations. Thus, a 22-fold increased incidence for pancreatic cancer was noted in the kindreds with *CDKN2* mutations (Goldstein et al., 1995). Germline mutations of *CDKN2* were also demonstrated in another family with squamous cell carcinoma of the pancreas, a rare subtype of this cancer, as well as adenocarcinoma of the pancreas, melanoma, and squamous cell carcinoma of the tongue. The ages of onset of the pancreatic tumors in this family were 45 and 56 (Whelan et al., 1995). Thus far, no obvious correlations of specific mutations of *CDKN2* and phenotypic expression have emerged.

OPTIONS FOR PREVENTION AND EARLY DETECTION

Careful surveillance offers the promise of cure for early stage lesions. Surveillance is generally accomplished by biannual total-body skin examination. Serial photography is useful in recording lesions being followed, and all suspicious lesions should be excised. Self-examination can play an important role in this process because individuals can gauge changes in size or color of existing lesions. Self-examination should be monthly. Children of affected individuals should be protected from sunburn and should receive their first skin exam by age 10. They should be monitored closely during puberty and also during pregnancy.

Of 116 patients with 3 or more dysplastic nevi who were examined and photographed every 3–6 months, the yield of newly diagnosed melanomas was highest among the subset of patients with a family history (MacKie et al., 1993). The ages of the four patients diagnosed with melanomas were 33, 37, 37, and 46 years. In this report, and in preliminary results of American Academy of Dermatology screening programs reported by Koh, the melanomas detected were thinner (earlier stage) than a comparison group of melanomas from population-based studies. These findings offer a strong rationale for regular skin examinations in these high-risk groups (Koh, 1993).

Prevention guidelines have traditionally stressed the importance of shielding, or applying sunscreen to sun-exposed skin. Although there is evidence linking sun exposure and melanoma risk, it is also clear that melanomas can arise in areas of the body that are protected from the sun. Tumors in such "protected" areas have been noted in families with multiple dysplastic nevi. In recent research studies of mice exposed to ultraviolet rays, sunscreens protected the mice from sunburn, but not from melanoma.

Case Example 5.2. A 39-year-old woman was admitted with metastatic melanoma. She explained that her family history was significant for "premalignant" pigmented skin lesions (dysplastic nevi) found in her sister, father, and paternal aunt. There was also a history of other tumor types, including pancreatic cancer and sarcoma, in more distant relatives. She had a 3-year-old son and was concerned that he would be at risk for cancer.

In this case, genetic testing for germline mutations in the *CDKN2* gene, as well as testing for *CDK4* and 1p linkage were discussed with the proband. The proband did not feel that genetic testing would add information to what she felt was an "obvious" familial clustering. In the meantime, the child, and other at-risk members, were counseled to undergo full dermatologic evaluation, including total body photography. The proband was concerned because of the history of other tumor types in her distant relatives. Although these tumors are not part of the recognized spectrum of the melanoma syndromes, this spectrum has not been fully established, and prudent preventive oncology practice seemed warranted. Pancreatic cancers have also been reported in *CDKN2*-associated kindreds, and the lack of proof of efficacy of radiographic surveillance was also discussed with the proband. The importance of avoiding sunburn in the 3-year-old son, and the need for regular dermatologic examination beginning at age 10, were discussed.

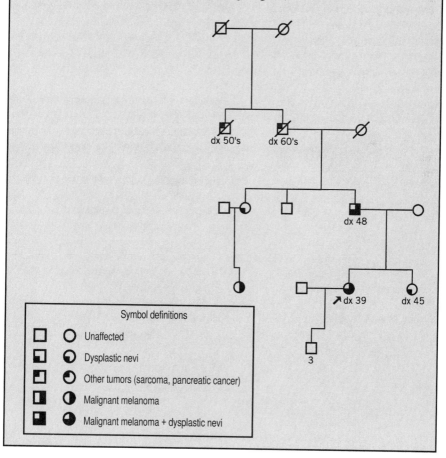

Symbol definitions

□	○	Unaffected
◨	◑	Dysplastic nevi
◪	◔	Other tumors (sarcoma, pancreatic cancer)
◧	◑	Malignant melanoma
■	●	Malignant melanoma + dysplastic nevi

As with the risk for visceral tumors in Li-Fraumeni syndrome, there are no clear guidelines for screening for the extradermatologic tumors associated with mutations of *CDKN2*. In families with cases of pancreatic cancer, annual CT or ultrasound examination may be offered on an investigational basis. The clinical role of genetic testing in melonoma-prone kindreds is still being defined. At present, clinical surveillance and management are based on family history, since the minority of melanoma-prone families will have identifiable *CDKN2* mutations (Goldstein and Tucker, 1997).

REFERENCES: PART B

Balch CM, Houghton AN, Peters LJ. 1993. Cutaneous melanoma. In: Devita VT, Hellman S, Rosenberg SA. Cancer: Principles and Practice of Oncology. Philadelphia: J.B. Lippincott, pp. 1612–44.

Bale SJ, Dracopoli NC, Tucker MA et al. 1989. Mapping the gene for hereditary cutaneous malignant melanoma-dysplastic nevus to chromosome 1p. New Eng J Med 320:1367–72.

Cannon-Albright LA, Goldgar DE, Meyer LJ et al. 1992. Assignment of a locus for familial melanoma, *MLM*, to chromosome 9p13-p22. Science 258:1148–52.

Cannon-Albright LA, Meyer LJ, Goldgar DE et al. 1994. Penetrance and expressivity of the chromosome 9p melanoma susceptibility locus (*MLM*). Cancer Res 54:6041–44.

CDC. 1995. Deaths from melanoma–United States, 1973–1992. Morbid Mortal Weekly Rep 44(337): 342–7.

Ford D, Bliss JM, Swerdlow AJ et al. 1995. Risk of cutaneous melanoma associated with a family history of the disease. Int J Cancer 62:377–81.

Frants RR, Van der Velden PA, Bergman W, Gruis NA. 1996. Melanocyte-stimulating hormone receptor (MC1R) variants modify melanoma risk in Dutch FAMM families. Am J Hum Genet 59:349 (abstr).

Ghiorzo P, Mantelli M, Ciotti P, et al. 1996. Italian melanoma-prone families: analysis of *CDKN2*/p16 mutations and linkage to 9p21. Am J Hum Genet 59:354 (abstr).

Goldgar DE, Cannon-Albright LA, Meyer LJ, Piepkorn MW, Zone JJ, Skolnick MH. 1991. Inheritance of nevus number and size in melanoma and dysplastic nevus syndrome kindreds. J Natl Cancer Inst 83:1726–33.

Goldstein AM, Dracopoli NC, Ho EC et al. 1993. Further evidence for a locus for cutaneous malignant melanoma-dysplastic nevus (CMM/DN) on chromosome 1p and evidence for genetic heterogeneity. Am J Hum Genet 52:537–50.

Goldstein AM, Fraser MC, Struewing JP et al. 1995. Increased risk of pancreatic cancer in melanoma-prone kindreds with p16[INK4] mutations. New Eng J Med 333:970–4.

Goldstein AM, Tucker MA. 1997. Screening for CDKN2A mutations in hereditary melanoma. J Natl Cancer Inst 89:676–8.

Greene MH, Clark WH Jr, Tucker MA et al. 1985. Acquired precursors of cutaneous malignant melanoma: the familial dysplastic nevus syndrome. New Engl J Med 312:91–7.

Gruis NA, van der Velden PA, Sandkuijl LA et al. 1995. Homozygotes for *CDKN2* (p16) germline mutation in Dutch familial melanoma kindreds. Nature Genet 10:351–3.

Hussussian CJ, Struewing JP, Goldstein AM et al. 1994. Germline p16 mutations in familial melanoma. Nature Genet 8:15–21.

Kamb A, Shattuck-Eidens D, Eeles R et al. 1994. Analysis of the p16 gene (*CDKN2*) as a candidate for the chromosome 9p melanoma susceptibility locus. Nature Genet 8:23–6.

Koh HK. 1991. Cutaneous melanoma. N Eng J Med 325:171–82.

Koh HK. 1993. Melanoma education and screening in the U.S.: third international conference on melanoma. Melanoma Res 3:7 (abstr).

Lynch HT, Fusaro RM, Danes BS et al. 1983. A review of hereditary malignant melanoma including biomarkers in familial atypical multiple mole melanoma syndrome. Cancer Genet Cytogenet 8:325–58.

MacKie RM, Freudenberger T, Aitchison TC. 1989. Personal risk-factor chart for cutaneous melanoma. Lancet 2:487–90.

Mackie RM, McHenry P, Hole D. 1993. Accelerated detection with prospective surveillance for cutaneous malignant melanoma in high- risk groups. Lancet 341:1618–20.

NIH Consensus Statement. 1992. Diagnosis and treatment of early melanoma. NIH Consensus Development Conference, January 27–29.

Parker SL, Tong T, Bolden S, Wingo PA. 1996. Cancer statistics, 1996 CA Cancer J Clin 46:5–27.

Platz A, Hansson J, Mansson-Brahme E et al. 1997. Screening of germline mutations in the CDKN2A and CDKN2B genes in Swedish familes with hereditary cutaneous melanoma. J Natl Cancer Inst: 697–702.

Reimer RR, Clark WH, Greene MH et al. 1978. Precursor lesions in familial melanoma: A new genetic preneoplastic syndrome. JAMA 239:744–6.

Skolnick MH, Cannon-Albright LA, Kamb A. 1994. Genetic predisposition to melanoma. Eur J Cancer 30A: 1991–5.

Stern RS, Weinstein MC, Baker SG. 1986. Risk reduction for nonmelanoma skin cancer with childhood sunscreen use. Arch Dermatol 122:537–45.

Tucker MA. 1988. Individuals at high risk of melanoma. Pigment Cell 9:95–109.

Tucker MA, Fraser MC, Goldstein AM et al. 1993. Risk of melanoma and other cancers in melanoma-prone families. J Invest Dermatol 100:S350–5.

Whelan AJ, Bartsch D, Goodfellow P. 1995. Brief report: a familial syndrome of pancreatic cancer and melanoma with a mutation in the *CDKN2* tumor suppressor gene. New Eng J Med 333:975–7.

Zuo L, Weger J, Yang Q et al. 1996. Germline mutations in the p16INK4a binding domain of *CDK4* in familial melanoma. Nature Genet 12:97–9.

PART C: MULTIPLE ENDOCRINE NEOPLASIAS (MEN)

CLINICAL AND PATHOLOGIC FEATURES

MEN 1

Although associations of pituitary tumors, parathyroid hyperplasia, and pancreatic islet cell tumors were described early in the century, it was not until 1954 that Wermer reported the familial nature of the syndrome. The most common feature of MEN1 is the *parathyroid adenoma,* seen in about 90% of cases. *Pancreatic islet cell tumors* are seen in about 50–75% of cases, and may present as gastrinoma, VIPoma, glucagonoma, or insulinoma. About a quarter of the pancreatic tumors are non-functional. *Pituitary adenomas* are seen in 25–65% of cases and may be nonfunctional or functional, most often as prolactinomas (Pang and Thakker, 1994; Thakker, 1993). Malignant neurendocrine tumors of thymic origin are also observed as part of the spectrum of MEN1 tumors.

Most patients with MEN1 will present with hypercalcemia by virtue of the parathyroid hyperplasia. The symptoms of the pancreatic tumor will depend on the ectopic hormone secreted. Zollinger-Ellison syndrome consists of peptic ulcer disease and gastric hyperacidity due to an excess of gastrin secretion by pancreatic D cells. Insulinoma commonly presents with symptoms of confusion, loss of consciousness, and dizziness due to hypoglycemia. Excess secretion of glucagon results in a characteristic *migratory necrolytic erythemia,* accompanied by weight loss and glucose intolerance. VIPomas commonly are diagnosed by a syndrome of watery diarrhea and hypokalemia. Functional pituitary adenomas may result in acromegaly or prolactinoma.

MEN 2

MEN2a is a syndrome, originally described by Sipple in 1961, in which there are multiple cases of endocrine tumors, particularly *medullary thyroid carcinoma* and *pheochromocytoma.* There is also *hyperplasia of the parathyroid* in 25% of cases.

The medullary thyroid carcinomas arise from parafollicular G cells and secrete calcitonin. Presentation is usually in the third or fourth decade, with diarrhea as the common symptom. Pheochromocytomas, arising from neural crest cells in the adrenal gland, are usually bilateral. Hypertension is the common presenting symptom, with diagnosis classically made by measurement of urinary vanillyl mandelic acid (VMA) and metanephrines. Routine screening for MEN2a has been directed to the thyroid medullary lesions, with a pentagastrin challenge given to measure calcitonin response (Telenius-Berg et al., 1984). Measurement of serum ionized calcium has also been performed in the diagnostic evaluation. In contrast to MEN1, only about 40% of individuals with MEN2a present clinically by age 50, although biochemical screening increases the ability to detect the MEN2a phenotype to over 90% by age 31 (Gagel et al., 1988; Telenius-Berg et al.,1984).

MEN2b is a variant of MEN2a characterized by an earlier age of onset, enlarged and nodular lips, a Marfanoid habitus, ganglioneuromatosis of the intestine, and a variety of other abnormalities (Vasen et al., 1992). This phenotype is also accompanied by medullary carcinoma of the thyroid, which may be more clinically aggressive, and pheochromocytoma. Parathyroid disease is less common than in MEN2a.

Familial Medullary Carcinoma of the Thyroid

Medullary carcinoma of the thyroid runs in families about 25% of the time, either as a syndrome of site-specific familial medullary carcinoma of the thyroid (FMCT), or as MEN2 (Farndon et al., 1986). The cases commonly present in the third and fourth decades, and are usually bilateral and multifocal. Diarrhea is a usual presenting symptom. It has been suggested that four cases of medullary carcinoma of the thyroid in the absence of the other hallmark tumors of MEN2a, are diagnostic for FMCT. Familial papillary thyroid cancer is distinct from FMCT and has been associated with an increased incidence of colorectal cancer (Stoffer et al., 1986) (see Appendix A).

GENETIC DIAGNOSIS AND OPTIONS FOR PREVENTION AND EARLY DETECTION

MEN1

About 75% of individuals with MEN1 develop symptoms by age 50, although with biochemical screening the estimated penetrance is 91% (reviewed in Pang and Thakker, 1994). In the absence of symptoms, extensive biochemical screening for the

Case Example 5.3. A 44-year-old man was referred for *"RET"* testing for a family history of thyroid cancer. In the process of documenting the pedigree, three cases of thyroid cancer were discovered in three generations. The thyroid cancers were all of papillary type. In examining the patient, a small nodule in the inferior pole of his gland was palpated.

This case illustrates the importance of documentation of histology. A syndrome of familial papillary thyroid cancer is distinct from the MEN2a-linked syndrome of hereditary medullary thyroid carcinoma. In the papillary thyroid cancer syndrome, germline mutations of *RET* are not observed. While being enrolled for research linkage studies, this family was also counseled to undergo physical examination by an endocrinologist, and a thyroid scan was ordered for the proband. In addition, as indicated in the Appendix A entry for this syndrome, there is an increased risk for colorectal malignancies (see also Stoffer et al., 1986). The age of onset for the colon cancers is not thought to be earlier than the general population. Therefore, baseline sigmoidoscopy or colonoscopy was rec-

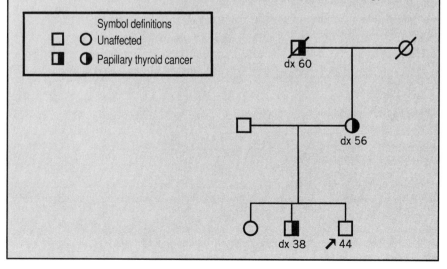

other component tumors is usually not informative. Nonetheless, in the setting of a family with documented MEN1, screening of offspring should begin at an early age (between ages 5 and 10) and be continued at regular intervals thereafter. Screening should include, at a minimum, serum ionized calcium and prolactin determinations. Many specialists recommend full screening with measurement of pituitary (GH, ACTH, FSH, TSH, prolactin), parathyroid (PTH), and pancreatic hormones (insulin, somatostatin, glucagon, pancreatic polypeptide, gastrin, VIP, neurotensin), as well as radiographic imaging to assess pituitary size (Vasen et al., 1989).

The *MEN1* gene was mapped to within a 2 Mb region at 11q13 (Debelenko et al., 1997), and *MEN1* was cloned in 1997 by Chandrasekharappa et al. The gene contained 10 exons. Analysis of 15 kindreds revealed 12 different mutations: 5 frameshift, 3 non-sense, 2 missense, and 2 in-frame deletions. Two mutations, 416delC, and 512delC were observed twice in unrelated families (Chandrasekharappa et al., 1997). Analysis of an additional 34 MEN1 kindreds identified eight mutations seen more than once (Agarwal et al., 1997). The presence of inactivating mutations in the *MEN1* gene and the detection of allelic deletions of linked markers in pancreatic and parathyroid tumors supports the role of the *MEN1* gene product as a tumor suppressor (Taggart et al., 1996). With the availability of direct mutation detection, more widespread genetic screening for this condition will be possible.

For the patient presenting with an isolated MEN1 type tumor, a detailed family history should be taken, with attention paid to clinical manifestations of the MEN1 phenotype (e.g., family members with renal stones due to hypercalcemia, or peptic ulcers due to gastrinoma). The absence of multicentricity in the tumor and the presence of normal serum calcium levels in first-degree relatives, are strong evidence against a hereditary syndrome. Individuals presenting with two component tumors, or with suggestive family histories, should receive more intensive biochemical screening. DNA should also be obtained for mutation analysis, preferably in the context of research studies.

Case Example 5.4. A visiting businessman came for a diagnostic procedure because of a low cervical neck mass. He had a history of hypercalcemia and surgical parathyroidectomy. As part of a fertility evaluation, elevated levels of prolactin had been found. On examination, he was noted to have a 3-cm right neck mass. Biopsy of the neck mass revealed a malignant neurendocrine tumor of unknown primary. An abdominal CT scan revealed a normal pancreas. Octreotide scan (Figure 5-3) showed an area of increased uptake in the right mediastinum. A CT-guided biopsy revealed a malignant neurendocrine tumor of presumed thymic origin. Surgery and chemotherapy were discussed as therapeutic approaches.

Family history was significant for "kidney stones" in multiple relatives. The diagnosis of Multiple Endocrine Neoplasia I was made. Affected family members consented to genetic testing so as to allow presymptomatic diagnosis for the proband's 5-year-old daughter.

This case illustrates presentation of MEN1 without a pancreatic islet cell tumor. Malignant neurendocrine tumors of thymic origin are a less frequent, but described, component of the syndrome.

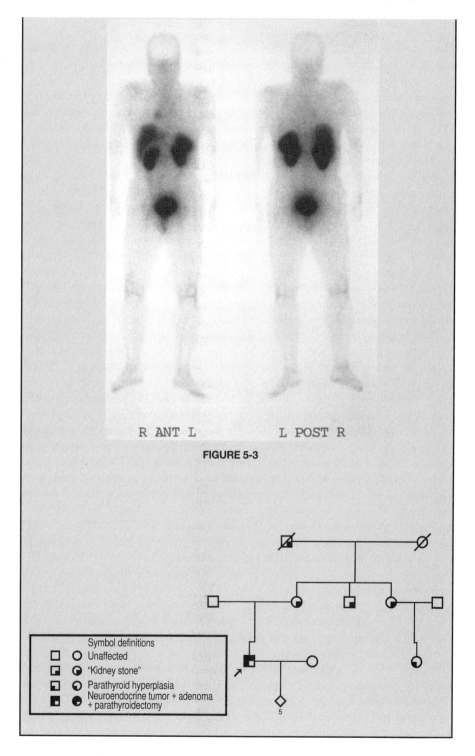

R ANT L   L POST R

FIGURE 5-3

MEN2a and MEN2b

The discovery in 1993 that mutations in the *RET* gene were associated with MEN2a and 2b changed the diagnostic evaluation of such families (Mulligan et al., 1993). Previously, all first-degree relatives of individuals with medullary carcinoma of the thyroid were recommended to receive pentagastrin stimulation tests, as noted above. *RET* testing of sporadic cases of medullary carcinoma of the thyroid yielded a relatively low (5%) rate of diagnosis of MEN2a in the absence of a family history of the disease, C cell hyperplasia, or multifocality (Eng, 1995c; Decker et al., 1995). Nonetheless, *RET* testing was more sensitive than traditional biochemical screening. In a study of 300 members of 4 large MEN2a families, 14 young individuals with *RET* mutations had normal plasma calcitonin levels. Thyroidectomy revealed small foci of medullary carcinoma of the thyroid in 8 of these 14, with the remaining 6 not having had surgery (Lips et al., 1994). A large study in the United States revealed medullary cancer in 6 *RET* heterozygotes in MEN2a families, although their calcitonin levels were normal (Wells et al., 1994).

These results have established *RET* testing as the gold standard for MEN2a screening and prophylactic thyroidectomy as the primary preventative intervention. The optimal age for performing surgery is as early as 5 years in some centers. Genetic testing should thus be undertaken by this age, and perhaps even before in families with MEN2b, because the thyroid cancers can occur at an earlier age. A review of 49 children with MEN2a or 2b, all receiving thyroidectomy before the age of 16 years, confirmed the somewhat more aggressive presentation of MEN2b (Skinner et al., 1996). Of 11 children with MEN2b, 10 had medullary cancer of the thyroid, with only 3 free of the disease at follow-up of 11 years. Of 24 children with MEN2a, in this historical series, 5 had recurrent medullary cancer of the thyroid at 9 years. Of 14 children diagnosed with MEN2a by *RET* testing, 11 were found to have medullary thyroid cancer (Skinner et al., 1996). Follow-up of these children will be necessary to substantiate an improved clinical outcome over time. These heterozygotes for *RET* mutations in the setting of MEN2a will continue to be screened for pheochromocytoma with abdominal ultrasound or CT, as well as 24-hour urine studies, through the adult years at least to age 35.

The *RET* proto-oncogene encodes a transmembrane-receptor kinase (Figure 5-4). A ligand for this receptor has been observed; gene targeting has identified a glial-cell-line derived neurotrophic factor (GDNF) as capable of activating *RET*. Although initial studies of mutations of GDNF have been directed primarily to Hirschsprung's disease (see following section) (Angrist et al., 1996), MEN2 and FMCT have clearly been associated with germline mutations of *RET*. MEN2a and FMCT were associated with mutations involving cysteine residues in the extracellular domain encoded by exons 10 and 11 of the gene. These included codons 609, 611, 618, and 620 in exon 10 and codon 634 in exon 11 (Mulligan et al., 1993; Mulligan et al., 1994; Donis-Keller et al., 1993). In MEN2a, preliminary genotype-phenotype correlations have associated codon 634 mutations in exon 11 with pheochromocytoma, and a TGC → CGC substitution at this same codon with parathyroid disease (Mulligan et al., 1994). These observations allow the directed use of single strand conformation polymorphism (SSCP) analysis (see Chapter 7) of these exons, followed by direct sequencing as a diagnostic

Case Example 5.5. Parents of three children ages 10 to 17 came for counseling regarding the risk for "family cancers." The father, age 41, was diagnosed the year before with medullary cancer of the thyroid. An abdominal CT scan and urine catecholamines were negative. His sister had a pheochromocytoma at age 36 as well as medullary thyroid cancer, both treated surgically. His father, the grandfather of the proband, had all three cardinal tumors of MEN2a. The proband had a paternal cousin with Hirschsprung's disease.

After extensive counseling, genetic testing was performed on the proband. A mutation in exon 10 of the *RET* gene was identified, and the same mutation was observed in another affected family member. Although biochemical testing for levels of PTH, urine catecholamines, and calcitonin were normal, this family member, a boy age 10, was referred for genetic testing. His parents gave consent and the boy agreed to the testing as well. The same mutation was identified in his blood sample. Prophylactic removal of his thyroid gland was discussed, consent obtained, and the procedure performed. The surgery was fully reimbursed by the insurer based on the genetic test results. The surgical specimen revealed a small focus of medullary cancer of the thyroid. The other members of the family were referred for mutation screening.

This case indicates the clinical application of genetic screening for MEN2a. Some surgeons feel that prophylactic thyroidectomy is indicated as early as age 5, while others prefer to wait until ages 12–13. Continued screening for additional manifestations of MEN2a in the 10-year-old boy included serum calcium, urine metanephrines, and abdominal ultrasound.

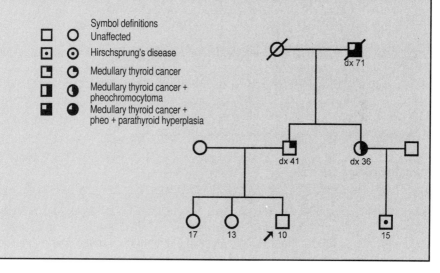

Symbol definitions

☐ ○ Unaffected

▣ ⊙ Hirschsprung's disease

◧ ◖ Medullary thyroid cancer

◪ ◕ Medullary thyroid cancer + pheochromocytoma

■ ● Medullary thyroid cancer + pheo + parathyroid hyperplasia

approach. Two missense mutations in exons 13 and 14, glu768asp and val804leu, have been associated with FMCT (Eng et al., 1995a; Bolino et al., 1995). These mutations affect the intracellular tyrosine kinase domain of *RET*, unlike the majority of FMCT mutations, which affect the extracellular domain. As many as 9% of all MEN2A and FMCT mutations may appear *de novo,* and were observed exclusively in the paternal allele. A preponderance of affected females was also observed in the offspring of probands, suggesting a role for genomic imprinting (Schuffenecker et al., 1997).

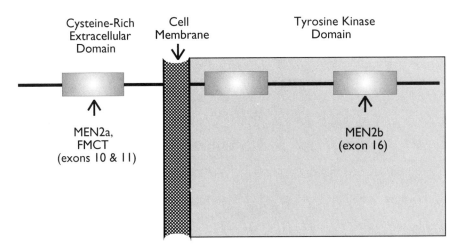

FIGURE 5-4   *The* RET *proto-oncogene encodes a transmembrane-receptor kinase. MEN2a and FMCT are associated with mutations involving cysteine residues in the extracellular domain encoded by exons 10 and 11 of the gene. FMCT also occurs as a result of mutations in the intracellular domain. MEN2b is associated with mutations affecting the intracellular tyrosine kinase domain, encoded by exon 16. A specific missense mutation at codon 918 in exon 16, met917thr, has been observed in over 90% of MEN2b cases.*

MEN2b is associated with mutations affecting the intracellular tyrosine kinase domain, encoded by exon 16 (Mulligan et al., 1994; Hofstra et al., 1994). A specific missense mutation at codon 918 in exon 16, met917thr, has been observed in over 90% of MEN2b cases (Hofstra et al., 1994; Carlson et al., 1994b). A high proportion of MEN2b cases appear to be the result of *de novo* germline mutations (Carlson, 1994a), with transmission through the paternal allele also observed.

Hirschsprung's Disease

Hirschprung's disease in many ways represents the anatomic inverse of MEN2b; instead of proliferation of autonomic ganglia in the gut, there is an absence of the enteric autonomic ganglion plexus. The disease results in intestinal obstruction in neonates and megacolon in adults. Significantly, mutations in both the extracellular as well as the tyrosine kinase domains of *RET* have been observed in this disease (Edery et al., 1994; Eng, 1996). Presumably these are inactivating mutations, in contrast to the mutations in MEN2b, MEN2a, and FMCT. This latter hypothesis is supported by experiments that demonstrate transformation of NIH 3T3 cells after transfection with constructs bearing *RET* genes with MEN2a mutations (Santoro et al., 1995). Some cases of familial Hirschsprung's disease, however, are not linked to the *RET* locus, and among those that are, linkage to other loci may also be evident (Bolk et al., 1996).

Isolated Pheochromocytoma

Since pheochromocytomas may be a component of MEN, should all patients with pheochromocytoma be screened for *RET* mutations? Only 1 of 48 cases of sporadic pheochromocytoma showed a germline *RET* mutation (Eng et al., 1995b). However, 2 cases with bilateral pheochromocytoma had germline *VHL* mutations. In another series, no germline mutations of *RET* and three germline mutations of *VHL* were observed in eight kindreds with familial pheochromocytoma (Woodward et al., 1997). Thus, the observation of familial pheochromocytomas or bilateral pheochromocytoma should lead to consideration of the diagnosis of von Hippel-Lindau syndrome (Crossey et al., 1995) (see Part G).

REFERENCES: PART C

Agarwal SK, Kester MB, Debelenko LV et al. 1997. Germline mutations of the *MEN1* gene in familial MEN1 and related states. Hum Molec Genet 6:1169–75.

Angrist M, Bolk S, Halushka M, Lapchak PA, Chakravarti A. 1996. Germline mutations in glial cell line-derived neurotrophic factor (GDNF) and *RET* in a Hirschsprung disease patient. Am J Hum Genet 59:1416 (abstr).

Bolino A, Schuffenecker I, Luo Y et al. 1995. *RET* mutations in exons 13 and 14 of FMTC patients. Oncogene 10:2415–9.

Bolk S, Angrist M, Croaker D, Krugylak L, Chakravarti A. 1996. Segregation of a chromosome 9q susceptibility gene in *RET*-linked Hirschsprung families. Am J Hum Genet 59:1221 (abstr).

Carlson KM, Bracamontes J, Jackson CE, Clark R, Lacroix A, Wells SA, Goodfellow PJ. 1994a. Parent-of-origin effects in multiple endocrine neoplasia type 2B. Am J Hum Genet 55:1076–82.

Carlson KM, Dou S, Chi D et al. 1994b. Single missense mutation in the tyrosine kinase catalytic domain of the *RET* proto-oncogene is associated with multiple endocrine neoplasia type 2B. Proc Natl Acad Sci 91:1579–83.

Chandrasekharappa SC, Guru S, Manickam P et al. 1997. Positional cloning of the gene for multiple endocrine neoplasia type 1. Science 276:404–7.

Crossey PA, Eng C, Ginalska-Malinowska M et al. 1995. Molecular genetic diagnosis of von Hippel-Lindau disease in familial pheochromocytoma. J Med Genet 32:885–6.

Debelenko LV, Emmert-Buck MR, Manickman P et al. 1997. Haplotype analysis defines a minimal interval for the multiple endocrine neoplasia type 1 (MEN1) gene. Cancer Res 57:1039–42.

Decker RA, Peacock ML, Borst MJ, Sweet JD, Thomson NW. 1995. Progress in genetic screening of multiple endocrine neoplasia type 2a: is calcitonin testing obsolete? Surgery 118:257–63.

Donis-Keller H, Dou S, Chi D et al. 1993. Mutations in the *RET* proto-oncogene are associated with MEN2a and FMTC. Hum Molec Genet 2:851–6.

Easton DF, Ponder BA, Cummings T et al. 1989. The clinical and screening age-at-onset distribution for the MEN-2 syndrome. Am J Hum Genet 44:208–15.

Edery P, Lyonnet S, Mulligan LM et al. 1994. Mutations of the *RET* proto-oncogene in Hirschsprung's disease. Nature 367:378–80.

Eng C, Smith DP, Mulligan LM et al. 1995a. A novel point mutation in the tyrosine kinase domain of the *RET* proto-oncogene in sporadic medullary thyroid carcinoma and in a family with FMTC. Oncogene 10:509–13.

Eng C, Crossey PA, Mulligan LM et al. 1995b. Mutations in the *RET* proto-oncogene and the von Hippel-Lindau disease tumor suppressor gene in sporadic and syndromic pheochromocytoma. J Med Genet 32:934–7.

Eng C, Mulligan LM, Smith DP et al. 1995c. Low frequency of germline mutations in the *RET* proto-oncogene in patients with apparently sporadic medullary thyroid carcinoma. Clin Endocrinol 43:123–7.

Eng C. 1996. The *RET* proto-oncogene in multiple endocrine neoplasia type 2 and Hirschsprung's disease. New Eng J Med 335:943–51.

Farndon JR, Dilley WG, Baylin SB et al. 1986. Familial medullary thyroid carcinoma without associated endocrinopathies: a distinct clinical entity. Br J Surg 73:278–81.

Forster-Gibson CJ, Mulligan LM. 1994. Multiple endocrine neoplasia type 2. Eur J Cancer 30A:1969–74.

Gagel RF, Tashjian AH Jr, Cummings T et al. 1988. The clinical outcome of prospective screening for multiple endocrine neoplasia type 2A. New Engl J Med 318:478–84.

Hofstra RM, Landsvater RM, Ceccherini I et al. 1994. A mutation in the *RET* proto-oncogene associated with multiple endocrine neoplasia type 2B and sporadic medullary thyroid carcinoma. Nature 367:375–6.

Larsson C, Shephard J, Nakamura Y et al. 1992. Predictive testing for multiple endocrine neoplasia type 1 using DNA polymorphisms. J Clin Invest 89:1344–9.

Lips CJM, Landsvater RM, Höppener JWM et al. 1994. Clinical screening as compared with DNA analysis in families with multiple endocrine neoplasia type 2A. New Engl J Med 331:828–35.

Mulligan LM, Kwok JB, Healey CS et al. 1993. Germ-line mutations of the *RET* proto-oncogene in multiple endocrine neoplasia type 2A. Nature 363:458–60.

Mulligan LM, Eng C, Healey CS et al. 1994. Specific mutations of the *RET* proto-oncogene are related to disease phenotype in MEN2A and FMTC. Nature Genet 6:70–74.

Pang JT and Thakker RV. 1994. Multiple endocrine neoplasia Type 1 (MEN 1). Eur J Cancer 30A:1961–8.

Santoro M, Carlomagno F, Romano A et al. 1995. Activation of *RET* as a dominant transforming gene by germline mutations of MEN2A and MEN2B. Science 267:381–3.

Schimke RN. 1990. Multiple endocrine neoplasia: how many syndromes? Am J Med Genet 37:375–83.

Schuffenecker I, Ginet N, Goldgar D et al. 1997. Prevalence and parental origin of de novo *RET* mutations in multiple endocrine neoplasia type 2A and familial medullary thyroid carcinoma. Am J Hum Genet 60:233–7.

Sipple JH. 1961. The association of pheochromocytoma with carcinoma of the thyroid gland. Am J Med 31:163–6.

Skinner MA, DeBenedetti MK, Moley JF, Norton JA, Wells SA Jr. 1996. Medullary thyroid carcinoma in children with multiple endocrine neoplasia type 2a and 2b. J Pediatric Surg 31:177–81.

Stoffer SS, Van Dyke DL, Bach JV, Szpunar W, Weiss L. 1986. Familial papillary carcinoma of the thyroid. Am J Hum Genet 25:775–82.

Taggart RT, Qian C, Mullins C, Slusher R, An Y, Richard CW. 1996. Multiple endocrine neoplasia type 1: identification of polymorphic markers and candidate genes. Am J Hum Genet 59:446 (abstr).

Telenius-Berg M, Berg B, Hamberger B et al. 1984. Impact of screening on prognosis in the multiple endocrine neoplasia type 2 syndromes: natural history and treatment results in 105 patients. Henry Ford Hosp Med J 32:225–31.

Thakker RV. 1993. The molecular genetics of the multiple endocrine neoplasia syndromes. Clin Endocrinol 38:1–14.

Vasen HFA, Lamers CBHW, Lips CJM. 1989. Screening for the multiple endocrine neoplasia syndrome type 1. A study of 11 kindreds in the Netherlands. Arch Intern Med 149:2717–22.

Vasen HF, van der Feltz M, Raue F et al. 1992. The natural course of multiple endocrine neoplasia type IIb. A study of 18 cases. Arch Intern Med 152:1250–2.

Wells Jr. SA, Chi DD, Toshima K et al. 1994. Predictive DNA testing and prophylactic thyroidectomy in patients at risk for multiple endocrine neoplasia type 2A. Ann Surg 220:237–47.

Wermer P. 1954. Genetic aspects of adenomatosis of the endocrine glands. Am J Med 16:363–71.

Woodward ER, Eng C, McMahon R et al. 1997. Genetic predisposition to pheochromocytoma: analysis of candidate genes *GDNF, RET* and *VHL*. Hum Molec Genet 6:1051–6.

PART D: NEUROFIBROMATOSIS

NF1: CLINICAL AND PATHOLOGIC FEATURES

Although it is one of the most common of the single gene disorders, with an incidence of approximately 1 in 3000, patients with neurofibromatosis 1 (NF1) have a small excess risk for malignancy. For this reason, the syndrome is not frequently encountered by cancer geneticists.

According to the 1988 NIH Consensus Conference, diagnostic criteria for NF1 include two or more of the following features: Six or more café au lait macules over 15 mm in size in adults and 5 mm in children; two or more neurofibromas or one plexiform neurofibroma; axillary or inguinal freckling; optic glioma; two or more hamartomas of the iris *(Lisch nodules);* characteristic osseous lesion (e.g., sphenoid dysplasia; long bone cortical thinning); or a first-degree relative with NF1.

The skin manifestations are readily apparent on physical examination. Most of the neurofibromas will be evident as dermal lesions, although they can also grow on nerve trunks. The plexiform neurofibromas present as large, sometimes disfiguring subcutaneous masses. Diagnosis of Lisch nodules generally requires a slit lamp examination by an ophthalmologist.

Although the penetrance of the disorder is 100%, there is a marked variability of expressivity that poses a special clinical challenge. Children may have very mild manifestations of the disease that will evolve over time. There is also a high rate of new mutations, which are estimated to account for half of cases.

The overall risk for malignancy in patients with NF1 is only slightly higher than the general population, but the distribution of tumors is unusual. Most of what is known of the tumor risk is derived from a prospective study of 212 individuals (Sorensen et al., 1986) and Welsh and Swedish population studies (Huson et al., 1988; Zoller et al., 1997). The tumor types observed are listed in Table 5-2.

NF1: GENETIC DIAGNOSIS AND OPTIONS FOR PREVENTION AND EARLY DETECTION

NF1 was cloned in 1990. A small amount of the protein product is a GTPase-activating protein (GAP), with the role of keeping RAS proteins in an inactive GDP-bound state (see Chapter 3). The very large size of the *NF1* gene, 57 exons over 350 kb of genomic DNA, has posed diagnostic difficulties. Mutational analysis is available from several commercial laboratories, although prenatal diagnosis utilizing closely linked markers has been available for several years. Approximately 100 germline mutations have been observed, with most predicted to result in premature translational truncation (Colman and Wallace, 1994). Mutation detection using standard techniques may miss large gene deletions, which have been documented as *de novo* events, and may be detected utilizing intragenic markers (Rasmussen et al., 1996) or FISH (Wu et al., 1996). A commercial assay utilizing protein truncation has been developed (Heim et al.,1994); however, positive results should be confirmed by sequencing.

Patients with NF1 are perhaps best managed in specialty clinics, although specific medical interventions are not necessary for many patients (Riccardi, 1992). In the absence of options for prevention of the central nervous system tumors, there remains a limited role for preventive oncologic counseling of patients. Baseline cranial imaging has been suggested, but is not practiced by most NF1 experts because the frequency of asymptomatic gliomas and other lesions needing intervention is quite low (Mulvihill, personal communication). The incidence of juvenile chronic myeloid leukemia, pheochromocytoma, and rhabdomyosarcoma is so low that routine presymptomatic screening for these tumors is not indicated (Guttman et al., 1997).

TABLE 5-2 Malignant Tumors Observed in Neurofibromatosis Type 1

Astrocytomas (cerebral and cerebellar)
Malignant peripheral nerve sheath tumors (neurofibrosarcomas and malignant schwannomas)
Rhabdomyosarcoma
Leiomyosarcoma
Pheochromocytoma
Optic glioma
Carcinoma of the ampulla of Vater
Juvenile chronic myeloid leukemia

REFERENCES: PART D—NF1

Colman SD, Wallace MR. 1994. Neurofibromatosis Type 1. Eur J Cancer 30A:1974–81.

Guttman DH, Aylsworth A, Carey JC et al. 1997. The diagnostic evaluation and multidisciplinary management of neurofibromatosis 1 and neurofibromatosis 2. JAMA 278:51–65.

Heim RA, Silverman LM, Farber RA, Kam-Morgan LNW, Luce M. 1994. Screening for NF1 truncating proteins. Nature Genet 8:218–9.

Huson SM, Harper PS, Compston DAS. 1988. Von Recklinghausen neurofibromatosis: a clinical and population study in South East Wales. Brain III:1355–81.

NIH Consensus Development Conference. 1988. Neurofibromatosis Conference Statement. Arch Neurol 45:575–8.

Rasmussen SA, Colman SD, Abernathy CR, Schwartz CE, Arn PH, Wallace MR. 1996. Prevalence of large NF1 gene deletions in neurofibromatosis type 1 (NF1). Amer J Hum Genet 59:37 (abstr).

Riccardi VM. 1992. Neurofibromatosis: Phenotype, Natural History, and Pathogenesis, 2ed. Baltimore: The Johns Hopkins University Press.

Sorensen SA, Mulvihill JJ, Nielsen A. 1986. Long-term follow-up of von Recklinghausen neurofibromatosis: survival and malignant neoplasms. New Eng J Med 314:1010–5.

Wu BL, Schneider GH, Boles RG et al. 1996. Characterization of NF1 mutations by FISH: Large deletions, somatic mosaicism, and translocation identified in sporadic or familial cases of NF1. Amer J Human Genet 59:764 (abstr).

Zoller MET, Rembeck B, Oden A, Samuelsson M, Angervall L. 1997. Malignant and benign tumors in patients with neurofibromatosis type 1 in a defined Swedish population. Cancer 79:2125–31.

NF2: CLINICAL AND PATHOLOGIC FEATURES

NF2 is a very rare disorder, with an incidence of approximately 1 in 35,000. The diagnostic criteria for NF2 include *bilateral vestibular schwannomas* (also called acoustic neuromas), or a first-degree relative with NF2 accompanied by a unilateral vestibular schwannoma or one additional feature: meningioma, glioma, neurofibroma, schwannoma, posterior subcapsular lenticular opacities, or cerebral calcification (Evans et al., 1992a,b). Although bilateral acoustic neuromas are the hallmark of this syndrome, the diagnosis can also be made when a unilateral tumor or multiple meningiomas are accompanied by any one of the additional features of the syndrome (reviewed in Guttman et al., 1997).

The growth of the tumor causes progressive compression of the VIII cranial nerve, producing progressive hearing loss and tinnitus. NF2 tumors can present in childhood or early adulthood, compared to a median age of 50 for sporadic unilateral cases. Lens opacities are found in 40–60% of patients, and may be diagnosed at an early age. Some manifestation of the disease will usually be evident by the age of 40 (Evans 1992c). A negative MRI scan at age 30 makes the inheritance of a mutated *NF2* gene highly unlikely (Guttman et al., 1997).

Gliomas and cutaneous tumors are much less common in NF2 than NF1, but meningiomas more common. Café au lait macules are also less frequent, but may occur. A useful diagnostic hallmark is the *NF2 plaque,* a pigmented, slightly raised, coarse lesion, sometimes with hair (Figure 5-5). The variability in expressivity of NF2 is manifest between families, but not between individuals in the same family. Two classes of severity of the NF2 phenotype have been described: the Wishart type with early onset, a rapid course, and multiple other tumors; and the milder Gardner type, with later onset, a more benign course, and few tumors other than the bilateral vestibular schwannomas. As in NF1, the new mutation rate for NF2 is estimated to be about 50%.

NF2: GENETIC DIAGNOSIS AND OPTIONS FOR PREVENTION AND EARLY DETECTION

In 1993, the *NF2* gene was independently identified by two groups. It has 16 exons and its protein product showed significant homology to moesin, ezrin, radixinlike proteins, hence the name "merlin" (Trofatter et al., 1993). These proteins are involved with the association of actin filaments to plasma membrane proteins. The *NF2* gene product is essential for extraembryonic development in animal models (McClatchey et al., 1997).

Utilizing DGGE and SSCP techniques (see Chapter 7), about 50 mutations of *NF2* were initially described (Thomas et al., 1994). Only 4 of these were missense mutations, with the remainder being large deletions or other mutations leading to a truncated protein. An analysis of 47 patients from 21 families associated nonsense and

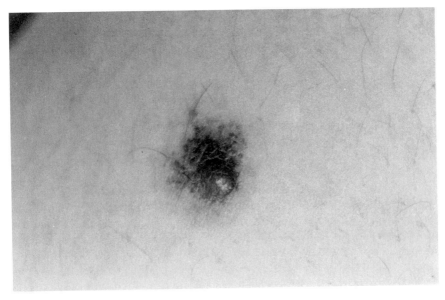

FIGURE 5-5 *An NF2 plaque.*

frameshift mutations with a younger age of onset and a greater number of tumors (Parry et al., 1996). Analysis of 59 unrelated NF2 patients in another series correlated frameshift and nonsense mutations with a severe phenotype (defined as two or more intracranial tumors or more than four spinal tumors). Missense mutations were found in both severe and mild forms of the disease (Kluwe et al., 1996). Because of the smaller size of the *NF2* gene, diagnostic screening for mutations is easier than for *NF1*. Because of the rarity of the syndrome, however, commercial availability of DNA testing is limited. Linkage analysis remains the method choice in many families.

Management of the NF2 patient is surgical and is best performed in large centers by experienced neurosurgeons and otolaryngologists. A multidisciplinary approach to the management of the deafness and other medical and emotional complications in these patients has been emphasized (Evans et al., 1993). Stereotactic radiosurgery (gamma knife) has been offered as a surgical alternative. Primary radiotherapy may actually induce tumors and is not generally recommended (reviewed in Guttman et al., 1997). Prior to genetic diagnosis, MRI scans with gadolinium enhancement were recommended at regular intervals between ages 10 and 40, with annual auditory brainstem

Case Example 5.6. A 10-year-old boy was scheduled for surgery for bilateral vestibular schwannomas detected by MRI scan. The child had undergone evaluation for increasing hearing impairment. His parents, both aged 45, and his 19-year-old sister came for counseling. On examination, he had several 1-cm raised lesions with hairs growing from them.

This case illustrates the variable age at onset for neurofibromatosis type 2. The diagnosis in the child was evident, and evaluation was completed with an axial MRI, which revealed abnormalities in the dorsal spine consistent with meningiomas. Suggested evaluation of the sister included cranio-axial MRI, brainstem auditory evoked potentials, ophthalmology evaluation for cataracts, and detailed skin examination. Identification of a germline mutation of the *NF2* gene (Merlin) was presented to the family as a potentially useful test for the sister, who could be spared the intrusion of the surveillance examinations if no mutation were found. Genetic testing of both parents was also offered, although it was indicated that most heterozygotes would have shown some signs of the disease by age 40. The possibilities of a new mutation or gonadal mosaicism (see Chapter 2) were discussed with the parents. A frameshift mutation of *NF2* was detected in the boy, consistent with the severe phenotype.

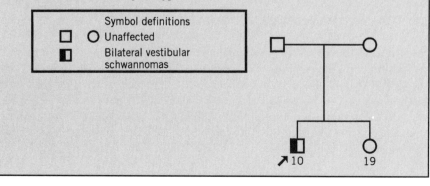

evoked responses. Genetic testing can now be considered at an early age, with a negative genetic test in an offspring of a family with a known mutation precluding the need for special surveillance.

REFERENCES: PART D—NF2

Evans DG, Huson SM, Donnai D et al. 1992a. A genetic study of type 2 neurofibromatosis in the United Kingdom. I. Prevalence, mutation rate, fitness and confirmation of maternal transmission effect on severity. J Med Genet 29:841–6.

Evans DG, Huson SM, Donnai D et al. 1992b. A clinical study of type 2 neurofibromatosis. Quart J Med 84:603–18.

Evans DG, Huson SM, Donnai D et al. 1992c. A genetic study of type 2 neurofibromatosis in the United Kingdom. II. Guidelines for genetic counseling. J Med Genet 29:847–52.

Evans DG, Ramsden R, Huson SM et al. 1993. Type 2 neurofibromatosis: the need for supraregional care? J Laryngol Otolaryngol 107:401–6.

Guttman DG, Aylsworth A, Carey JC et al. 1997. The diagnostic evaluation and multidisciplinary management of neurofibromatosis 1 and neurofibromatosis 2. JAMA 276:51–65.

Kluwe L, Bayer S, Baser ME, Hazim W, Haase W, Funsterer C, Mautner VE. 1996. Comparison of NF2 germ-line mutations with neurofibromatosis 2 phenotypes. Amer J Hum Genet 59:526 (abstract).

McClatchey AI, Saotome I, Ramesh V, Gusella JF, Jacks T. 1997. The NF2 tumor suppressor gene product is essential for extra embryonic development immediately prior to gastrulation. Genes and Devel 11:1253–65.

Parry DM, MacCollin MM, Kaiser-Kupfer MI et al. 1996. Germ-line mutations in the neurofibromatosis 2 gene: correlations with disease severity and retinal abnormalities. Am J Hum Genet 59:529–39.

Thomas G, Merel P, Sanson M et al. 1994. Neurofibromatosis type 2. Eur J Cancer 30A:1981–7.

Trofatter JA, MacCollin MM, Rutter JL et al. 1993. A novel moesin-, ezrin-, radixin-like gene is a candidate for the neurofibromatosis 2 tumor suppressor. Cell 72:791–800.

PART E: NEVOID BASAL CELL CARCINOMA SYNDROME

CLINICAL AND PATHOLOGIC FEATURES

Basal cell carcinomas are the most common malignancy in humans, with three quarters of a million cases occurring each year. Most of these are sporadic tumors in sun-exposed areas of middle-aged or older individuals. In a small subset of families, basal cell carcinomas occur at early age and in great numbers. The nevoid basal cell carcinoma (NBCC) syndrome is quite rare (1 in 70,000). It consists of multiple basal cell carcinomas, usually presenting after puberty, accompanied by odontogenic jaw cysts, congenital skeletal abnormalities, ectopic calcification of the falx cerebri, and characteristic "pits" in the skin of the palms and soles (Gorlin and Goltz, 1960). Only about

50% of patients 20 years of age or older were affected by basal cell carcinomas. In his review of 53 cases in 1987, Gorlin defined the cardinal features of the syndrome that bears his name (Gorlin, 1987). (The author added in a footnote that he was "personally opposed to eponyms since they say nothing about the disorder . . . and may be chauvinistic.")

In his original description of the syndrome, Gorlin warned clinicians not to be frustrated by the difficulty in establishing the diagnosis because of variability in expressivity. For example, such features as medulloblastoma, meningioma, short fourth metacarpal, cleft lip and/or palate, congenital cataract, glaucoma, coloboma, and cardiac fibroma were observed in 10% or less of cases. The diagnosis may be suspected at birth in any infant with an enlarged head circumference and a family history of the disorder. Because a significant proportion of cases are new mutations, the diagnosis of NBCC syndrome often have to be made without benefit of the family history, based solely on the constellation of findings.

One of the hallmarks of the syndrome is the increased susceptibility of the skin to the damaging and tumor-inducing effects of ionizing radiation (Strong, 1977). Multiple basal cell carcinomas have developed within 6–36 months following radiation therapy. Unlike Bloom syndrome or ataxia telangiectasia, there is no *in vitro* evidence of chromosome fragility.

GENETIC DIAGNOSIS AND OPTIONS FOR TREATMENT AND PREVENTION

Linkage analysis of 137 individuals from 8 multiplex families followed at the National Institutes of Health localized the NBCC gene to band 9q22.3-9q31. Maximal lod scores were in the range of 3–6, with three linked markers showing no significant recombination. This allowed localization of the gene to a 10 cM region. Inherited as a dominant trait, NBCC syndrome is almost completely penetrant (Gailani et al., 1992). Previously, loss of heterozygosity at 9q22-31 had been demonstrated in basal cell cancers, suggesting that the NBCC gene acts as a tumor suppressor along the model of Knudson.

In 1996, Johnson and coworkers found mutations in exon 15 of the human homolog of the Drosophila *patched* gene (called *PTH* or *PTCH)* in two of 60 typical NBCC kindreds. One kindred had a 9 base pair duplication (2445ins9) and the other an 11 base pair deletion (2442del11). In addition, an exon 3 missense mutation was found in 1 of 12 sporadic basal cell carcinomas, and not in the germline of this individual, suggesting that mutations of *PTCH* could also occur as a tumor-related change (Johnson et al., 1996). Overexpression of *PTCH* mRNA was confirmed in both sporadic and hereditary basal cell carcinomas (Unden et al., 1997), and somatic mutations of *PTCH* were observed at low frequency in a variety of extracutaneous tumors (Xie et al., 1997). An analysis of 71 unrelated individuals with NBCCS revealed 26 with mutations scattered throughout the 23 exons of the gene. In 86% the mutations caused a truncated protein. There was no evidence of genotype–phenotype associations; three families with the same mutation (244delCT) had variable phenotypes (Wicking et al., 1997). Further studies will resolve the sensitivity of the SSCP and sequencing techniques that have been used to find *PTCH* mutations in these studies. The existence of a significant number of NBCC families in which *PTCH* mutations have not been detected suggests that routine DNA diagnosis of the syndrome is yet at hand.

A multidisciplinary approach to the evaluation of NBCC kindreds has been employed (Evans et al., 1993). Workup of members of NBCC kindreds should include, in addition to skin examination and measurement of head circumference, radiographic examination of the skull, spine, ribs, and jaws. In addition, ophthalmologic and dental examination and radiographic monitoring of the jaw cysts (oropantomography) may be performed on affected individuals. MRI scans of at-risk children is a means to diagnose medulloblastomas, although it is unclear if this will improve outcome. If no physical or radiographic stigmata are noted by 5 years of age in the child of an affected patient, the chances that the child is a heterozygote are minimal.

Options for primary prevention are limited. Sunscreens and limitation of sun exposure can be recommended, although it is not clear that there is an association between the numbers of basal cell carcinomas in NBCC kindreds and sun exposure (Goldstein et al., 1993).

In affected individuals, the treatment of the jaw cysts is surgical enucleation; how-

---

Case Example 5.7. A 26-year-old woman was referred for counseling prior to radiation therapy for a large basal cell tumor near the pinna of the ear. The patient gave a history of multiple basal cell carcinomas and removal of a "jaw cyst" when she was a child. On examination, she demonstrated multiple small pits in the skin of her palms. Her family history was significant for relatives with basal cell carcinomas.

The diagnosis of nevoid basal cell carcinoma syndrome was suggested by the clinical presentation. Additional workup included radiographic examination of the jaw, skull, spine, and hands (to detect phalangeal pseudocysts). It was suggested that radiotherapy was not the option of choice for the basal cell carcinomas, given the radiation sensitivity demonstrated in this condition. A plastic surgeon was able to perform the resection. Genetic diagnosis may be undertaken on a research basis following the identification of mutations of the gene *PTCH* in some NBCC families.

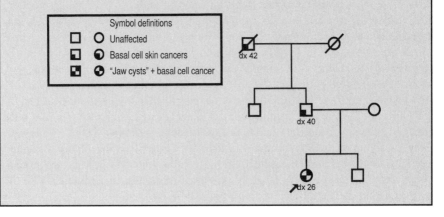

ever recurrence rates are high. Similarly, the basal skin cancers may be present in extremely high number, and sometimes may require treatment with topical chemotherapy in addition to local surgery or cryotherapy. The psychological sequelae of disfigurement and continual outpatient visits to multiple specialists are real burdens for members of NBCC kindreds. The existence of a well-organized NBCC support group is a valuable resource for patients and clinicians.

REFERENCES: PART E

Evans DGR, Ladusans EJ, Rimmer S et al. 1993. Complications of the naevoid basal cell carcinoma syndrome: results of a population based study. J Med Genet 30:460–4.

Gailani MR, Bale SJ, Leffell DJ et al. 1992. Developmental defects in Gorlin syndrome related to a putative tumor suppressor gene on chromosome 9. Cell 69:111–17.

Goldstein AM, Bale SJ, Peck GL, DiGiovanna JJ. 1993. Sun exposure and basal cell carcinomas in the nevoid basal cell carcinoma syndrome. J Am Acad Dermatol 29:34–41.

Gorlin RJ, Goltz RW. 1960. Multiple nevoid basal-cell epithelioma, jaw cysts and bifid rib syndrome. New Engl J Med 262:908–12.

Gorlin RJ. 1987. Nevoid basal-cell carcinoma syndrome. Medicine 66:98–113.

Johnson RL, Rothman AL, Xie J et al. 1996. Human homolog of patched, a candidate gene for the basal cell nevus syndrome. Science 272:1668–71.

Strong LC. 1977. Genetic and environmental interactions. Cancer 40:1861–6.

Unden AB, Zaphiropoulos PG, Bruce K, Toftgard R, Stahle-Backdahl M. 1997. Human *patched (PTCH)* mRNA is overexpressed consistently in tumor cells of both familial and sporadic basal cell carcinoma. Cancer Res 57:2336–40.

Wicking C, Shanley S, Smyth I et al. 1997. Most germ-line mutations in the nevoid basal cell carcinoma syndrome lead to a premature termination of the PATCHED protein, and no genotype-phenotype correlations are evident. Amer J Hum Genet 60:21–26.

Xie J, Johnson R, Zhang X et al. 1997. Mutations of the PATCHED gene in several types of sporadic extracutaneous tumors. Cancer Res 57:2369–72.

PART F: RETINOBLASTOMA

CLINICAL AND PATHOLOGIC FEATURES

Although it is the most common tumor of the eye in children, retinoblastoma (RB) accounts for only 1% of pediatric malignancies. About 200 cases are diagnosed each year and, of these, 20 will be associated with a family history of the disease. Of the remaining 180 tumors, 40–50 (25%) will be bilateral and are presumed to be heritable. Of the 130–140 unilateral tumors, an additional 10% will be heritable, with the remainder sporadic. Overall, this translates to about 70 heritable retinoblastomas of 200 diagnosed each year.

The tumor is generally diagnosed before the age of 4 years, with the median age of diagnosis at a year and a half. Unilateral tumors present around 2 years of age, whereas bilateral tumors are diagnosed at a median age of 8 months. Affected children present with strabismus, visual abnormalities, or leukocoria ("white eye"), in which the pupil appears whitish instead of black. Most tumors are restricted to the eye and orbit, although the tumor can gain access to the meninges via the optic nerve. A number of staging systems, based on size or extent of tumor involvement, have been developed. In general, patients with limited disease can be treated with cryotherapy or photocoagulation, whereas patients with advanced disease require enucleation and radiation therapy. Patients with bilateral disease are also usually treated with radiation therapy in an attempt to preserve vision. In hereditary cases, where there is a known risk of bilateral disease, it is usually possible to preserve both eyes. The critical importance of early diagnosis is a strong justification to offer genetic counseling to all affected patients (Gallie et al., 1991).

GENETIC DIAGNOSIS AND OPTIONS FOR EARLY DETECTION AND PREVENTION

In 1971, based on the observation of an earlier age of onset in heritable retinoblastomas, Knudson derived the two-hit model of tumorigenesis (see Chapter 3). The observation of deletions of chromosome 13q14 in retinoblastoma tumors was consistent with the loss of one allele in the Knudson model. The detection of homozygous deletions in two RB tumors led to the identification of an anonymous DNA fragment from 13q14 that localized to the region of deletion. These studies led to the molecular cloning of the RB gene *(RB1)* and the identification of germline mutations of the gene in lymphocytes of a child with bilateral disease (Friend et al., 1986).

RB1 spans 27 exons and 180 kb of genomic DNA. This large size and the lack of hotspots in the more than 100 known mutations, complicate routine analysis. About 5% of RB patients have cytogenetically visible deletions in peripheral lymphocytes. Approximately 20% of RB tumors reveal rearrangements by Southern analysis. A variety of techniques, including isotopic and nonisotopic SSCP, DGGE, and heteroduplex analysis can serve as useful screens for mutations. Direct sequencing remains the gold standard, although this will not detect mutations in promotor regions, splice sites, etc. Availability of tumor-derived RNA greatly facilitates mutation detection because it allows screening of 3000 bp of coding transcript, rather than studying the 27 exons of genomic DNA. These mutations can be screened for in the germline to establish if a case is truly hereditary. In many cases, however, tumor material is not available for analysis, and this constitutes a significant barrier to the widespread clinical utilization of predictive *RB1* testing.

A survey of germline mutations in 119 patients with bilateral or hereditary retinoblastoma revealed germline mutations in 99 (83%). These included large deletions, small length alterations, and base substitutions. There was no correlation between location of frameshift or nonsense mutations and phenotypic features, including age at diagnosis, number of tumor foci, or occurrence of secondary neoplasms (Lohmann, 1996). Missense mutations affecting *RB1*, which are much less common, appear to cluster around exon 20. These mutations have often been associated with a

Case Example 5.8. A 20-year-old woman came for counseling because of a history of retinoblastoma. Her own history was notable for curative treatment for bilateral retinoblastoma at 4 months of age. She desired to learn of options for genetic testing and risks to potential offspring. Although her father was not affected, her paternal grandfather had retinoblastoma at age 7 years. An extended family history revealed that distant paternal relatives also had retinoblastoma.

This unusual pedigree illustrates a putative "low penetrance" *RB1* mutation. Missense mutations in exon 20 of the gene have been associated with pedigrees similar to this one. Testing for *RB1* mutations was discussed as a means to preclude medical screening, which would involve retinal examinations under general anesthesia for the probands' future children. The proband was also counseled regarding her own risks for secondary cancers (see text) and was offered participation in a research surveillance study.

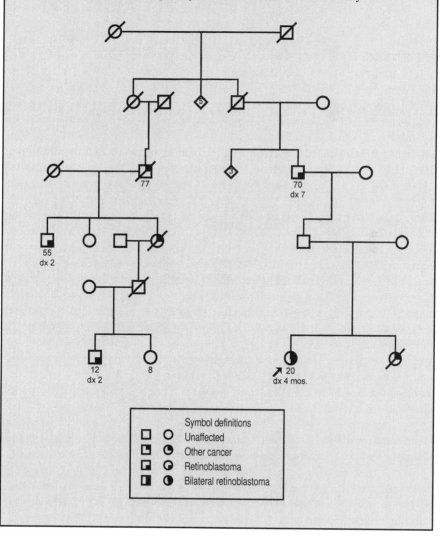

Symbol definitions

□	○	Unaffected
◧	◔	Other cancer
⊡	◑	Retinoblastoma
■	◐	Bilateral retinoblastoma

lower penetrance variant of the syndrome, characterized by unilateral tumors, or regressed tumors (Yandell et al., 1991). One mutation associated with this subset, arg881trp, has been repeatedly seen. In these families, unilateral tumors and unaffected gene carriers have been observed. A "low penetrance" family has also been associated with deletions of exons 24 and 25 of *RB1* (Bremner et al., 1997). Recent series have documented germline *RB1* mutations in up to 17% of unilateral cases (reviewed in Gallie, 1997) and germline mosaicism in several families with mutations (Sippel et al., 1997).

In the absence of genetic markers, counselors have had to rely on empiric risks. Such estimations are affected by the small proportion of hereditary unilateral cases which will be missed even by careful pedigree documentation. In the setting of a child with unilateral retinoblastoma, parents have been counseled that the recurrence risk to the second child was 1%. This increased to 2–6% if the first child had bilateral disease. In clearly hereditary cases, the risk was cited as 50%. This decreases to 45% if the assumption of 90% penetrance is taken into account (Draper et al., 1992). Genetic diagnosis can serve as a critical resource in the counseling of these families.

Within a short time of the identification of *RB1*, presymptomatic diagnosis was performed on 19 kindreds (Wiggs et al., 1988). Molecular screening was carried out utilizing polymorphic markers within the gene. DNA diagnosis offers the advantage of more precisely refining cancer risk. In the event that a child of an affected parent tests negatively, an enormous saving in cost as well as medical risk will result from the cancellation of the routine examinations under general anesthesia that these children require. As an example, the 3-year cost for conventional screening for seven at-risk relatives was over $25,000, compared to about $7,000 for screening utilizing mutation detection (Noorani et al., 1996). In the setting of a positive test, early diagnosis can lead to treatments that preserve the eyes.

Early diagnosis at the time of detecting a mutation generally calls for a rigorous set of ophthalmologic exams. One schedule of surveillance consists of retinal examination at birth and monthly for 3 months when an examination under general anaesthesia is performed. These examinations are continued every 3 months, until age 2, every 4 months until age 3, then examination without anesthesia every 6 months until age 5, and every 12 months until age 11. Physical examinations through the teen years should be focused on possible manifestations of secondary tumors, particularly sarcomas.

The detection of germline *RB1* mutations increases the vigilance for second primary tumors. In these patients the risk can approach 26% with occurrence from 1 to 40 years posttreatment (Sanders et al., 1989; Eng et al., 1993). The tumors include osteosarcoma and other types of sarcoma, malignant melanoma, brain tumors, and possibly other common tumors such as breast cancer or leukemia. Osteosarcomas in a patient who has received radiation therapy can present outside of the radiation field of the primary tumor, with the femur a common site. Surveillance for the osteosarcomas with bone scans has been suggested, but may itself increase cancer risk. It is also observed that children treated with radiation therapy for their primary tumor(s) had the highest risk for a second tumor. In a follow-up of 1458 patients, the cumulative mortality from second neoplasms at 40 years of follow-up was over 30% in the radiotherapy group compared to 6% in the group that did not receive radiotherapy (Eng et al., 1993). These findings have added to the rationale for reserving radiation treatment only for those cases when it is necessary to preserve vision. In addition, radiation therapy, especially in the infant, causes cosmetic deformity. In newborns, chemotherapy with vincristine or teniposide has been used to shrink tumors to make the tumor more amenable to cryotherapy or photocoagulaton.

In addition to soft-tissue sarcomas and osteosarcomas, adult-onset lipomas have also been observed at increased frequency in survivors of hereditary retinoblastoma. The detection of lipomas in these patients may predict the occurrence of other secondary tumors (Li et al., 1997).

The detection of *RB1* mutations in utero is possible; it has been carried out successfully with chorionic villous sampling and amniocentesis (Onadim et al., 1992b). If found, mutation detection in the fetus can lead to earlier delivery and a better chance at curative therapy. However, this is not fail-safe since at least one newborn with metastatic retinoblastoma has been reported. Another option is therapeutic termination of the pregnancy. This option raises ethical issues (see Chapter 9) which have led to the limited utilization of prenatal diagnosis of RB in some centers.

Despite the technical feasibility of testing for *RB1* mutations, clinical utilization of DNA diagnosis has largely been confined to research studies. This has been due to various factors including limited commercial availability of mutation testing, high cost and complexity of tests, uncertain negative predictive value for differing testing methodologies, requirement for tumor-derived DNA, and lack of perceived benefit for many patients. Increasing availability and demonstrated cost benefit of *RB1* testing (Noorani et al., 1996) should lead to the better integration of *RB1* testing into clinical management of affected families (Gallie, 1997).

REFERENCES: PART F

Bremner R, Du D, Connolly-Wilson MJ et al. 1997. Deletion of *RB* exons 24 and 25 causes low penetrance retinoblastoma. Amer J Hum Genet 61:556–70.

Draper GJ, Sanders BM, Brownbill PA, Hawkins MM. 1992. Patterns of risk of hereditary retinoblastoma and applications to genetic counseling. Br J Cancer 66:211–9.

Eng C, Li FP, Abramson DH et al. 1993. Mortality from second tumors among long-term survivors of retinoblastoma. J Natl Cancer Inst 1993; 85:1121–8.

Friend SH et al. 1986. A human DNA segment with properties of the gene that predisposes to retinoblastoma and osteosarcoma. Nature 323:643–6.

Gallie BL. 1997. Predictive testing for retinoblastoma comes of age. Amer J Hum Genet 61: 279–81.

Knudson AG. Jr. 1971. Mutation and cancer: statistical study of retinoblastoma. Proc Natl Acad Sci 68:820–3.

Li FP, Abramson DH, Tarone RE, Kleinerman RA, Fraumeni JF Jr., Boice JD Jr. 1997. Hereditary retinoblastoma, lipoma, and second primary cancers. J Natl Cancer Inst 89:83–4.

Lohmann DR, Brandt B, Hopping W, Passarge E, Horsthemke B. 1996. The spectrum of *RB1* germ-line mutations in hereditary retinoblastoma. Amer J Hum Genet 58:940–9.

Noorani HZ, Khan HN, Gallie BL, Detsky AS. 1996. Cost comparison of molecular versus conventional screening of relatives at risk for retinoblastoma. Am J Hum Genet 1996; 59:301–7.

Onadim Z, Hungerford J, Cowell JK. 1992. Follow-up of retinoblastoma patients having prenatal and perinatal predictions for mutant gene carrier status using intragenic polymorphic probes from the *RB1* gene. Br J Cancer 65:711–6.

Sanders BM, Jay M, Draper CJ, Roberts EM. 1989. Non-ocular cancer in relatives of retinoblastoma patients. Br J Cancer 60:358–65.

Sippel DC, Fraioli RE, Smith GD et al. 1997. Frequent somatic and germline mosaicism in retinoblastoma. Am J Hum Genet 61:75 (abstr).

Wiggs J, Nordenskjöld M, Yandell D et al. 1988. Prediction of the risk of hereditary retinoblastoma, using DNA polymorphisms within the retinoblastoma gene. N Engl J Med 318:151–7.

Yandell DW, Herrera GE, Dayton SH, Dryja TP, Ludeke BI. 1991. Penetrance of RB mutations: two families with a low-penetrance form of hereditary retinoblastoma carry the same missense mutation. Am J Hum Genet 49:45.

PART G: VON HIPPEL-LINDAU SYNDROME AND OTHER HEREDITARY RENAL CELL CARCINOMA SYNDROMES

CLINICAL AND PATHOLOGIC FEATURES

Renal cell carcinomas are relatively rare in the United States, with about 30,000 cases occurring each year. Renal cell carcinomas comprise about 85% of kidney tumors, with the remainder consisting of transitional cell tumors of the renal pelvis and nephroblastoma (Wilms' tumor) in children. The most important environmental association with renal cell carcinoma is cigarette smoking, which is thought to explain the preponderance of male cases. About 10% of the tumors are of papillary type, based on cell type and growth pattern. A large case control study by McLaughlin showed that about 2% of renal cell cancer patients had a family history of the disease (McLaughlin et al., 1984). The two common hereditary forms of renal cell carcinoma in adults are von Hippel-Lindau (VHL) syndrome and a hereditary syndrome of site-specific renal cell carcinoma (SSRC) (Maher et al., 1991a; 1991b). In rare instances, the hereditary tumors may be limited to the papillary type (Zbar et al., 1994).

VHL syndrome is an extremely rare hereditary syndrome associated with both cancer predisposition and a tendency to form cysts (Maher, 1994). Its incidence is probably less than 1 in 36,000. In 1926 Lindau associated retinal angiomas and cerebellar hemangiomas with visceral cysts. Although there are at least 25 manifestations of the syndrome, 6 are associated with the greatest clinical morbidity. These include the cerebellar, spinal, and medullary hemangioblastomas, retinal angiomas, renal cell carcinomas, and pheochromocytomas. Of these, the retinal and cerebellar lesions are the most common, seen in the majority of cases. They generally present at early age (25–30 years) with symptoms of visual abnormalities or occipital or frontal headaches. The hemangioblastomas may also present with symptoms of polycythemia.

Of tumors associated with VHL syndrome, the renal cell carcinomas are observed in about 25% of cases. The renal tumors present around age 45, compared to 62 years of age in the general population. These tumors commonly, but not always, appear in the presence of renal cysts. The majority of VHL patients will probably develop renal cell carcinoma if they survive the other manifestations of the syndrome. The renal tumors are frequently multifocal, bilateral, and recurrent. The pheochromocytomas are less common, observed in about 10% of cases, but also may be multifocal. As noted in the section on MEN2, the observation of familial pheochromocytoma should lead to the consideration of the diagnosis of VHL (Crossey et al., 1995; Woodward et al., 1997). Pancreatic tumors are also observed, but are much less common. The penetrance of the syndrome is high, with 90% of individuals affected by age 45 and 99% affected by age 65 (Maher et al., 1990; Maher, 1994). Tumors more rarely seen in VHL syndrome include meningiomas, testicular tumors, papillary adenocarcinomas of the endolymphatic sac (causing hearing loss), and lung cancers (reviewed in Decker et al., 1997). Endolymphatic sac tumors (ELSTs) may be more common than originally suspected. MRI scanning detected ELSTs in 13 of 121 (11%) VHL patients (Manski et al., 1997).

GENETIC DIAGNOSIS AND OPTIONS FOR EARLY DETECTION AND PREVENTION

In 1993, positional cloning strategies led to the identification of the *VHL* gene (Latif et al., 1993). As predicted by the Knudson model, a series of small (1 to 10 nucleotide) deletions causing frameshift mutations were noted in both sporadic renal cell tumors and in the germline DNA of VHL families. Neither the nucleotide nor the predicted amino acid sequences showed significant homology to known genes. The function, and even the location, of the *VHL* protein (PVHL) is not understood. Interestingly, it was shown that the nuclear localization of PVHL was determined by the degree of confluence of the cell in culture (Lee et al., 1996), with a region of nuclear localization identified that is not mutated in patients with VHL or in renal tumors. Although data on growth suppression by *VHL* have been contradictory, restoring *VHL* in a renal cancer cell line suppressed its tumorigenicity, consistent with the model of a tumor suppressor gene (Iliopoulos et al., 1995). Work by Klausner and colleagues indicated that the protein product of the *VHL* gene controlled transcription by binding to two components of a transcriptional elongation factor complex (Duan et al., 1995), which, in turn, bound a member of the "cullin" gene family (Pause et al., 1997). This is of interest because the cullins are involved in cell cycle regulation, and 70% of predisposing *VHL* mutations disrupt the PVHL-elongin-cullin interaction. The *VHL* protein also appears to play a role in angiogenesis, possibly related to the vascular nature of VHL cysts and tumors (summarized by Decker et al., 1997).

The *VHL* gene was also shown to be mutated in 56 of 98 sporadic nonpapillary renal tumors and 0 of 12 papillary cases (Gnarra et al., 1993).

The availability of a molecular diagnostic marker for VHL syndrome allows a more precise risk determination than the Mendelian estimates previously offered. Mutations appeared to be scattered across the three exons of this relatively small gene, with the first 300 nucleotides on the 5' end generally not affected (Figure 5-6). About 40% of

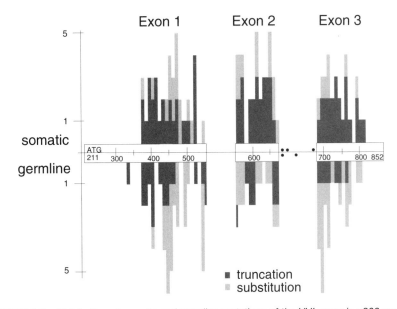

FIGURE 5-6 *Distribution of somatic and germline mutations of the VHL gene in >300 sporadic renal carcinomas (above) and >360 VHL kindreds (below). Germline mutations are more likely to be missense mutations affecting exons 1 and 3. No mutations have been observed in the 5' portion of exon 1. (Redrawn from Decker et al., 1997.)*

mutations resulted in a truncated protein, while the remainder were missense mutations (Decker et al., 1997). Genotype–phenotype correlations have been preliminary. Pheochromocytoma appeared to be more common in patients with missense mutations, compared to those with deletions, insertions, or nonsense mutations (Crossey et al., 1994). Over 250 mutations of the gene have been described (Decker et al., 1997). There does not appear to be a relationship between mutation type and disease severity, as measured by number of hemangioblastomas (Maher et al., 1996).

The sensitivity of available techniques for detection of *VHL* mutations has remained an issue. The sensitivity of Southern blot techniques (to detect rearrangements) combined with direct sequencing has been estimated to be only 65%. This figure has been improved to 90% by the addition of a Southern blot measurement for gene dosage (Stolle et al., 1996). In practice, some combination of PCR/SSCP/direct sequencing and Southern blot (to detect large deletions missed by PCR/SSCP) is recommended (Decker et al., 1997).

Molecular diagnosis of VHL has profound clinical consequences, because the surveillance for VHL syndrome is onerous. According to the Cambridge screening regimen suggested by Maher (Maher et al., 1990), screening for the at-risk relative should consist of annual physical exam, urine cytology, direct and indirect ophthalmologic exam from age 5, with fluorescein angioscopy or angiography from age 10 until age 60, MRI of the brain every 3 years from age 15 to 40, then every 5 years until age 60, annual renal ultrasound, abdominal CT every 3 years from age 20 to 65, and annual

Case Example 5.10. A 47-year-old man presented with a 6-month history of palpitations and headaches and high blood pressure refractory to calcium channel blockers and beta blockers. Urine studies showed elevated catecholamines and a CT revealed bilateral 6-cm adrenal masses. His past medical history was significant for retinal hemangioma in the right eye. His family history was significant for a father and aunt who died of adrenal tumors. His aunt also had retinal hemangiomas.

At surgery, bilateral pheochromocytomas were resected.

This case illustrates the presentation of familial pheochromocytoma, a described but atypical presentation of von Hippel-Lindau disease (Crossey et al., 1995). The major counseling issues in this case related to the patient's children, who required screening according to the Maher regimen (see text). Molecular diagnosis was offered to the family as a means of tailoring the children's screening regimens.

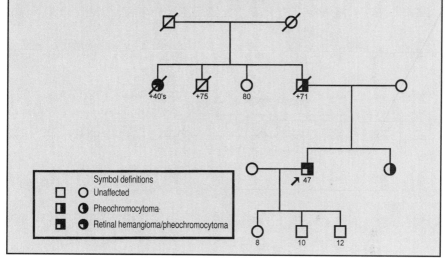

24-hour urine collection for VMA and metanephrine. These studies may be ordered more frequently, depending on symptoms and findings of previous examinations. Unfortunately, it may be extremely difficult to recover costs for these expensive radiographic procedures in the absence of a referable symptom.

When the renal tumors are diagnosed at an early stage, partial nephrectomy may preserve some renal function. Early surgery may also be curative for the other component tumors.

Although the majority of site-specific hereditary renal cell carcinomas (SSRC) did not carry constitutional chromosomal translocations (Kantor et al., 1982), a kindred with multiple SSRC in three generations was associated with a constitutional t(3;8)(p14;q24) (Cohen et al., 1979). Other translocations involving 3p13-4 have been observed in sporadic renal tumors. DNA analysis revealed loss of heterozygosity at 3p13-4 and 3p21, loci distinct from *VHL* at 3p25-6 (Yamakawa et al., 1991). Germline mutations of the *MET* proto-oncogene were detected in four of seven familes with

Case Example 5.11. A 49-year-old male sought counseling because of a family history of renal cell cancer. The family was enrolled in a research study with the goal of identifying a mutation of the *VHL* tumor suppressor gene. No mutations were detected, and linkage analysis was not informative. There were no constitutional chromosome abnormalities. During the past year, the proband's sister had been diagnosed with metastatic renal cell carcinoma at another institution. On review of the clinical materials, a hyperechoic area was noted on the sister's renal sonogram performed two years earlier. Based on this information, sonograms or CT scans were recommended for the consultand on a yearly basis. The insurance carrier informed the consultand that these procedures were "preventive" and would not be covered.

This example illustrates that many cases of familial renal cancer will not have a means for molecular diagnosis. Sonograms or CT scans are a logical screening measure because the prognosis for this tumor is stage dependent. In these and other circumstances, it may be necessary for the cancer genetics consultant to serve as the family's advocate in appealing insurance decisions.

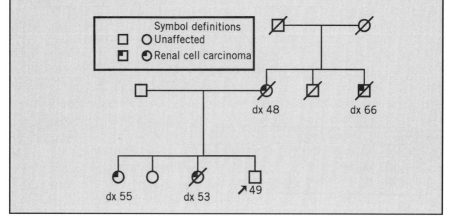

hereditary papillary renal carcinomas. Of interest, these mutations were in regions homologous to *C-KIT* and *RET*. Obligate heterozygotes were also affected by carcinomas of the breast, pancreas, and bile duct, as well as squamous cell carcinoma of the lung (Schmidt et al., 1997). In the absence of genetic markers for other kindreds with SSRC, counseling utilizing Mendelian principles and modifications of the screening regimens for VHL seem most prudent.

REFERENCES: PART G

Cohen AJ, Li FP, Berg S et al. 1979. Hereditary renal cell carcinoma associated with a chromosomal translocation. New Engl J Med 301:592–5.

Crossey PA, Richards FM, Foster K et al. 1994. Identification of intragenic mutations in the von Hippel-Lindau disease tumor suppressor gene and correlation with disease phenotype. Hum Molec Genet 3:1303–8.

Crossey PA, Eng C, Ginalska-Malinowska M et al. 1995. Molecular genetic diagnosis of von Hippel-Lindau disease in familial pheochromocytoma. J Med Genet 32:885-6.

Decker HJH, Weidt EJ, Brieger J. 1997. The von Hippel-Lindau tumor suppressor gene. Cancer Genet Cytogenet 93:74–83.

Duan DR, Pause A, Burgess WH et al. 1995. Inhibition of transcription elongation by the VHL tumor suppressor protein. Science 269:1402–6.

Gnarra JR, Glenn GM, Latif F et al. 1993. Molecular genetic studies of sporadic and familial renal cell carcinoma. Urol Clin N Amer 20(2):207–16.

Iliopoulos O, Kibel A, Gray S, Kaelin WG Jr. 1995. Tumour suppression by the human von Hippel-Lindau gene product. Nature Med 1:822–6.

Kantor AF, Blattner WA, Blot WJ et al.1982. Hereditary renal carcinoma and chromosomal defects. New Engl J Med 307:1403–4.

Latif F, Tory K, Gnarra J et al. 1993. Identification of the von Hippel-Lindau disease tumor suppressor gene. Science 260:1317–20.

Lee S, Chen DYT, Humphrey JS, Klausner RD. 1996. Nuclear/cytoplasmic localization of the von Hippel-Lindau tumor suppressor gene product is determined by cell density. Proc Natl Acad Sci 93:1770–5.

Maher ER, Yates JRW, Harries R et al. 1990. Clinical features and natural history of von Hippel-Lindau disease. Quart J Med. 77:1151–63.

Maher ER, Yates JRW. 1991a. Familial renal cell carcinoma: clinical and molecular genetic aspects. Br J Cancer 63:176–9.

Maher ER, Iselius L, Yates JRW et al. 1991b. Von Hippel-Lindau disease: a genetic study. J Med Genet 28:443–7.

Maher ER. 1994. Von Hippel-Lindau Disease. Eur J Cancer 30A (13):1987–90.

Maher ER, Webster AR, Woodward ER, Richards FM, Moore AT. 1996. Allelic heterogeneity and modifier effects determine expression in von Hippel-Lindau disease. Am J Hum Genet 59:394 (abstr).

Manski T, Heffner DK, Glenn GM et al. 1997. Endolymphatic sac tumors. A source of morbid hearing loss in von Hippel-Lindau disease. JAMA 277:1461–6.

Martz CH. 1992. von Hippel-Lindau Disease: a genetically transmitted multisystem neoplastic disorder. Sem in Onc Nursing 8:281–7.

McLaughlin JK, Mandel JS, Blot WJ, Schuman LM, Mehl ES, Fraumeni JF Jr. 1984. A population-based case-control study of renal cell carcinoma. J Natl Cancer Inst 72:275–84.

Pause A, Lee S, Worrell R et al.1997. The von Hippel-Lindau tumor suppressor gene product forms a stable complex with human CUL-2, a member of the Cdc53 family of proteins. Proc Natl Acad Sci 94:2156–61.

Schmidt L, Duh FM, Chen F et al. 1997. Germline and somatic mutations in the tyrosine kinase domain of the MET proto-oncogene in papillary renal carcinomas. Nature Genet 16:68–73.

Stolle CA, Spinner NB, Stump TS et al. 1996. Deletion of the entire *VHL* gene is a common mutation in patients with von Hippel-Lindau disease. Amer J Hum Genet 59:1658 (abstract).

Woodward ER, Eng C, McMahon R et al., Genetic predisposition to phaeochromocytoma: analysis of candidate genes GDNF, RET, and UHL. Hum Molec Genet 6:1051–6.

Yamakawa K, Morita R, Takahashi E et al. 1991. A detailed deletion mapping of the short arm of chromosome 3 in sporadic renal cell carcinoma. Cancer Res 51:4707–11.

Zbar B, Tory K, Merino M et al. 1994. Hereditary papillary renal cell carcinoma. J Urol 151:561–6.

PART H: WILMS' TUMOR SYNDROMES

CLINICAL AND PATHOLOGIC FEATURES

One child in 10,000 develops Wilms' tumor. This corresponds to approximately 450 cases a year in the United States (Breslow et al., 1993). Of these, only 4 or 5 cases will occur in the setting of a family history of the disease, usually in autosomal dominant fashion. About 30 of the 450 Wilms' tumors diagnosed each year in the United States will be bilateral. The median age of diagnosis is 39 months for patients with unilateral tumors and 26 months for the bilateral tumors.

Wilms' tumors are derived from metanephric blastema or mesenchymal renal stem cells. There is a characteristic triphasic histologic pattern of blastemal, epithelial, and stromal components. The tumors usually present as an asymptomatic mass, detected on a routine examination by the pediatrician or the parents when bathing the child. If localized at the time of surgical resection, the prognosis is excellent. In 15% of patients, metastatic disease is present at time of diagnosis and the outcome is less favorable. A series of national trials, combining surgery with adjuvant chemotherapy, and including radiation therapy for later stage disease, have led to an overall "cure" rate of 80% for this disease.

The bilateral Wilms' tumors are more commonly associated with a host of congenital abnormalities (Clericuzio et al., 1993). These include the *WAGR* syndrome in which the Wilms' tumors are accompanied by aniridia, genitourinary abnormalities, and mental retardation. Separate from WAGR is an association of Wilms' tumor and sporadic aniridia (absence of the iris), noted by Miller in 1964. For patients with sporadic aniridia, the risk of Wilms' tumor may be as high as 1 in 3. Wilms' tumor is also a component in the *Beckwith-Wiedemann syndrome* (BWS), an extremely rare (1 in 14,000) hereditary syndrome characterized by asymmetric organomegaly, often involving the tongue and abdominal viscera, umbilical hernia, and neonatal hypoglycemia. In this syndrome there is also a predisposition to adrenocortical carcinoma and hepatoblastoma (Sotelo-Avila et al., 1980). Although fitting a dominant pattern of inheritance, cases of transmitting males were noted to be rare in BWS, suggesting genomic imprinting.

Other rare Wilms' tumor syndromes include *Denys-Drash syndrome* (DDS), in which the tumors are accompanied by male pseudohermaphroditism and a progressive glomerulonephritis ending in renal failure. Even rarer is *Perlman syndrome,* a recessive disorder in which there are renal hamartomas, macrosomia, visceromegaly, and other associated congenital abnormalities.

GENETIC DIAGNOSIS AND OPTIONS FOR PREVENTION AND EARLY DETECTION

Although the various syndromes of Wilms' tumor predisposition are quite rare, they served as a model system for Knudson and Strong in their 1972 development of the two-hit hypothesis (see Chapter 3), and for Stanbridge and Saxon in their classic experiments supporting the notion of the tumor suppressor gene. In these experiments, the tumorigenicity of cultured Wilms' tumor cells was reversed by introducing normal copies of chromosome 11. As indicated above, there are very few extended pedigrees of familial Wilms' tumor that can serve to illustrate these models. The number of bilateral cases is greater than the proportion with a family history, suggesting that *de novo* germline mutations may occur.

The Wilms' tumor syndromes provide a vivid illustration of the principle of genetic heterogeneity. There appear to be at least four separate loci associated with the Wilms' tumor syndromes.

The identification of constitutional visible cytogenetic deletions at 11p13 in patients with WAGR and the demonstration of loss of heterozygosity at this same locus in Wilms' tumor specimens led to the narrowing of the region of a candidate gene. The ultimate cloning of *WT1* at 11p13 led to the description of a zinc finger-containing transcription factor with presumed function as a tumor-suppressor gene (Call et al., 1990; Gessler et al., 1990). *WT1* mutations were subsequently identified in the germline of rare families with WAGR as well as Denys-Drash syndrome, although the types of mutations appeared different.

In WAGR, the mutations of *WT1* were commonly deletions, with some presumably involving a contiguous aniridia gene. Whether the associated genitourinary abnormalities of WAGR were due to other contiguous genes or dominant negative effects remained unclear. In Denys-Drash syndrome, on the other hand, the mutations were commonly point mutations in the second or third zinc finger domain, resulting in amino acid substitutions or truncation of the protein (Figure 5-7). However, the most common mutation of Denys-Drash syndrome was observed in a patient with Wilms' tumor without the stigmata of Denys-Drash syndrome (Akasaka et al., 1993). Several models have been proposed to account for the spectrum of genotype–phenotype correlations observed in WAGR and Denys-Drash syndrome (Van Heyningen et al., 1990; Little et al., 1993).

A second Wilms' tumor susceptibility locus at 11p15 was implicated by loss of heterozygosity (LOH) studies of other Wilms' tumors and by demonstration of 11p15 linkage of familial BWS (Moutou et al., 1992). In a subset of Wilms' tumors, the 11p13 locus for *WT1* was not affected, suggesting the presence of an 11p15 tumor suppressor gene. In these cases the lost allele was of maternal derivation, suggesting a role for genetic imprinting. Analysis of children with BWS revealed cases of rearrangements and duplications of 11p15. These rearrangements resulted in increased "doses" of the paternal 11p15 locus. This occurred either by partial trisomy, with the duplicated chromosomal fragment derived from the father, or by uniparental disomy, in which both copies of chromosome 11 were shown to be paternal in origin by molecular analysis. A gene localized at 11p15, insulin-like growth factor 2 (*IGF2*), was known to be inactive (imprinted) on the maternal allele in humans. *IGF2* overexpression in BWS was proposed as a pathogenetic model (Ohlsson et al., 1993). The pattern of imprinting for *IGF2* is opposite that for other candidate genes in the region, however, suggesting that contiguous genes may be involved in the syndrome.

Familial Wilms' tumor is characterized by early onset, bilateral presentation, and

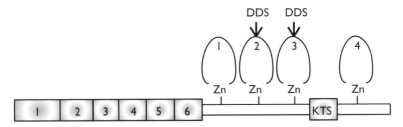

FIGURE 5-7 *Mutations in the WT1 gene. In WAGR syndrome most mutations are deletions. In Denys-Drash syndrome (DDS) mutations are commonly point mutations in the second or third zinc finger domains, as shown, resulting in amino acid substitutions or truncation of the protein. "KTS" is an alternative splice site between the third and fourth zinc fingers.*

absence of congenital abnormalities. In three families with true dominant transmission of Wilms' tumor, it was not possible to demonstrate linkage to either of the two loci on chromosome 11, and a locus on chromosome 16 was implicated (Huff et al., 1988). Although linkage to 16q has not been demonstrated in families, linkage to a novel Wilms' tumor susceptibility locus on chromosome 17q12-21 was demonstrated in a large Canadian family (Rahman et al., 1996). Interestingly, loss of heterozygosity at this locus was not observed in 13 tumors studied. In those rare families with familial WAGR or Denys-Drash syndrome, molecular diagnosis based on *WT1* mutations can be utilized to inform risk counseling. Most familial Wilms' tumors, however, are not associated with *WT1* mutations. Analysis of six WT pedigrees failed to reveal linkage to either *WT1* or 17q12-21, suggesting genetic heterogeneity (Huff et al., 1997).

In practice, genetic counseling is prompted by the identification of sporadic cases with associated anomalies, or bilateral or multifocal Wilms' tumors. In the presence of any of the syndromic manifestations in which there are congenital abnormalities associated with susceptibility to Wilms' tumor (e.g., aniridia), a surveillance schedule should be set in place. As with von Hippel-Lindau syndrome, and most of the screening recommendations for cancer predisposition syndromes, there is presumed but unproven efficacy for these strategies. One approach to Wilms' tumor susceptibility is renal imaging, either by ultrasound, CT, or MRI on a frequent basis (e.g., every few months) during the period of greatest risk (birth to age 5–8) and then less frequently thereafter. It is unclear if true "downstaging" can be accomplished by such screening (Green et al., 1993). In BWS, there should also be screening for the other related neoplasms, including serum alpha-feto protein for the associated hepatomas.

Unlike the risk in hereditary retinoblastoma, the risk for secondary neoplasms after Wilms' tumor does not appear to be particularly high (Hawkins et al., 1987). Radiotherapy may be implicated in many of the cases reported. However, a case of secondary leukemia with mutated *WT1* has been reported in a WAGR survivor (Pritchard-Jones et al., 1994); and four cases of pleural mesothelioma have also been observed in the same setting (Austin et al., 1986).

REFERENCES: PART H

Akasaka Y, Kikuchi H, Nigai T et al. 1993. A point mutation found in the *WT1* gene in a sporadic Wilms' tumor without genitourinary abnormalities is identical with the most frequent point mutation in Denys-Drash syndrome. FEBS Lett 317:39–43.

Austin MB, Fechner RE, Roggli VL. 1986. Pleural malignant mesothelioma following Wilms' tumor. Am J Clin Path 86:227–30.

Breslow N, Olshan A, Beckwith JB et al. 1993. Epidemiology of Wilms' tumor. Med Pediatr Oncol 21:172–81.

Call KM, Glaser T, Ito CY et al. 1990. Isolation and characterization of a zinc-finger polypeptide gene at the human chromosome 11 Wilms' tumour locus. Cell 60:509–20.

Clericuzio CL. 1993. Clinical phenotypes and Wilms' tumor. Med Pediatr Oncol 21:182–7.

Gessler M, Poustka A, Cavenee W et al. 1990. Homozygous deletion in Wilms' tumors of a zinc finger gene identified by chromosome jumping. Nature 343:774–8.

Green DM, Breslow NE, Beckwith JB et al. 1993. Screening of children with hemihypertrophy, aniridia and Beckwith-Wiedemann syndrome in patients with Wilms' tumor: a report from the national Wilms' Tumor Study. Med Pediatr Oncol 21:188–92.

Hawkins M, Draper G, Kingston J. 1987. Incidence of second primary tumours among childhood cancer survivors. Br J Cancer 56:339–47.

Huff V, Compton DA, Chao LY et al. 1988. Lack of linkage of familial Wilms' tumor to chromosomal band 11p13. Nature 336:377–8.

Huff, V, Amos C, Douglass EC et al. 1997. Evidence for genetic heterogeneity in familial Wilms' tumor. Cancer Res 57:1859–62.

Knudson AG Jr, Strong LC. 1972. Mutation and cancer: a model for Wilms' tumor of the kidney. J Natl Cancer Inst 48:313–24.

Little MH, Williamson KA, Mannens M et al. 1993. Evidence that *WT1* mutations in Denys-Drash syndrome patients may act in a dominant-negative fashion. Hum Mol Genet 2:259, 264.

Moutou C, Junien C, Henry I et al. 1992. Beckwith-Wiedemann syndrome: a demonstration of the mechanisms responsible for the excess of transmitting females. J Med Genet 29:217–20.

Ohlsson R, Nystrom A, Pfeifer-Ohlsson S et al. 1993. IGF2 is parentally imprinted during human embryogenesis and in the Beckwith-Wiedemann syndrome. Nature Genet 4:94–7.

Pelletier J, Bruening W, Kashtan CE et al. 1991. Germline mutations in the Wilms' tumor suppressor gene are associated with abnormal urogenital development in Denys-Drash syndrome. Cell 67:437–47

Pritchard-Jones K, Renshaw J, King-Underwood L. 1994. The Wilms' tumor (*WT1*) gene is mutated in a secondary leukemia in a WAGR patient. Hum Molec Genet 3:1633–7.

Rahman N, Arbour L, Tonin P et al. 1996. Evidence for a familial Wilms' tumor gene (*FWT1*) on chromosome 17q12-21. Nature Genet 13:461–2.

Sotelo-Avila C, Gonzolez-Crussi F, Fowler JW. 1980. Complete and incomplete forms of Beckwith-Wiedemann syndrome: their oncogenic potential. J Pediatr 96:47–50.

van Heyningen V, Bickmore WA, Seawright A et al. 1990. Role for the Wilms' tumor gene in genital development? Proc Natl Acad Sci 87:5383–6.

PART I: OTHER FAMILIAL CANCERS

In addition to the syndromes discussed in Chapter 4 and the first part of this chapter, there are cancer predisposition syndromes that have not yet been fully characterized. In some cases, the familial clustering of cancers has been observed for centuries (e.g. familial gastric cancer) while in other cases registries have recently been established to allow future studies (e.g. familial gliomas, pancreatic carcinomas). In contrast to the syndromes described in the remainder of this chapter, there are rarer syndromes in which cancers may occur, but may not be the predominant features. These syndromes are included in Appendix A.

BLADDER CANCER

In 1967, Joseph F. Fraumeni, Jr. and Louis B. Thomas reported a kindred in which a 57 year old man and his three sons were each affected by bladder cancer (Fraumeni and Thomas, 1967). In an effort to document an environmental sensitivity, metabolites of tryptophan were measured in the urine. Levels were normal. All four men were smokers. Subsequent reports documented another family with 6 cases in two generations (McCullough et al., 1975). A review of the literature in 1981 revealed 5 familial bladder cancer clusters (Mahboubi et al., 1981). An epidemiologic analysis of 2,982 bladder cancer cases and 5,782 controls confirmed a relative risk of 1.45 for individuals with a family history of bladder cancer (Kantor et al., 1985). Because of its links to occupational exposures, a number of genes involved in xenobiotic metabolism have been implicated as potential markers for risk of bladder cancer. These include the "slow acetylator" phenotype, *CYP2D6* (debrisoquine hydroxylase), *NAT1,* and *NAT2* (see Table 2-6, and review by d'Errico et al., 1996).

With the possible exception of hereditary retinoblastoma (Sanders et al., 1989), bladder cancer is not a component in hereditary cancer syndromes (Appendix A). When encountered in a pedigree, it is important to look for occupational exposures (see the third case example in Chapter 2). At-risk individuals can be screened with urine cytologies, or entered into trials utilizing PCR-based molecular markers (see Table 8-3).

REFERENCES

d'Errico A, Taioli E, Xiang C, Vineis P. 1996. Genetic metabolic polymorphisms and the risk of cancer: a review of the literature. Biomarkers 1:149–73.

Fraumeni JF, Jr, Thomas LB. 1967. Malignant bladder tumors in a family. JAMA 201:507–9.

Kantor AF, Hartge P, Hoover RN, Fraumeni JF. 1985. Familial and environmental interactions in bladder cancer risk. Int J Cancer 35:703–6.

Mahboubi AO, Ahlvin RC, Mahboubi EO. 1981. Familial aggregation of urothelial cell carcinoma. J Urol 126:691–2.

McCullough DL, Lamm DL, McLoughlin AP, Gittes RF. 1975. Familial transitional cell carcinoma of the bladder. J Urol 113:629–35.

Sanders BM, Jay M, Draper CJ, Roberts EM. 1989. Non-ocular cancer in relatives of retinoblastoma patients. Br J Cancer 60:358–65.

BRAIN TUMORS

A registry of families with two or more first degree relatives, or a single spouse pair affected by brain tumors, has been established at the John Hopkins University (Grossman et al., 1995). The registry excludes acoustic neuromas and meningiomas, and includes 127 cases from 59 families. The registry includes 30 parent-child pairs, 27 sib pairs, and 9 husband-wife pairs. Multiple generations are not affected, and cases tend to be diagnosed within two years of one another, suggesting an environmental etiology. The most common histology is high grade astrocytoma, although all types of gliomas have been observed. Subsequent reports have documented 2 cases of triple primary tumors, including glioblastoma (Nagane et al., 1996), four siblings with glioblastoma multiforme (Dirven et al., 1995), and three cases of medulloblastoma in two generations (Offit, unpublished).

Of 22 adult gliomas, somatic *p53* mutations were found in 8 cases, and germline mutations in 2 cases, both less than 35 years of age (Chen et al., 1995). In another series, germline *p53* mutations were found in one out of 80 unselected cases of glioma, and one out of 20 cases selected for family history (Li et al., 1995).

These findings, in addition to numerous other case reports, clearly document the existence of a familial glioma syndrome. A small proportion of these cases may be variants of Li-Fraumeni syndrome, and demonstrate germline *p53* mutations. The vast majority, however appear to be due to other genetic or environmental factors. Brain tumors may also be components in a number of hereditary syndromes (see Appendix A). Of these, Turcot syndrome must be considered when there is also a family history of polyposis (see Chapter 4 and review by Paraf et al., 1997).

REFERENCES

Chen P, Ivarone A, Fick J et al. 1995. Constitutional *p53* mutations associated with brain tumors in young adults. Cancer Genet Cytogenet 82:106–15.

Dirven CM, Tuerlings J, Molenaar WM, Go KG, Louis DN. 1995. Glioblastoma multiforme in four siblings. J Neuro Oncol 24:251–8.

Grossman SA, Osman M, Hruban RH, Piantadosi S. 1995. Familial gliomas: the potential for environmental exposure. Proc Amer Soc Clin Oncol 14:A291 (abstr).

Li YJ, Sanson M, Hoang-Xuan K et al. 1995. Incidence of germ-line *p53* mutations in patients with gliomas. Int J Cancer 64:383–7.

Nagane M, Shibui S, Nishikawa R et al. Triple primary malignant neoplasms including a malignant brain tumor: report of two cases and a review of the literature. Surg Neurol 45:219–29.

Paraf F, Jothy S, Van Meir EG. 1997. Brain tumor polyposis syndrome: two genetic diseases? J Clin Oncol 15:2744–58.

CHEMODECTOMA

Chemodectomas are also known as glomus tumors or paragangliomas of the head and neck. These tumors are formed from neuroectodermal and mesodermal origins and most frequently are observed in the carotid, aortic, jugular or vagal bodies. Of 30 cases reviewed in one series, about half were bilateral, with a family history of chemodectoma in about a third of these cases (Milanesi et al, 1994; Netterville et al, 1995). A greater proportion of the familial cases presented with multiple tumors. The remarkable feature about hereditary chemodectomas is the evidence of imprinting (Chapter 3); children of affected fathers develop chemodectomas, but the children of affected mothers do not (van der May et al., 1989).

Treatment is surgical. Minimal morbidity occurs with small tumors, but once the size is greater than five centimeters, cranial nerve loss and baroreceptor failure may be postoperative sequelae.

REFERENCES

Milanesi U, Mangili F, Milanesi I. 1994. Flow cytometric study of paraganglionomas of the carotid body. Acta Otorhinolaryngologica Italica 14:439047.

Netterville JL, Reilly KM, Robertson D, Reiber ME, Armstrong WB, Childs P. 1995. Carotid body tumors: a review of 30 patients with 46 tumors. Laryngoscope 105:115—26.

van der May, AGL, Maaswinkel-Mooy PD, Cornelisse CJ et al. 1989. Genomic imprinting in hereditary tumors: evidence for a new genetic theory. Lancet 2:1291–4.

GASTRIC CANCER

The incidence of gastric cancer is eight-fold higher in Japan compared to the United States. There is a well-documented increased relative risk of gastric cancer in relatives of those affected by the disease (see Table 6-1). In addition to the well known family of Napoleon Bonaparte, there have been numerous families with dominant inheritance of gastric cancer (Creagen and Fraumeni, 1973).

Along with IgA deficiency and other disorders (see Appendix A), gastric cancer is a feature of familial adenomatous polyposis as well as hereditary non-polyposis colorectal cancer. Microsatellite instability was observed in 14 of 30 patients with gastric cancer, three of whom had a strong family history of the disease, and one of whom carried a germline missense mutation of *hMLH1* (Keller et al., 1996).

In Japan, a relative risk of 2.3 was associated with a parental history of gastric cancer, with a risk of 6.0 if a mother was affected (Nagase et al., 1996). Significantly, in a study of relatives of patients with gastric dysplasia, risk was nearly doubled if a sibling or spouse had this pre-cancerous lesion (Zhao et al., 1994). This suggests important acquired or environmental exposures as well as genetic factors. For example, infection with H. Pylori, as well as atrophic gastritis have been associated with an increased risk for gastric cancer. In Japan, where gastric cancer rates are the highest in the world, invasive screening by endoscopy may be warranted. In kindreds with HNPCC, screening for upper gastrointestinal tumors is often considered when such cases have been documented in the family.

REFERENCES

Creagen ET, Fraumeni JF, Jr. 1973. Familial gastric cancer and immunologic abnormalities. Cancer 23:1325–31.

Keller G, Grimm V, Vogelsang H, Bischoff P, Mueller J, Siewert JR, Hofler H. 1996. Analysis foe microsatellite instability and mutations of the DNA mismatch repair gene *hMLH1* in familial gastric cancer. Int J Cancer 68:571–6.

Nagase H, Ogino K, Yoshida I et al. 1996. Family history related risk of gastric cancer in Japan: a hospital based case-control study. Jap J Cancer Res 87:1025–8.

Zhao L, Blot WJ, Liu WD et al. 1994. Familial predisposition to precancerous gastric lesions in a high-risk area of China. Cancer Epidem Biomar Preven 3:461–4.

LEUKEMIA AND LYMPHOMA

In a comprehensive review of the literature in 1996, ten families with multi-generational transmission of acute myeloid leukemia (AML), and nine families with chronic lymphocytic leukemia (CLL) were identified (Horwitz et al., 1996). Twenty additional families were documented with combinations of different types of leukemia. In each of these subsets there was evidence of anticipation (see Chapter 2). The median age of diagnosis decreased from 57 years in the grandparental generation of AML patients to 13 years of age in the grandchildren's generation, and from 66 years in the parental CLL generation to 51 in the children's generation. Among several explanations for this phenomenon, there exists the possibility of a common environmental exposure at a fixed point in time. Alternatively, mechanisms involving unstable repetitive DNA elements were postulated (Horwitz et al., 1996).

Familial myeloproliferative disease (Gilbert, 1995) and a family with a syndrome of platelet disorders and AML linked to chromosome 21q (Ho et al., 1996) have also been reported. Two families with familial myeloid leukemia or erythroleukemia and deletions of the long arm of chromosome 5 have been documented (Olopade et al., 1996; Siebert et al., 1995). Linkage analysis including eight relatives affected by leukemia or myelodysplasia revealed a lod score of 2.82 for markers linked to chromosome 16q22 (Horwitz et al., 1997).

There have been numerous reports of familial lymphoproliferative disorders, including cases of acute lymphocytic leukemia, Hodgkin's and non-Hodgkin's lymphoma (reviewed by Linet and Pottern, 1992), and familial hairy cell leukemia (reviewed in Gramatovici et al., 1990).

With the exception of X-linked lymphoproliferative syndrome (Purtilo, 1977), Bloom syndrome, and ataxia telangiectasia, lymphomas are infrequently observed in cancer predisposition syndromes. Both leukemias and lymphomas are components of a number of less common syndromes (see Appendix A). Importantly, a population-based assessment of cancer risk in first-degree relatives of affected patients revealed an increased risk for both Hodgkin's and non-Hodgkin's lymphoma (Goldgar et al., 1994). Hodgkin's disease has been documented in families, usually in siblings, where a relative risk of 7.1 was observed for young adult cases (Grufferman et al., 1977). Concordance of Hodgkin's disease has also been observed in identical twins (Mack et al., 1995). Thus, the patterns of inheritance of Hodgkin's (HD) and non-Hodgkin's lymphomas (NHL) in families appear distinct, suggestive of an age-specific genetic susceptibility to HD, with a time-specific exposure in some NHL families (Siebert et al., 1997).

Germline mutations of *p53* were not detected in 35 individuals from 19 lymphoma-prone kindreds (Weintraub et al., 1996). There was no excess of Epstein Barr Virus RNA expression in the tumors of familial Hodgkin's disease patients (Lin et al., 1996).Germline mutations of the *FAS* gene were observed in a family with a pediatric autoimmune disease (Canale-Smith syndrome); however, this was believed to be a relatively rare genetic syndrome of lymphoma predisposition (Drappa et al. 1997).

REFERENCES

Drappa J, Vaishnaw AK, Sullivan KE, Chi JL, Elkon KB. 1997. FAS gene mutations in the Canale-Smith syndrome, an inherited lymphoproliferative disorder associated with autoimmunity. New Engl J Med 335:1643-9.

Gilbert HS. 1995. Familial myeloproliferative disease. In: Wasserman BB (ed). Polycythemia vera and the myeloproliferative disorders. WB Saunders, New York, pp 222–5

Goldgar DE, Easton DF, Cannon-Albright LA, Skolnick MH. 1994. Systematic population-based assessment of cancer risk in first-degree relatives of cancer probands. J Natl Cancer Inst 86:1600–8.

Gramatovici M, Bennett JM, Hiscock JG, Grewal KS. 1990. Three cases of familial hairy cell leukemia. Am J Hematol 42:337–9.

Grufferman S, Cole P, Smith PG, Lukes RJ. 1977. Hodgkin's disease in siblings. New Engl J Med 296:248–50.

Ho CY, Otterud B, Legare RD et al. 1996. Linkage of a familial platelet disorder with a propensity to develop myeloid malignancies to chromosome 21q22.1-22.2. Blood 87:5218–5224.

Horwitz M, Goode E, Jarvik GP. 1996. Anticipation in familial leukemia. Amer J Hum Genet 59:990–8.

Horwitz M, Benson K, Li F et al. 1997. Genetic heterogeneity in familial AML: evidence for a second locus at chromosome 16q21-23.2. Am J Hum Genet 61:873–81.

Lin A, Kingman DW, Lennette ET et al. 1996. Epstein-Barr Virus and Familial Hodgkin's Disease. Blood 88:3160–5.

Linet MS, Pottern LM. 1992. Familial aggregation of hematopoietic malignancies and risk of non-Hodgkin's lymphoma. Cancer Res 52:5468s-5473s.

Mack TM, Cozen W, Shibata DK et al. 1995. Concordance for Hodgkin's disease in identical twins suggesting genetic susceptibility to the young-adult form of the disease. New Engl J Med 332:413-18.

Olopade OI, Roulston D, Baker T et al. 1996. Familial myeloid leukemia associated with loss of the long arm of chromosome 5. Leukemia 10:669–74.

Purtilo DT. 1977. Opportunistic non-Hodgkin's lymphoma in X-linked recessive immunodeficiency and lymphoproliferative syndromes. Semin Oncol 4:335–343.

Siebert R, Jhanwar S, Brown K, Berman E, Offit K. 1995. Familial Acute Myeloid Leukemia and DiGuglielmo Syndrome. Leukemia 9:1091–94.

Siebert R, Louie D, Lacher M, Schluger A, Offit K. 1997. Familial Hodgkin's and non-Hodgkin's lymphoma: different patterns in first-degree relatives. Leukemia and Lymphoma (in press).

Weintraub M, Lin AY, Franklin J, Tucker MA, Magrath IT, Bhatia KG. 1996. Absence of germline *p53* mutations in familial lymphoma. Oncogene 12:687–91.

LUNG CANCER

Lung cancer is the most common cause of cancer death for both men and women. Over 170,000 cases are diagnosed each year. As introduced in Chapter 2, lung cancer remains the model for an environmentally induced neoplasm; the disease was virtually unknown a century ago and has become an epidemic as a result of global tobacco use.

Postoperative survival for patients with early stage disease less than 3 cm in size (T1N0M0) is excellent, and is comparable to the survival of patients with the earliest stage breast cancer. Unlike breast cancer, however, a small minority of lung cancer patients, about 20,000, will be diagnosed with early stage disease.

Lung cancers fall into two categories: small cell and non-small cell. The non-small cell tumors are the most common and are comprised of adenocarcinomas, epidermoid carcinomas, and large cell carcinomas. The small cell lung cancers (oat cell type) account for about 20% of the total, and are of neurendocrine origin. They are also more responsive to systemic chemotherapy.

Since the early 1960s there have been reports of familial aggregations of lung cancer (Tokuhata and Lilienfeld, 1963). These observations have been limited by the tendency of smoking also to run in families. When smoking rates were adjusted in the analysis, the increased risk for lung cancer in relatives of affected probands was confirmed. A segregation analysis of 3276 individuals from 337 lung cancer families resulted in a "best fit" for a Mendelian codominant model. The estimated gene frequency was .05, implying that 10% of the population carried a putative lung cancer susceptibility gene (Sellers et al., 1990). Limiting the analysis to nonsmoking cases and controls also suggested a codominant model of inheritance. Genomic search and candidate gene studies are in progress utilizing markers identified in somatic genetic studies of lung cancer tumors.

Although it was initially reported that variations in the genetic factors that control the metabolism of carcinogens were correlated with lung cancer risk, these associations have not been clear-cut. The activity of the aryl hydrocarbon hydroxylase enzymes and slow metabolizers of the drug debrisoquine (CYP206) were correlated with significantly increased risk for lung cancer (d'Errico et al., 1996). Subsequent genetic studies of the polymorphisms of the genes encoding these and other cytochrome p450 enzymes have not established these markers in the clinical assessment of lung cancer risk (Shaw et al., 1995). Further analysis of polymorphisms of the genes encoding these metabolic pathways are in progress (Law, 1990; Gonzolez, 1995; d'Errico et al., 1996) and this constitutes an area of active research in lung cancer epidemiology.

Thus, the recognition of a familial cluster of lung cancers should be accompanied by risk counseling based on principles of Mendelian dominant inheritance. First-degree relatives of individuals affected with lung cancer at an early age may be at greater risk for lung cancer based on increased susceptibility to environmental carcinogens. Genetic testing outside the research context of linkage and association studies is not available.

Screening for lung cancer by serial chest radiographs and sputum cytology has not been shown to decrease mortality due to lung cancer. This conclusion emerged from three large screening trials sponsored in the 1970s. In these studies the mortality rates in populations receiving chest radiographs and/or sputum cytologies at intervals varying from 4 to 12 months was no different in one trial compared to the other (Miller, 1986). Conspicuously, none of these studies compared screening with no screening at all. Also, these studies were performed on males, many of whom had other smoking-related lung diseases. These are important points to keep in mind when counseling an individual at increased hereditary risk for lung cancer. Yearly chest radiographs will diagnose some lung tumors at an early stage. To be visible on a chest radiograph, the tumor has to be about one centimeter in size, and at that point resection can lead to a cure. Such screening recommendations, although not proven in high-risk settings, have a presumed benefit.

A number of novel approaches have the potential to be utilized in the screening of individuals at increased hereditary risk for lung cancer. In the late 1980s, Tockman showed the effectiveness of monoclonal antibody staining of sputa preserved from one of the large trials of the 1970s. In this study it was possible to predict which patients went on to develop lung cancer by analyzing specimens collected over a year before the tumors clinically presented (Tockman et al., 1988). A 1990s version of this study was performed, analyzing *K-RAS* mutations in some of the same archived sputum specimens. In this study, 10 patients with *K-RAS* mutations in their lung cancers had detectable *K-RAS* mutations in their sputum before the onset of clinical disease (Mao et al., 1994). These studies need to be repeated in the setting of prospective trials. An evaluation of monoclonal antibody-based methodologies has been included in the ongoing Lung Cancer Early Detection Working Group trials.

The case for retinoid-based chemoprevention of lung cancer was not supported by a 1994 study of beta carotene, alpha tocopherol, and isotretinoin in patients at high risk for lung cancer (Lee et al., 1994). In the 29,133 patients in a joint U.S.–Finnish study, incidence of lung cancer was actually higher in the group randomized to receive beta carotene (The Alpha-Tocopheral Beta Carotene Cancer Prevention Study Group, 1994). Further studies of other chemopreventive agents are in progress, including an NCI-sponsored trial of 13-cis-retinoic acid in patients already treated for early stage lung cancer.

REFERENCES

d'Errico A, Taloli E, Chen X, Vineis P. 1996. Genetic metabolic polymorphisms and the risk of cancer: a review of the literature. Biomarkers 1:149–73.

Gonzolez F. 1995. Genetic polymorphisms and cancer susceptibility. Cancer Res 55:710–5.

Law MR. 1990. Genetic predisposition to lung cancer. Br J Cancer 61:195–206.

Lee JS et al. 1994. Randomized placebo-controlled trial of isotretinoin in chemoprevention of bronchial squamous metaplasia. J Clin Oncol 12:937–45.

Mao L, Hruban RH, Boyle JO et al. 1994. Detection of oncogene mutations in sputum precedes diagnosis of lung cancer. Cancer Res 54:1634–7.

Miller A. 1986. Lung cancer screening: summary. Chest 89:325s.

Sellers TA, Bailey-Wilson JE, Elston RC et al. 1990. Evidence for Mendelian inheritance in the pathogenesis of lung cancer. J Natl Cancer Inst 82:1272–9.

Shaw GL, Falk RT, Deslauriers J et al. 1995. Debrisoquine metabolism and lung cancer risk. Cancer Epidemiol Biomar 4:41–8.

The Alpha-Tocopheral Beta Carotene Cancer Prevention Study Group. 1994. The effect of vitamin E and beta carotene on the incidence of lung cancer and other cancers in male smokers. New Engl J Med 330:1029–35.

Tockman MS, Gupta PK, Myers JD et al. 1988. Sensitive and specific monoclonal antibody recognition of human lung cancer antigen on preserved sputum cells: a new approach to early lung cancer detection. J Clin Oncol 6:1685–93.

Tokuhata GK, Lilienfeld AM. 1963. Familial aggregation of lung cancer in humans. J Natl Cancer Inst 30:289–312.

NEUROBLASTOMA

Neuroblastomas are the most common solid malignant tumor of early childhood. When diagnosed early after discovery by a pediatrician or a parent) these tumors can be cured by surgical excision. The vast majority (over 95%) of neuroblastomas are not hereditary. The risk of disease in a sibling of a child with neuroblastoma is less than six per cent (Kushner et al., 1986). However, a number of extended pedigrees with neuroblastoma have been described, including one family with seven affected members (Maris et al., 1997). In these families, high penetrance of the phenotype was the rule.

Although cytogenetic abnormalities affecting band 1p36 were frequently observed in neuroblastoma tumors, no linkage to this locus was found after analysis of three neuroblastoma kindreds (Maris et al., 1996). For such rare families, careful physical examination and screening of the urine for catecholamines should be performed. As discussed in Chapter 8, analysis of gene amplification is part of the basic evaluation of newly diagnosed patients, since *NMYC* copy number directly correlates with prognosis.

REFERENCES

Kushner BH, Gilbert F, Helson L. 1986. Familial neuroblastoma: case reports, literature review, and etiologic considerations. Cancer 57:1887–93.

Maris JM, Kyemba SM, Rebbeck TR et al. 1996. Familial predisposition to neuroblastoma does not map to chromosome band 1p36. Cancer Res 56:3421–5.

Maris JM, Chatten J, Meadows AT, Biegel JA, Brodeur GM. 1997. Familial neuroblastoma: a three generation pedigree and a further association with Hirschsprung disease. Med Ped Oncol 28:1–5.

PANCREATIC CANCER

The lifetime risk for pancreatic cancer is one in 150. Most patients are diagnosed with advanced disease, and the five year survival is less than 5%. Epidemiologic studies have shown that about 8 percent of individuals with pancreatic cancer have a family history of the disease, compared to 0.6 per cent of controls (Lynch, 1994). Syndromes associated with an increased risk of pancreatic cancer include hereditary non-polyposis colorectal cancer (HNPCC), hereditary breast-ovarian cancer, dyskeratosis congenita, hereditary pancreatitis, Li-Fraumeni syndrome, MEN1 (islet cell tumors of the pancreas), Peutz-Jegher syndrome, von Hippel-Lindau syndrome, hereditary melanoma, and site-specific pancreatic cancer (See Appendix A). In hereditary pancreatitis, there is a pre-existing setting of early-onset chronic pancreatitis. Pancreatic cancer is also considered part of the spectrum of HNPCC tumors (Chapter 4), although there has been relatively scant documentation of microsatellite instability in pancreatic carcinomas (Han et al., 1993; Lumadue et al., 1995).

As noted earlier in this chapter, pancreatic cancers have been observed in rare families with malignant melanoma. Investigators who are documenting kindreds affected by pancreatic cancer for epidemiologic or genetic studies include J.J. Mulvihill at the University of Pittsburgh, H. Lynch at Creighton University, and J. Lumadue and colleagues at Johns Hopkins (see Lumadue et al., 1995 for the address of the National Familial Pancreatic Tumor Registry). Experimental methods for the monitoring of individuals at the highest familial risk include endoscopic obtaining of pancreatic secretions for PCR analysis of gene mutations (e.g. *RAS*), and possibly PCR analysis of peripheral blood as well (Tada et al., 1993).

REFERENCES

Han HJ, Yanagisawa A, Yo K et al. 1993. Genetic instability in pancreatic cancer and poorly differentiated type of gastric cancer. Cancer Res 53:5087–9.

Lumadue JA, Groggin CA, Osman M, Hruban RH. 1995. Familial pancreatic cancer and the genetics of pancreatic cancer. Surg Clin N Amer 75:845–55.

Lynch HT: Genetics and pancreatic cancer. 1994. Arch Surg 129:266–8.

Tada M, Omaata M, Kawai S et al. 1993. Detection of *RAS* gene mutations in pancreatic juice and peripheral blood of patients with pancreatic adenocarcinoma. Cancer Res 53:2472–4.

TESTICULAR CANCER

Testicular cancer is the most commonly diagnosed malignancy among young adult males. Familial clustering has been reported. A 1990 review of the literature documented 24 father-son pairs, 45 brother pairs, and 12 pairs of identical twins (Patel et al., 1990). The tumors were bilateral in 4% of the cases. A family with 5 affected brothers was subsequently reported (Cooper et al., 1994).

A population-based study of 2,113 index cases from the Danish tumor registry found a two-fold relative risk for fathers of affected individuals, with an increased risk of cancers of the lung and digestive tract also noted (Westergaard et al., 1996). In contrast, a study of Swedish and Norwegian relatives of testicular cancer patients revealed fewer than expected cases of prostate and gastrointestinal cancer cases in the parents of the index cases (Heimdal et al., 1996).

A segregation analysis of 978 Scandinavian patients with testicular neoplasms was suggestive of an autosomal recessive model of inheritance with an estimated gene frequency of 3.8%, and a lifetime penetrance for homozygotes of 43% (Heimdal et al., 1997). Mutations of the *p53* gene were not observed in 32 patients with bilateral familial germ cell tumors (Heimdal et al. 1993), excluding *p53* as a candidate gene.

Options for early detection of testicular cancer include physical examination and ultrasound of suspicious masses. Cryptorchidism, which may also be familial, is associated with a marked increase in risk for testicular cancer. In these instances, orchidopexy should be performed in early childhood in order to decrease the risk.

REFERENCES

Cooper MA, Fellows J, Einhorn LH. 1994. Familial occurrence of testicular cancer. J Urol 151:1022–3.

Heimdal K, Lothe RA, Lystad S, Holm R, Fossa SD, Brresen AL. 1993. No germline T*P53* mutations detected in familial and bilateral testicular cancer. Genes, Chrom, Cancer 6:92–7.

Heimdal K, Olsson H. Tretli S, Flodgren P, Brresen AL, Fossa SD. 1996. Risk of cancer in relatives of testicular cancer patients. Br J Cancer 73:970–3.

Heimdal K, Olsson H, Tretli S, Fossa SD, Brresen AL, Bishop DT. 1997. A segregation analysis of testicular cancer based on Norwegian and Swedish families. Br J Cancer 75:1084–7.

Patel SR, Kvols LK, Richardson RI. 1990. Familial testicular cancer: report of six cases and review of the literature. Mayo Clin Proc 65:804–8.

Westergaard T, Olsen JH, Frisch M et al. 1996. Cancer risk in fathers and brothers of testicular cancer patients in Denmark. A population-based study. Int J Cancer 66:627–31.

6

Quantitative Methods in Cancer Risk Assessment

In counseling a member of a cancer-prone family, a basic requirement is an estimate of the risk to that individual. The level of detail in explaining the risk will vary according to the needs and interests of the individual seeking counseling. A body of literature in reproductive genetic counseling has questioned the desire or ability of clients to receive quantitative risk information. This was not found to be an issue in the early cancer prevention clinics, where it was observed that individuals often desired quantitative risk information. Increasingly, families and health-care professionals are also requesting explanations for cancer risk estimates and recommendations for making these estimates more precise. A relatively small increment in risk may make the difference when considering, for example, preventive surgical options.

A number of approaches may be employed in the derivation of cancer risk figures. These include population-derived (*epidemiologic*) risks, pedigree-derived (*genetic epidemiologic*) risks, and risks deduced by direct genetic testing. Although risks derived from direct testing are the most accurate, this chapter emphasizes that the sensitivity, specificity, and predictive value of the testing methodology must be considered. It is possible to infer risks to family members by modifying their probability depending on such factors as age and the relationship to other family members who have been tested.

In addition to estimating cancer risks associated with documented mutations of genes, individuals will seek to understand the meaning of negative test results. They will request reassurance that their cancer risk is no higher than that of the general population. To address these issues, providers of genetic testing services must be able to frame test results in a clinical context. As will be seen, to calculate the negative predictive value of a given test, the clinician needs to consider such factors as the probability of mutations in other genes and the performance characteristics (*analytic sensitivity*) of the test that was carried out. Although the responsibility (and liability) for the technical performance of the test rests with the laboratory, the interpretation of test results remains the task of the provider of these services.

This chapter highlights the statistical concepts that underlie familial cancer risk calculations. Examples are drawn largely from breast cancer risk counseling and genetic testing, although the same concepts can be applied to other cancer susceptibility syndromes.

EPIDEMIOLOGIC METHODS

As a discipline, epidemiology originated in the study of the great contagions, or epidemics, that have characterized world history. Even in the absence of an understanding of the pathogenesis of individual infectious diseases, interventions based on epidemiologic observations saved many lives. Methods to statistically define causal associations of disease were developed by epidemiologists. From their perspective, genetic predisposition was just one of a myriad of constitutional and environmental factors that cause cancer. For this reason, epidemiologic methodology offers useful approximations of the relative risk of various causal factors that can be utilized in routine clinical counseling. Epidemiologically derived risk estimates, based on population-based studies, can reflect quite accurately the multigenic as well as multifactorial nature of such complex traits as cancer.

Measures of Disease Prevalence

The *prevalence* of a disease is defined as the existing cases of that disease at a point in time. The *incidence* of a disease is the number of newly diagnosed cases of a diseases in an at-risk population over a given interval in time. Incidence (I) and prevalence (P) are related by the duration of the disease (D), so that: $P = I \times D$. For example, a disease of lesser incidence may have a very high prevalence if the patients survive for many years with the disease (e.g., diabetes). Similarly, the incidence may be very high but the prevalence may be low because the course of the disease is rapid (e.g., influenza), the treatments are highly effective (bacterial infections), or the disease is rapidly fatal.

Cumulative incidence is a measure of probability that a given individual will develop a disease over a given period of time. For breast cancer, the cumulative incidence of 11% means that about one in nine women will develop the disease in her lifetime (one in eight for a cohort of women who live past 100 years of age).

Relative Risks

The early studies of familial cancer were descriptive. The frequencies of cancers within affected families were compared to frequencies expected in the general population. Cancer risks in these families were expressed as observed-to-expected ratios. In general, these studies showed a two- to threefold increase in the frequency of the same type of cancer in first-degree relatives (mother, father, brothers, sisters, children) of an individual affected by a malignancy of the breast, colon, stomach, lung, or prostate.

Although these studies constituted first approximations of possibly inherited cancer risks, they were methodologically limited. Clustering of cases could have been due, for example, to different environmental exposures or common diets, rather than genetic factors.

The basic tools of analytic epidemiology, *cohort* and *case control* studies, did not emerge until the second half of the twentieth century. A cancer-associated exposure (cigarette smoking) served as the stimulus for many of these advances. Each of these two types of epidemiologic methods have been utilized in cancer genetic studies; each has distinct advantages and limitations.

Cohort studies are perhaps the most direct, and least sensitive to bias, of epidemiologic studies. One begins with populations exposed or not exposed to a given agent and then measures the incidence of disease in each group. Epidemiologists consider family history of a disease as one of a number of possible risk factors. The relationship between the risk factor and the disease is expressed by the following 2 × 2 table:

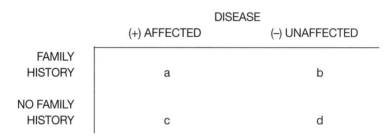

In cohort studies the *relative risk* (RR) represents the risk of a disease in a population exposed to a risk factor relative to the risk in a population unexposed to that factor. If data is given in a 2 × 2 table, then it is expressed as:

$$\text{Relative Risk} = \frac{\text{Incidence in those with family history of disease}}{\text{Incidence in those with no family history}}$$

$$= \frac{a/(a + b)}{c/(c + d)}$$

An advantage of cohort studies is that they start with participants free of disease and thus can look at multiple effects of a single exposure. Disadvantages are that cohort studies require many subjects and can take a lot of time for follow-up. They are also quite expensive. For these reasons, there are relatively few ongoing large-scale cohort studies.

One cohort study, started after World War II, was based in Framingham, Massachusetts. The Framingham Heart Study revealed to epidemiologists most of what we now know about the risk factors for cardiovascular disease. One of the largest ongoing cancer epidemiology cohort studies is the Nurses' Health Study, based in Boston and started in 1976. It involves over 100,000 registered nurses who have been followed for a number of health-related endpoints.

When the risk of breast cancer was compared in individuals in the Nurses' Health Study with and without a family history of breast cancer, the ratio of the breast cancer incidence rates in the two groups was 2.5 (Colditz et al., 1993). When this same study population was used to measure the risk of dietary fat and breast cancer, the relative risk was not significantly elevated above 1.0, signifying no effect. A second follow-up was performed 8 years after the initiation of the study. By then, 1439 cases of breast cancer had been documented in the study population. It was possible to categorize the women according to the percentage of calories consumed as fat. Again, no effect was found (Willett et al., 1992).

A *confounding variable* in an epidemiologic study is a factor associated with the exposure that also has a causal relationship with the outcome. The hidden effects of confounding variables are the bane of the epidemiologist, because they can compromise a study and cause misleading results. In the breast cancer-dietary studies, frequency of mammographic examination met the criteria of a potential confounder. It would be expected that individuals who ate more fat might have mammograms performed more frequently (i.e., because these individuals were wealthier and could afford them). It is known that mammograms can diagnose breast cancers. This could lead to a false association between increased dietary fat and breast cancer incidence. It could also mask such an association if the high fat group did not receive regular mammograms. One way to take potential confounders into account in epidemiologic studies is to be sure that both exposed and unexposed groups are *stratified* (have known proportions) of individuals with the confounding exposure. When the Nurses' Health Study results were statistically adjusted to take into account the frequency of mammography in groups at varying levels of intake of dietary fat, there was still no significant interaction with breast cancer incidence. Ten other cohort studies with 50 or more cases of breast cancer have also failed to document this association. Some argue, however, that the range of fat consumed by participants in these studies was insufficient to see the association with risk of breast cancer.

The second major method for epidemiologic analysis is the case control study. In these studies, individuals with disease (cases) and without disease (controls) are compared with respect to their relative exposures. The measure of risk derived is called the *odds ratio*,

$$OR \text{ (odds ratio)} = \frac{a/c}{b/d} = \frac{ad}{bc}$$

The derivation of odds ratio can be thought of as the approximation of the relative risk when the disease is quite rare ($a \gg b$, and $d \gg c$). Advantages of case control studies are that they can yield results more rapidly than cohort studies, because the disease has already occurred. They are also well suited for rare diseases. However, case control studies are also quite vulnerable to bias in the method of measurement of the exposure and in the selection of both case and control group.

In case control studies, the frequency of an exposure is compared in groups with and without disease. Studies have compared the frequency of a family history of cancer in an individual affected by cancer to the frequency of a family history of cancer in a control group. In some studies, the control group had a history of another type of cancer. These designs were able to match for common environmental backgrounds in both cases and controls, which were not accounted for in the earlier descriptive studies. The odds ratios derived from these studies are generally explained to patients as the risk of a cancer given an exposure (family history) compared to the risk if there were no exposure. However, as mentioned previously, odds ratios are technically derived in inverse fashion, i.e., odds of exposure (family history) in cancer cases compared to controls. This literature has documented significant associations between a family history of cancer and the occurrence in individuals of malignancies of breast, colon, stomach, ovary, prostate, and malignant melanoma. Selected risk ratios for various constellations of familial cancer are shown in Table 6-1.

Absolute Risk

The risk ratios shown in Table 6-1 are the results of an extensive epidemiologic literature. However, they are, in general, poorly translated to the clinic. Relative risk ratios are of limited utility in clinical counseling for a number of reasons. The magnitude of the relative risk varies depending on the control group chosen and reflects the methodologic limitations and biases of an individual study. Thus, relative risks from one study may not be comparable to estimates derived from another study. This can prove frustrating to individuals interested in comparing the risk of cancer due to family history to other known risk factors. Relative risks correspond to a time interval, which may also vary between studies, and relative risks may themselves change over time. Individuals seeking to make decisions based on risk tend to be more interested in their actual likelihood of contracting the disease (*absolute risk*) than in their relative risk compared to some other person.

While relative risk is expressed as an increased risk compared to a control population (e.g., "4 times more likely"), absolute risk is expressed as a probability of an event over a period of time (e.g., "a 15-year risk of 20%"). The absolute risk can be explained as "gambler's odds." For example, the 15-year risk of 20% can be explained as "One woman out of five with your risk factors will get breast cancer over the next 15 years." An advantage of absolute risk data is that they can be compared to other statistical risks. For example, a woman's risk of developing breast cancer before the age of 25 is the same as the risk of drowning in a year. Additional comparisons can be made with statistical probabilities of other catastrophes (for example, car accidents) or to other unexpected health events. Such comparisons prove useful for many individuals seeking a frame of reference during genetic counseling sessions (Table 6-2).

The relationship between relative risk and absolute risk is evident in the following example (see Figure 6-1). Assume that the risk of a type of cancer between ages 40 and 43 increases from 1% to 4%, and then flattens out to approach 5% by age 80. If the relative risk is 5, due to, for example, a family history or a positive genetic test, then the risk (the annual cancer incidence rate) would increase from 5% to 20% during the ages 40–43. Let us assume that in this population the probability of surviving free from

TABLE 6-1   Selected Lifetime Risk Ratios for Adult Malignancies

Relative Affected	Risk Ratios
Breast Cancer	
Mother affected (any age)	1.7–4
Sister affected (any age)	2–3
Sister premenopausal	3.6–5
Sister postmenopausal	2
Sister bilateral, <age 40	11
Sister and mother	2.5–14
Sister and mother premenopausal, bilateral disease	39
Second-degree relative	1.4–2
Third-degree relative	1.35
Colon Cancer	
Mother or father	3–4
Brother or sister	3–7
First-degree relative with adenomatous polyp	1.8
First-degree relative <60 with polyp	2.6
First-degree relative with polyp and parent with colon cancer	3.3
Gastric Cancer	
First-degree relative	2–3
Ovarian Cancer	
First-degree relative	3.9–4
Prostate Cancer	
First-degree relative	2–5
Malignant Melanoma	
First-degree relative	2.7

Source: Data reviewed in Offit K, Brown K. Quantitative risk counseling for familial cancer: a resource for clinical oncologists. J Clin Oncol 1994; 12: 1724–36.

cancer is 100% at age 40, but drops 5% a year to 85% by age 43. To calculate the absolute risk of cancer by a certain age, one multiplies the chances of being alive without cancer at that age by the risk (incidence of cancer) at that age (Dupont and Plummer, 1996). These absolute risks are shown by the dotted bars in the second part of Figure 6-1. The sum of these bars is the cumulative risk from ages 40–43, or $5 + 9 + 13.5 + 17 = 44.5\%$.

This example also illustrates the important concept that, in general, relative risks should not be multiplied by absolute risks in the general population to give absolute

TABLE 6-2   Comparison of Lifetime Risks

Being diagnosed with cancer	1 in 3
Being diagnosed with breast cancer (women)	1 in 9
Being diagnosed with ovarian cancer (women)	1 in 70
Being diagnosed with a germ cell cancer (male)	1 in 500
Dying in a fire	1 in 800
Being electrocuted	1 in 5000
Being killed in a motor vehicle accident	1 in 10,000
Dying in a tornado	1 in 60,000
Being diagnosed with neuroblastoma	1 in 500,000
Food poisoning by botulism	1 in 3 million

Source: Data from Desonie D. Table "Chances of dying from selected causes" in Cosmic Collisions, New York, Henry Holt, 1996, p. 105; and American Cancer Society, 1997, Cancer Facts and Figures.

risk in the cohort being counseled. Thus, it is misleading for the individual who is 41 in the prior example simply to multiply 5 by the 5% risk by age 80. In this example, the actual cumulative risk over that interval is much greater. In fact, when the absolute risk of developing a disease is very low, it may be accurate to multiply the relative risk by the population absolute risk but this should not be relied upon in counseling settings (DuPont and Plummer, 1996).

Case Example 6.1. An individual was concerned about the risks of breast cancer following a biopsy showing atypical hyperplasia. She was 40 years old, her age of menarche was 14, age at first live birth was 27 and she had one biopsy showing atypia. She had no family history of cancer and no other known risk factors. She had read that the relative risk following a biopsy showing atypical lobular hyperplasia was 5.0. She also knew that the lifetime risk for developing breast cancer is 10%. She was concerned that her risk for developing breast cancer was 50%.

As explained in the text, the absolute risk is calculated by multiplying the age-specific breast cancer incidence rate by the cumulative breast cancer-free survival probability in that age group. It would not be correct to multiply an interval-specific relative risk by the population risk of cancer. For a 40-year-old woman the relative risk of 5.0 translates to a 9% chance of breast cancer over the next 20 years. In contrast, for a 60-year-old woman, for whom the baseline breast cancer risk is higher, the 20-year risk is 25%. Significantly, it appears that increased relative risk—and hence the absolute risk—for breast cancer following a biopsy showing atypical hyperplasia is greatest during the first 10 years following diagnosis. If no breast cancer has occurred by that time, the relative risk decreases by half (Dupont and Plummer, 1996).

Another approximation of risk for this individual was provided by the BDDP model (Gail et al., 1989) (see Appendix C). For the risk factors given (e.g., age of first birth, age of menarche, number of biopsies), the 30-year cumulative risk for breast cancer was about 8%.

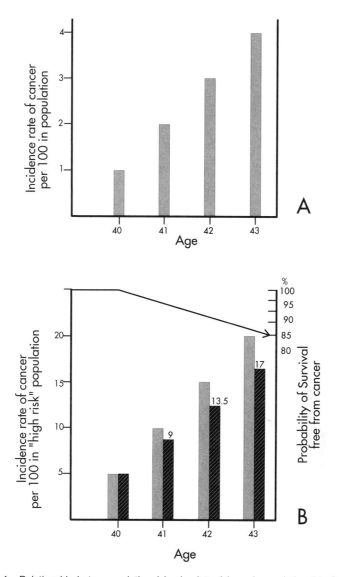

FIGURE 6-1 *Relationship between relative risk, absolute risk, and cumulative risk. See text for explanation of example. A. Baseline risk increases from 1% at age 40 to 4% at age 43. B. Assuming relative risk of 5, risk increases from 5% at age 40 to 20% at age 43 (gray bars). Scale on right of graph refers to probability of survival free from cancer. Note that this decreases from 100% at age 40 to 85% by age 43. Bars with stripes represent absolute risk of cancer, the product of the age specific incidence and the probability of being alive free from cancer.*

The relative risk for breast cancer in a *BRCA1* heterozygote actually changes over time, from around 30 at age 40 to less than 20 at age 55, and even lower at later age. These changes are reflected in the shifting absolute risks for breast cancer over time (see Table 4-2). These absolute risk tables, rather than relative risk approximations, are most useful in counseling settings.

A large relative risk may be of lesser concern to the individual being counseled if the baseline absolute risk is low. This principle is illustrated by the contrast in risks due to estrogen replacement, where a lesser increase in breast cancer risk may be offset by a greater decrease in cardiovascular risk (discussed in Offit and Brown, 1994).

Absolute risk data, derived empirically, are available for individuals at familial risk for a number of malignancies (Tables 6-3 and 6-4). Four independent data sets can be applied for routine clinical counseling for women at familial risk for breast cancer. These include: data derived by Anderson and colleagues based on 556 carefully verified pedigrees with breast cancer probands (Anderson and Badzioch, 1993); data based on 2852 cases and 3146 matched controls in the Breast Cancer Detection and Demonstration Project (BCDDP) (Gail et al., 1989); data derived from 4730 breast cancer cases, ages 20 through 54, and 4688 controls in the Cancer and Steroid Hormone study (CASH) (Claus et al., 1994); and data derived from a prospective study of 117,998 registered nurses followed since 1976 (Colditz et al., 1993). In general, risk estimates from these models agree. A special appeal of the BCDDP model is that it is available on a computer disc or in graphical charts and was utilized to determine eligi-

TABLE 6-3 Cumulative Risk (percentage) to Individuals with First-Degree Relatives with Cancers of Breast, Colon, or Ovary, Compared to Individuals with No Family Histories of These Malignancies

	Breast Cancer[a]			Colon Cancer[b]			Ovarian Cancer[c]	
	Age of Relative Affected			Age of Relative Affected				
Age	30–39	60–69	Control	<55	≥55	Control	All Ages	Control
29	.5	.2	.02	—	—	—	.25	—
39	1.7	.6	.45	.2	.1	0.0	.5	.1
49	4.4	1.8	1.6	.9	.5	.1	.5	.4
59	8.6	4.0	2.9	2.8	1.0	.6	1.0	.5
69	13.0	7.0	4.6	5.0	2.2	1.3	3.0	1.0
79	16.5	9.6	7.3	8.4	4.4	2.4	4.7	1.2

Source: Offit K, Brown K. Quantitative risk counseling for familial cancer; a resource for oncologists. J Clin Oncol 1994; 12: 1724–36.

[a]Claus et al., 1994; controls are "mother controls" from Claus et al., 1990, Table 1. Note: cumulative probability of breast cancer in controls was 9.0 by age 89 and 11.4% by age 94.

[b]St. John et al., 1993; derived from an Australian population, where the colon cancer incidence in spouse controls (2.4%) is lower than that of 5.2% in women and 4.4% in men in the United States.

[c]Amos et al., 1992; risks approximated from Figure 1.

Key: Cumulative risks are expressed as percentages. Data are interpreted as the percentage of individuals with or without (control) a family history of cancer who will develop that same malignancy by the age shown in the left-hand column.

Case Example 6.2. A 51-year-old woman considering postmenopausal hormone replacement was advised by her gynecologist that this option was contraindicated due to her family history of breast cancer. Her mother and maternal aunt both had postmenopausal breast cancer. There were also multiple individuals with atherosclerotic heart disease, including cases of myocardial infarction at an early age. The proband had a history of hypertension, and brought with her bone densitometry results that reported moderate to high risk of new vertebral fracture, a right femoral neck bone density that was 60% of normal, and a battery of blood tests revealing an elevated serum low density lipoprotein.

There were no living relatives with breast cancer available for testing. Because of the late age of onset in the two sisters, the prior probability of linkage to *BRCA1* in this family was quite low. Considering this woman had a relative risk of breast cancer of approximately 2.0 and was at moderate to high risk for both hip fracture and cardiovascular disease, data from the metanalysis by Grady and colleagues was applied (Grady et al., 1992). Based on these data, it was possible to provide this woman with the following guidelines: Should she begin use of unopposed estrogen at age 50, her risk of breast cancer would increase 5% over her lifetime while her risk of coronary artery disease and hip fracture would decrease 11% and 5% respectively. Addition of progesterone would presumably abrogate the predicted 16% increase in risk for endometrial cancer, but would not impact on the breast cancer risk. Overall, it could be estimated that a half to a full year of life would be gained by hormone replacement therapy (Grady et al., 1992).

For this individual, these data and her menopausal symptoms led her to decide to begin hormonal replacement. Another woman with similar medical and family history felt that *any* increased risk of breast cancer was completely unacceptable. The range of breast cancer screening procedures was recommended for both women, with follow-up by the gynecologist/endocrinologist for monitoring of hormone replacement and consideration of treatment with Fosamax, and by the internist for dietary modification and risk reduction based on the lipid profile and family history of heart disease.

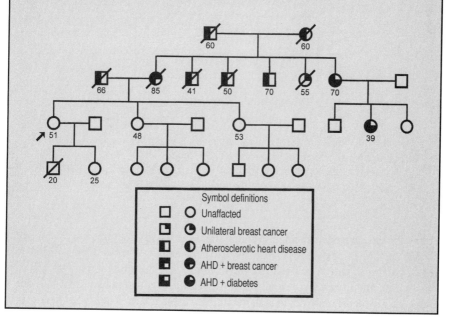

Case Example 6.3. Two women, Jean and Lynn, came for cancer risk counseling. Both were 30 years old, both had menarche at age 13, had no children, and had had no breast biopsies. Jean's mother had breast cancer at age 39, Lynn's at age 59. They desired to know their risk of developing breast cancer.

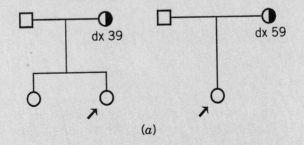

(a)

By the Gail model, both had the same risk: 16.6% lifetime. By the CASH model (Appendix C) Jean's lifetime risk was 16.5%, Lynn's 11.0%. This demonstrates the insensitivity of the Gail model to age at diagnosis.

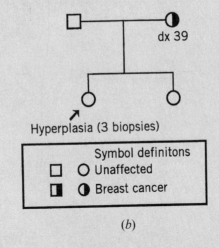

(b)

Jean's sister also had menarche at age 13. She had a child at age 24, but had three breast biopsies, one showing hyperplasia. By the Gail model her risk increased to 29.4%. This change in risk was not reflected in the CASH model.

bility for the tamoxifen chemoprevention trial. The variables utilized in the model include: current age, age at first live birth, age at menarche, number of first-degree relatives with breast cancer, and number of prior biopsies. The limitation of family history ascertainment to first-degree relatives with breast cancer and potential for bias due to unnecessary biopsies are obvious shortcomings of this model. The CASH dataset is by

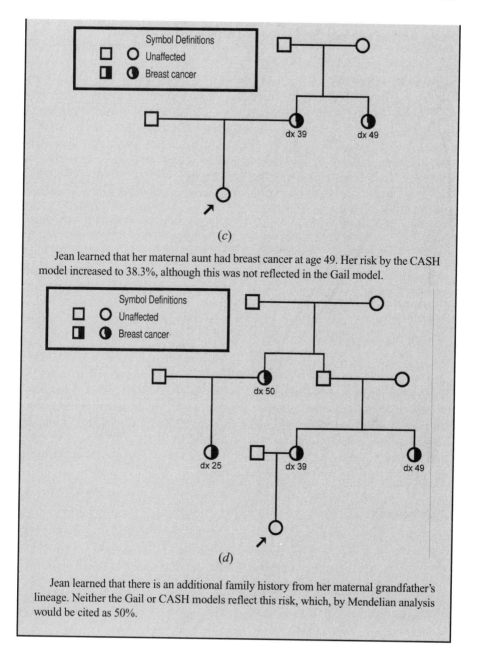

(c)

Jean learned that her maternal aunt had breast cancer at age 49. Her risk by the CASH model increased to 38.3%, although this was not reflected in the Gail model.

(d)

Jean learned that there is an additional family history from her maternal grandfather's lineage. Neither the Gail or CASH models reflect this risk, which, by Mendelian analysis would be cited as 50%.

far the most extensively analyzed and has been compiled by Claus and colleagues as tabular risk data that can readily be applied by clinical oncologists to most commonly encountered counseling scenarios (see Appendix C).

Absolute risk data for family history of colon cancer have been published and show

TABLE 6-4 Comparison of Cumulative Risks (percentage) for a Woman with Sister and Mother Affected by Breast Cancer According to Three Different Models

| Age | Nurses' Health Study[a] | Anderson[b] | | CASH[c] |
		Unilateral Disease	Bilateral Disease	
30	—	—	—	.71
40	1.5	1.0	7.0	5.0
50	5.0	8.0	13.0	12.2
60	10.1	15.0	21.0	15.9
70	17.4	18.0	25.0	25.3[d]

Source: Offit K, Brown K. Quantitative risk counseling for familial cancer: a resource for oncologists. J Clin Oncol 1994; 12: 1724–36.

Note: "Gail model" derived from the BCDDP (Gail et al, 1989; 1992) predicts a cumulative risk of approximately 29.0% from age 30–80 for an individual having two first-degree relatives with breast cancer (assuming no biopsies, age of menarche 12, and age of first live birth 29.0 years).

[a]Colditz et al., 1993 Table 5.
[b]Anderson et al., 1985 Table 2; note that bilateral disease refers to risk to sisters of patients affected with bilateral breast cancer.
[c]Claus et al., 1990 Table 3.
[d]To age 64.

the same dependence on age of onset as do the CASH breast cancer data (St. John et al., 1993). An increased risk of colorectal cancer has also been observed in first-degree relatives of probands with adenomatous polyps (Winawer et al., 1996). Age-specific absolute risk data according to age of onset of adenomatous polyps in the proband have been derived and are directly applicable to counseling and screening recommendations. Absolute risk by age can also be derived for relatives of those affected by ovarian cancer (Table 6-4). Similar empiric data are not yet available for individuals at familial risk for other common adult malignancies.

PAR Percent

Another useful statistical invention of epidemiologists is the *population attributable risk (PAR) percent*. This figure represents the amount of a disease in a population that is attributable to a given exposure. It is the amount of disease that would presumably be eliminated if the exposure could be removed. This calculation tends to be of more interest in the newsroom than in the clinic, because it reflects the public health impact of specific exposures. It is commonly derived by the *Levin formula*, utilizing the odds ratios (or relative risks) that have been calculated from epidemiologic studies:

$$\text{PAR\%} = \frac{p(RR-1)}{p(RR-1)+1} \times 100$$

where p is the proportion of total population that has been exposed and RR is the relative risk for exposed versus nonexposed.

To cite an example of the calculation of PAR%, a publication noted a 27-fold increased risk for early-onset breast cancer in Jewish women carrying the 185delAG mutation of *BRCA1* (i.e., RR = 27) (Fitzgerald et al., 1996). Since 1% of Ashkenazi Jews carry the 185delAG mutation, from the Levin formula we calculate that the PAR% is (.01)(26)/(.01)(26) +1 which is equal to .26/1.26, or 20%. Thus, about 20% of early onset breast cancer in Jewish women is due to the 185delAG mutation. Confidence limits should also be included in PAR% calculations.

GENETIC EPIDEMIOLOGIC METHODS

Viewed from the perspective of the geneticist, calculation of odds ratios and relative risks, taking into account environmental differences, is just one of many strategies to study the influence of genes in human diseases. Genetic approaches to studying hereditary risks for disease include twin studies, adoption studies, and segregation and linkage analysis.

Twin and Adoption Studies

Discordance rates among monozygotic (identical) twins and comparisons of disease concordance rates between monozygotic and dizygotic twins have been historical approaches to the inference of genetic influences on disease expression. Such studies are particularly prone to ascertainment bias, because, in general, disease occurrences in monozygous twins are more likely to be reported in the literature. Nonetheless, studies utilizing twin registries can provide a first approximation of the heritability of traits. An analysis of over 20,000 twin pairs from The Swedish Twin Registry revealed a significant genetic susceptibility to cancers of the colon, breast, cervix and prostate (Ahlbom et al., 1997). Adoption studies can derive the frequency of a disease among the biologic and adopted relatives of both adopted cases and adopted controls. A higher frequency of disease among biologic relatives of cases constitutes evidence for genetic transmission of disease susceptibility.

Segregation Analysis

A statistical means to analyze the mode of inheritance of a trait is *segregation analysis*. In segregation analysis, the pattern of disease in a family is fitted to Mendelian patterns of inheritance of a putative susceptibility allele. Data are collected on family structure, phenotype, and age at onset. Phenotypic data may be qualitative (e.g., whether the individual has the diagnosis of Bloom's syndrome) or quantitative (e.g., the degree of chromosome fragility in a patient). These data are utilized to test various models. The test of the model proceeds in several stages. First is the computation of a goodness-of-fit parameter, such as a probability (*P*) associated with a chi-squared statistic. A large *P* (e.g., 0.5) means a good fit, and a low *P* value means that the model can be rejected with that level of confidence. Analysis of various models can be made by comparisons of their goodness-of-fit values. Genetic goodness-of-fit tests have been derived for a number of models of inheritance including: the single gene, polygenic, multifactorial, mixed (multifactorial plus major locus), two-locus, and other models. Computerized software is available to test these models. It is also necessary to make an appropriate adjustment in the model to account for the manner in which the pedigrees were ascertained.

Most cancer susceptibility syndromes thus far identified have demonstrated a dominant pattern of inheritance with high penetrance, although instances of recessive inheritance have also been documented. These pedigrees will be amenable to analysis by a single gene model. *Polygenic* traits are those due to a large number of genes with small, or possibly additive effects. *Multifactorial* disorders are caused by multiple genetic and environmental factors, each of which contributes in a small way. Some multifactorial traits, like congenital abnormalities, appear to be the result of an underlying continuous variation in phenotype, which becomes a "disease" when the patient's "liability" exceeds a "*threshold*." In this model, the threshold is that point on the disease liability scale beyond which the disease trait develops. These concepts are particularly relevant to tumors with strong environmental components and distinct stages of malignant progression (e.g., head and neck tumors).

A particular challenge in the genetic epidemiologic analysis of common adult malignancies is the variability in age at onset. By utilizing the presence of precursor lesions, segregation analyses defined highly penetrant dominant genes associated with proliferative breast disease and adenomatous colon polyps (Chapter 4). A two-locus model for a common recessive locus provided a statistical fit with the patterns of inheritance of pigmented nevi in an analysis of Utah pedigrees (Chapter 5).

Linkage Analysis

After it has been determined that a cancer predisposition syndrome fits with a single gene model, that gene can be mapped by linkage analysis. Genetic markers are analyzed to see which most often cosegregate with the disease phenotype in an extended pedigree (see Figure 3-6). The closer the marker and the gene in question are located, the more frequently they will be transmitted together. The closer the distance between the disease gene and the marker, the smaller the probability of crossing over during meiosis. The recombination fraction is measured as the *centimorgan*. Genetic linkage is thus related to physical linkage: one hundredth of a Morgan (cM) represents the distance over which recombination occurs 1% of the time, which is equal to about 1 million base pairs.

In the odds ratio method of linkage analysis, the likelihood of obtaining data collected at two loci is determined. The likelihood that loci are linked at a specific recombination frequency (θ) is compared to the likelihood that they are not linked. The log of the ratio of the two likelihoods is the *odds for linkage (lod score)*. A lod score $\leqslant 0$ is evidence against linkage, while a value $\geqslant 1$ suggests linkage. When the lod score is 3, the odds of linkage is $10^3 : 1$, and the hypothesis is accepted.

Starting in the 1970s, and continuing over 20 years, Mary Claire King collected blood specimens from 100 families with breast cancer. Linkage analysis in those early years utilized about 30 protein markers, but in the 1980s Southern blot analysis of regions with *variable numbers of tandem repeats (VNTRs)* in the human chromosome allowed identification of about 100 markers. In 1985, the polymerase chain reaction (PCR) technique allowed the detection of short repeated sequences (e.g., CACACA-CA), which varied in length from one individual to the other. For several years, King and colleagues performed one negative linkage study after another, until in August of 1990, on their 183rd attempt, linkage was found to a marker on the long arm of chromosome 17. Detected in only 7 of 23 families, the calculated lod score was 5.98. When these data were pooled with 57 families with both breast and ovarian cancer, and 153 families with breast cancer alone, the lod score jumped to 26, indicating a 10^{26} odds in favor of linkage.

Linkage analysis is currently performed utilizing banks of polymorphic di-, tri-, and tetranucleotide repetitive elements (microsatellites) scattered throughout the human genome. A panel of 300–400 such markers constitutes a genomic search. Such searches can now be performed in a matter of weeks.

In general, the generation of a lod score occurs in the setting of a research study aimed at positional cloning of a disease susceptibility gene. In special circumstances, the results of linkage studies have been shared with families to inform their medical management. This sharing has taken place in the research phases of positional localization of cancer predisposition genes, but may also be necessary when mutations of known genes cannot be detected. In cancer genetics, linkage-based risk assessment has been offered to some families with hereditary breast cancer, retinoblastoma, familial polyposis, neurofibromatosis, and other hereditary syndromes. In some of these families, high lod scores have indicated linkage, but for various reasons (e.g. mutations outside coding regions), direct testing was unsuccessful. The clinical translation of the lod score in these settings is specific to the family under study and the hereditary syndrome.

A recent analytical advance has allowed linkage studies to be performed when multiple members of several generations are not available for testing. In *nonparametric* methods of linkage analysis, the ascertainment is directed toward affected sib pairs. The notion is that affected sib pairs share a genotype identical by descent from the parents of the siblings (except when the parents carry more than one disease-associated allele). Linkage is determined by a shift in the random distribution of alleles, resulting in an excess of affected sib pairs with 1 (or 2) alleles identical by descent. This method of analysis may be utilized in the initial mapping of cancer susceptibility genes.

PROBABILITY LAWS IN CANCER RISK COUNSELING

Law of Multiplication

One of the basic laws of probability relates to outcome of two or more independent events. In this circumstance, the probabilities are multiplied together to determine the chances of both events occurring. This simple calculation is relevant to a common question asked by affected and carrier mothers in breast/ovarian cancer families who have *BRCA1* or *BRCA2* mutations: "What is the chance that all of my three children will carry the same mutation?" Since the risk for each child is 0.5, the probability that all of her three children would be *BRCA1* carriers is $1/2 \times 1/2 \times 1/2$, or 1 chance in 8. The risk for each child, however, remains 50%.

The Summation Principle

The sum of all probabilities of a chance event equals one. If a woman with a particular mutation has three children, what is the chance that there will be at least one mutation carrier and one without the mutation? The probability that all three will be mutation carriers is $1/8$ and the probability that none will be mutation carriers is $1/8$. The only other outcomes left are that at least one child will be a carrier and one a noncarrier. Therefore, since the sum must be 1, the answer is $1 - 1/8 - 1/8 = 3/4$.

The Binomial Distribution and the Hardy-Weinberg Principle

The *binomial distribution* states that given two alternative events with probability p and q (where $q = 1 - p$), the frequencies of the possible combinations of p and q in n trials are equal to $(p + q)^n$. In a family of 2 children, this is $(p + q)^2 = p^2 + 2pq + q^2$. In the example where p is the probability of a *BRCA1* mutation in a child of an affected parent:

$p^2 = 1/4$ of all sibships will have both sibs with *BRCA1* mutations
$q^2 = 1/4$ of all sibships will contain no *BRCA1* carriers
$2pq = 1/2$ of sibships will have one carrier and one noncarrier

In the previous example of three children, the binomial expansion is

$$(p + q)^3 = p^3 + 3p^2q + 3pq^2 + q^3$$

that is,

$p^3 = 1/8$ of sibships will have all three as *BRCA1* carriers
$q^3 = 1/8$ of sibships will have none as *BRCA1* carriers
$3p^2q = 3/8$ of sibships will have 2 *BRCA1* carriers and 1 noncarrier
$3pq^2 = 3/8$ of sibships will have 1 *BRCA1* carrier and 2 noncarriers

Thus, in $3/8 + 3/8 = 3/4$ of sibships, at least one sib will be a carrier and one will be a noncarrier, as previously derived using the summation principle.

Hardy-Weinberg distributions of genotypes in populations are binomial distributions where p and q represent frequencies of wild-type and mutant alleles at a given locus. The major use of the Hardy-Weinberg law is for calculating gene frequencies. For a dominant trait, the incidence of the phenotype is the sum of the homozygotes with the mutant allele (q^2) plus the heterozygotes ($2pq$). For dominant traits, this incidence rate is often approximated as the *carrier frequency*. For this approximation, one takes the frequency of the (rare) homozygotes to be zero and the frequency of the normal allele (p) to be about equal to one. Thus, the carrier frequency is approximately equal to $2q$. Carrier frequency is not to be confused with the *gene frequency*, which is q. Thus, segregation analysis predicted a gene frequency for *BRCA1* of .003, which means that six per thousand in the population would be a carrier. Similarly, the carrier frequency for the 185delAG mutation is 1 per 100; the gene frequency would be half this value.

Bayes' Rule: General Notation

The theorem introduced by the mathematician Reverend Thomas Bayes in 1763 has had enormous impact on the refinement of risk calculations in both genetics and epidemiology. In its most general form, the value of Bayes' theorem is its ability to modify a prior probability of an event by taking into account conditional circumstances.

In cancer risk counseling, Bayes' formula is most commonly used in two circumstances. In the first instance, it is used to estimate the risk that an individual is or is not harboring a mutation of a cancer predisposition gene given that she or he is disease free at a given age. In the second circumstance, it is used to estimate the risk of a disease, or a genotype, given a specific genetic test result. The theorem is also utilized in genetic risk calculation in a number of other settings, for example, the calculation of risk to individuals based on lod score determinations from linkage studies.

While it is possible to make these calculations simply by inserting numbers into established equations, this section presents a simplified derivation of the general form of the theorem (Young, 1991; Weinstein and Feinberg, 1980).

Bayes' Theorem

The expression $p(A|B)$ signifies the probability of A contingent upon the presence of B. It is called a *conditional probability*. The expression $p(A$ and $B)$ is a *joint probability*. It is the probability of the joint occurrence of A and B. In a common example in cancer genetic testing, $p(G|O)$ is the probability of being a gene carrier contingent on, or given the fact that, one is unaffected by cancer. Alternatively, $p(G|C)$ would be the probability of being a gene carrier given that one is affected by breast cancer. To derive the relationship between conditional and joint probabilities, we look at the following hypothetical example:

	Cancer	No Cancer	Total
Gene mutation	3	3	6
No gene mutation	1	13	14
Totals	4	16	20

In this example, $p(G$ and $C)$ would be $3/20 = 0.15$, $p(G|C)$ would be $3/4 = .75$, and $p(C)$ would be $4/20 = 0.2$. Their relationship is: $p(G|C) = p$ (G and C) / $p(C)$, or $.75 = 0.15/0.2$

Case Example 6.4. A family with multiple cases of breast cancer was tested with markers closely linked to *BRCA1*. Multiple affected and unaffected members of the family were tested, and a lod score of 0.5 was derived. The sister designated with an arrow in the pedigree on the next page came for counseling. It was noted from her haplotype that she was carrying the marker associated with the cancers in her family. Analysis of the *BRCA1* gene failed to reveal a mutation within the coding region of the gene. Should the results be divulged? What further workup could be considered at this point?

A Bayesian adjustment is performed to accurately assess the probability of linkage in this kindred. Letting p equal the probability that the family is linked to the locus (in this case, *BRCA1* on chromosome 17q), and $1-p$ equal the probability that it is not, then the lod score is $\log_{10}(p/1-p)$. From other linkage studies, the proportion of families with four or more cases of breast cancer (one bilateral) that are linked to *BRCA1* is s. The Bayesian construction for this family is:

Prior probability	p	$1-p$
Conditional probability	s	$1-s$
Joint probability	sp	$(1-p)(1-s)$

The posterior probability of linkage is

$$\frac{sp}{sp + (1-p)(1-s)}$$

If we divide by $1-p$, this is equal to

$$\frac{s(p/1-p)}{s(p/1-p)+(1-s)}$$

where $(p/1-p) = 10^{\text{lod score}}$, in this case, where lod $= 0.5$, $10^{0.5} = 3.16$.

Thus, expressed in general terms, the rule relating conditional probabilities and joint probabilities is:

$$p(A|B) = \frac{p(A \text{ and } B)}{p(B)} \qquad (6\text{-}1)$$

The definition of the relationship of joint and conditional probabilities is:

$$p(A \text{ and } B) = p(A|B)p(B) \text{ [or} = p(B|A)p(A)] \qquad (6\text{-}2)$$

Thus,

$$p(A|B) = p(B|A)p(A)/p(B) \qquad (6\text{-}3)$$

From early reports, s was estimated to be 45% in families with four or more cases of breast cancer. Thus, the posterior probability of linkage was $(.45)(3.16)/(.45)(3.16 + .55)$ $= 0.72$. This translated to a 72% probability for linkage to the markers of the gene being tested. With appropriate confidence intervals, the range was 51% to 85%.

Because analysis failed to reveal a mutation of *BRCA1*, the family was counseled that these extensive efforts had not improved their risk estimation beyond the 50% Mendelian risk originally given. This case illustrates the limitations of linkage-based counseling for the average size families encountered in practice. In other circumstances, with larger families and higher conditional probabilities of linkage, lod scores have successfully been utilized in cancer genetic counseling. In this case, a blood sample for RNA extraction was obtained to look for a possible regulatory mutation in *BRCA1* that might have been missed by DNA analysis (see Chapter 4).

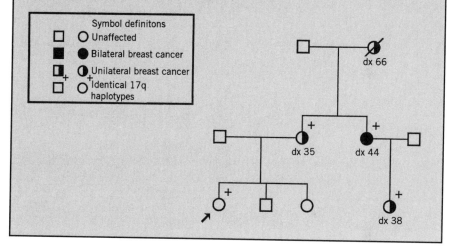

Often, event A is comprised of two mutually exclusive events, A1 or A2. In common examples, these could be the probabilities of being a gene carrier [$p(G)$] or not being a gene carrier [$p(NG)$]; or probabilities of the disease being positive [$p(D+)$] or not [$p(D–)$]. The summation rule for mutually exclusive events is:

$$p(B) = p(B \text{ and } A1) + p(B \text{ and } A2)$$ (6-4)

Rewriting (6-3) by substituting (6-4) for the denominator:

$$p(A|B) = \frac{p(B|A)p(A)}{p(B \text{ and } A1) + p(B \text{ and } A2)}$$ (6-5)

and utilizing the summation rule for mutually exclusive events:

$$p(A|B) = \frac{p(B|A)p(A)}{p(B|A1)p(A1) + p(B|A2)p(A2)}$$ (6-6)

Equation 6-6 is the general formula for Bayes' theorem. In a common example, it is desired to derive the *posterior probability* of being a gene carrier given that one is unaffected, [$p(G|O)$]. The posterior probability reflects the conditions that have been taken into account in deriving the joint probabilities. The posterior probability is derived as:

$$p(G|O) = \frac{p(O|G)(G)}{p(O|G)p(G) + p(O|NG)p(NG)} \quad (6\text{-}7)$$

where $p(NG)$ is probability of being a noncarrier.

In a second common application of Bayes' theorem, $p(D+|T+)$ is the probability of a disease being present if a test is positive. This latter term is also referred to as the *predictive value* of a test. It is the probability that the disease is present given a positive test result [$p(D+|T+)$], and is derived as:

$$p(D+|T+) = \frac{p(T+|D+)p(D+)}{p(T+|D+)p(D+) + p(T+|D-)p(D-)} \quad (6\text{-}8)$$

Applications of Bayes' Theorem

Pedigree Analysis Utilizing Age-Specific Penetrance   In pedigree analysis, the value of Bayes' theorem is its ability to modify a prior probability of a Mendelian event by taking into account conditional circumstances. While these relationships were formally defined above, it is possible to describe their meaning here. In Bayesian analysis, "anterior" information allows determination of a *prior probability,* which is then modified, or "conditioned" by additional information, resulting in a *joint probability,* which is the product of the prior and conditional probabilities. The *posterior probability* is obtained by dividing the joint probability of the event by the sum of the joint probabilities of the event occurring or not occurring.

Thus, for example, we consider a Mendelian dominant scenario where a daughter in a family affected by multiple cases of breast and ovarian cancer knows that one of the relatives in her family has tested positive for a *BRCA1* mutation. She finds that she has reached a mature age unaffected by cancer. It is less likely that her risk of inheriting the cancer susceptibility gene is 50% as predicted by Mendel. Her risk has been conditioned by the observation that most women her age who inherited the mutation would have developed breast cancer early in their lives.

As an example, in the pedigree shown on page 233, when the daughter of a woman affected by breast and ovarian cancer is alive at age 70 and free of disease, it becomes less likely that she has inherited her mother's cancer susceptibility. But how much less than the Mendelian estimate of 50% is her risk of inheriting this altered gene? We first establish that it is appropriate in this "highly penetrant" family to use the age-specific cumulative probabilities of breast cancer for *BRCA1* heterozygotes shown in the middle column of Table 4-2. (If family history were not known, it might be more appropriate to use the figures in the right-hand column of Table 4-2.) We see that, by age 70,

Case Example 6.5. A 70-year-old woman and her 42-year-old daughter sought consultation regarding cancer risk. They reported that the niece of the mother, recently affected by ovarian cancer, tested "positive" for *BRCA1*, but did not want to discuss any of the details of the testing or the specific results. The woman and her daughter who sought consultation could not afford to pay out of pocket for *BRCA1* testing, which was not covered by their insurance.

Counseling in this case utilized and extended the example of Bayesian analysis given in the text. Since a mutation of *BRCA1* was responsible for the breast and ovarian cancers in this family, it was possible to utilize published age-specific penetrance data for *BRCA1* (Table 4-2). Because of the clearly hereditary nature of the highly penetrant trait in this family, the cumulative probabilities derived from linkage families were utilized (center column of data in the table). The probability that the mother was a gene carrier was 16%. A similar Bayesian calculation for the daughter revealed only a 6.8% probability of being a gene carrier, considerably less than the 25% Mendelian risk calculated without Bayesian inference.

The mother and daughter were counseled to observe breast cancer screening recommendations consisting of annual mammography, breast self-examination, and physician exam.

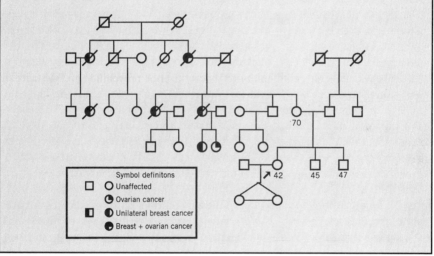

82% of carriers (heterozygotes) will have developed breast cancer, compared to the general population, in which only 7% will have developed breast cancer. But how can these figures be utilized to modify the risk estimates for the mother and her daughter? A Bayesian table is constructed listing the prior probability of being a gene carrier $p(G)$ and the prior probability of not being a gene carrier $p(NG)$. This is modified by the conditional probability of being unaffected if a gene carrier $p(O|G)$, and the probability of being unaffected if not a gene carrier $p(O|G)$. These are multiplied together to give the joint probabilities:

	Being a Gene Carrier	Not Being a Gene Carrier
Prior probability	$p(G)$	$p(NG)$
Conditional probability	$p(O|G)$	$p(O|NG)$
Joint probability	$p(G)\,p(O|G)$	$p(NG)\,p(O|NG)$

Finally, the posterior probability of being a gene carrier is equal to the expression that was derived as equation (6-7) in the preceding section

$$\frac{p(G)\,p(O|G)}{[p(G)\,p(O|G)] + [p(NG)\,p(O|NG)]}$$

In this example $p(G)$ and $p(NG)$ would be 0.5, while $p(O|G)$ would be $1 - .82$, or .18. Similarly $p(O|NG)$ would be $1 - .07$, or .93. The joint probabilities would be .09 and .465, respectively. The posterior probability would be $.09/[.09 + .465]$, or 16%. Thus, we have modified probability of inheriting a mutant *BRCA1* allele from a prior estimate of 50% to a posterior probability of only 16%. Her daughter's risk would be half of this, or 8%. [A Bayesian adjustment can also be performed for this 42-year-old daughter, yielding a posterior probability of 6.8%.]

These types of Bayesian adjustments are appropriate when (1) the age-specific penetrance of specific genes, or specific mutations of genes, is known; and (2) when it is known that a specific gene, or specific mutation, is segregating in the family. This latter assumption can be tested by direct mutation analysis of an affected family member. Bayesian adjustments are common in many genetic counseling situations where prior information is combined with conditional (observed) information. They may apply to families with dominant syndromes such as breast-ovarian and hereditary colon cancer, or Li-Fraumeni syndrome, where prior information is modified by knowledge of unaffected siblings or children, or where risk is modified by knowledge of age-at-onset, as in the foregoing examples. Similar adjustments in risk can be made for recessive traits and are routinely utilized in counseling for such diseases as cystic fibrosis.

Risks Deduced from Direct Testing   The basic attributes of a genetic test, or any medical screening test, are its *reliability* and its *validity*. Reliability can be maximized by quality assurance procedures, training of the technical staff performing the test, and monitoring of the professionals who interpret the results. Validity is a more complex measure and is generally defined as consisting of two major components: sensitivity and specificity. In the context of cancer genetic testing, sensitivity refers to the ability of a genetic test to identify those with the cancer susceptibility, and specificity refers to the ability of the test to identify those without the susceptibility.

Expressing these concepts in the form of the 2×2 table:

	CANCER SUSCEPTIBILITY	
	(+) INCREASED RISK	(−) AVERAGE RISK
TEST +	*a*	*b*
TEST −	*c*	*d*

In this notation, *a* would be the true positives, *b* the false positives, *c* the false negatives, and *d* the true negatives. *Sensitivity* would be the individuals with the susceptibility who test positive (*a/a+c*); and *specificity* would be the individuals at average risk who test negative (*d/b+d*). The lower the false negatives, the better the sensitivity; the lower the false positives, the better the specificity. Another concept, of great relevance to the clinician, is the *(positive) predictive value*, or the probability that an individual with a positive test will be susceptible. This is given by (*a/a+b*).

It is inherent in these definitions that the sensitivity and specificity are not impacted by the prevalence of the disease, whereas the predictive value will be affected by a shift in the prevalence (*a+c/a+b+c+d*). A decrease in the prevalence rate results in a decrease in the predictive value. In equation (6-8) in the preceding section, this relationship was depicted in the formula for the predictive value of a test $p(D+|T+)$

$$p(D+|T+) = \frac{p(T+|D+)p(D+)}{p(T+|D+)p(D+) + p(T+|D-)p(D-)} \tag{6-8}$$

In this equation $p(D+)$ represents the prevalence of the disease. Similarly, $p(T+|D+)$ is another way of defining the sensitivity and $p(T+|D-)$ is the false positive rate. Since $p(T+|D-)$ must be equal to $(1 - [p(T-|D-)])$, and since $p(T-|D-)$ is the definition of specificity, the predictive value can be expressed as:

$$p(D+|T+) = \frac{(\text{sensitivity})(\text{prevalence})}{(\text{sensitivity})(\text{prevalence}) + (1 - \text{specificity})(1 - \text{prevalence})} \tag{6-9}$$

Applications of Sensitivity and Specificity in Cancer Genetic Testing

As defined previously, sensitivity refers to the number of individuals with a disease who test positive for a given assay. The notion of clinical sensitivity and the related concept of positive predictive value are helpful in interpreting the results of any medical test. *Analytic sensitivity* and *analytic specificity* refer to the ability of a laboratory procedure to detect an established analytic standard (an *analyte*); for example, the ability of a new technique to detect a certain mutation. In general, while commercial laboratories may emphasize the excellent analytic sensitivity of a testing methodology, the cancer genetic counselor focuses on its clinical sensitivity. For example, the gold standard for mutation detection has been direct sequencing. As novel methods to detect mutations have been introduced, they have been compared to direct sequencing. Judged against this standard, certain techniques (e.g., chemical cleavage methodologies) may have excellent analytic sensitivities and specificities (see Chapter 7). However, direct sequencing, whether done manually or by automated fluorescent machines, will not detect very large deletions, duplications, or insertions, and will also not detect mutations in regulatory regions that affect transcription or translation. Thus, even direct sequencing for detection of mutations will not have 100% clinical sensitivity.

Similarly, some mutations detected by sequencing will be false positives. This may be the case for some missense mutations, which may represent normal variants, or polymorphisms. As an example, one large series (Shattuck-Eidens et al., 1995) tested 372 samples for *BRCA1* mutations. This study documented a number of both false negatives and false positives for the reasons mentioned. However, the methods of mutation analysis were not uniform in this combined series. A report of 60 families analyzed uniformly detected mutations in 32 families, of which 49 would have been predicted to carry mutations based on linkage estimates (Gayther et al., 1995). An allele-specific expression assay documented absence of a transcript in one case, confirming a presumed regulatory mutation. A number of mutations could have been missed in this series simply because the individual tested in the family was a phenocopy. But assuming there were no phenocopies, the clinical sensitivity of this strategy of *BRCA1* mutation detection in this European population was only 67%. The absence of missense mutations in this series increased specificity but decreased sensitivity. In a subsequent analysis in 1997 by Shattuck-Eidens et al., automated sequencing of *BRCA1* was utilized. A very high proportion (38 of 166) mutations were missense mutations of unknown significance. Sensitivity was increased, but specificity was decreased, thus complicating the clinical interpretation (Shattuck-Eidens et al., 1997).

Similarly, reports of screening for mutations of genes associated with hereditary nonpolyposis colon cancer HNPCC reveal that about 70% of cases meeting strict criteria for HNPCC had mutations in the coding regions of the five genes associated with the syndrome. As was the case for hereditary breast cancer, there were hereditary colon cancer families linked to the loci of *hMSH2* and *hMLH1* for which mutations could not be detected. As discussed in Chapter 4, methylation of promotor regions may provide part of the explanation for the seemingly low sensitivity of sequencing of coding regions of these genes. In addition, large deletions may also have been missed by sequencing, leading to decreased clinical sensitivity. Missense mutations, as in other hereditary syndromes, may have been normal variants, decreasing specificity. *In vitro* protein assays (see Chapter 7) may improve specificity, but seem to lower sensitivity.

In the absence of uniform guidelines or regulatory standards governing cancer genetic testing, it will be left to the clinician to choose among contrasting testing strategies with varying levels of sensitivity and specificity, and to interpret these findings for patients and their families. This may require quantitative derivations. For example, without functional assays for the protein products of most of the cancer predisposition genes, missense mutations of unknown significance will be investigated by establishing if the mutation cosegregates with the disease (linkage analysis), or if it has been observed previously in a high proportion of the general population (epidemiologic analysis). The development of functional assays should improve clinical sensitivity and specificity, and the development of automated or chip-based approaches to mutation detection (Chapter 7) may improve the analytical sensitivity of current modes of molecular diagnosis.

Applications of Predictive Value   Determinations of predictive value are relevant to clinical counseling. The probability of a disease given a positive test is of paramount interest in cancer genetic testing. However, the concept of disease probability by a given age can be confused with the notion of age-specific penetrance. In most cancer genetic counseling, the latter approach will be more appropriate to convey to patients.

For example, a young Jewish woman desires an explanation of the positive predictive value associated with the detection of a 185delAG mutation. She has been told by her physician that the figure 9% is cited in a publication, meaning that the chances of developing early onset breast cancer if she has positive test are 9% (Fitzgerald et al., 1996). How this figure was derived must be considered.

Values can be plugged into equation (6-9) to make the derivation. The prevalence of breast cancer by age 40 in Jewish women can be estimated by the population value, which is 1 in 217. Similarly, $p(T+|D+)$ can be estimated as 8/39 from the Fitzgerald data. Other studies confirmed that about 20% of early onset breast cancer in Jewish women was due to the 185delAG mutation. How was (1-sensitivity), or the false positive rate estimated? In the derivation of a 9% predictive value in this report, the false positive rate was estimated as the 1% (8/858) frequency of the mutation in a large population series. But are these really false positives? In fact they may not be, because some of the women in this anonymous population series may have had prior histories of breast cancer, and others may have harbored undetected disease. These considerations could substantially increase the estimate of the predictive value from the published value (Offit, 1996).

Whether the positive predictive value is 9% or higher, what does it mean? It refers to the chances of getting early onset (before age 40) breast cancer if one carries the 185delAG mutation. But what about the chances of breast cancer after age 40? The period from age 40 to 60 is, in fact, the greatest period of risk for a *BRCA1* heterozygote. For this counseling scenario, the genetic concept of age-specific penetrance is most relevant. Counseling utilizing data such as that depicted in Table 4-2 may be the more useful way for an individual to visualize the distribution of risk over a lifetime.

More commonly, the predictive value of a genetic test is used to estimate its usefulness in population screening.

Predictive Value of a Genetic Test in Population Screening

POSITIVE PREDICTIVE VALUE   An illustration of predictive value is based the use of a test in population screening. For the sake of illustration, if one assumes a 1% false negative rate, and a 1% false positive rate, how is the predictive value of the *BRCA1* direct mutation test impacted by varying the underlying prevalence? In this example, we assume a prevalence for *BRCA1* mutations in the general population of 1 in 300. Assuming that 30,000 individuals are screened, one will detect 99 of the 100 mutations (sensitivity of 99%). Similarly, of the remaining 29,900, a 1% false positive rate (specificity of 99%) will give 299 false positives, and 29,601 true negatives. This translates into a predictive value of 99/398, or about 25%. If instead, one screens 30,000 women who were members of families with at least three cases of breast cancer diagnosed before age 50, the prevalence would be 4 in 10 (Shattuck-Eidens et al., 1995). Thus, of the 12,000 mutation carriers, 11,880 would be detected, with 120 false negatives (sensitivity 99%). Similarly, there would be 180 false positives among the 18,000 at normal susceptibility (specificity 99%). This would yield an impressive predictive value of 11,880/12,060, or 98.5%.

At the lower population prevalence, for every mutation detected, there would be three false positives, whereas in the higher prevalence group the proportional yield of true positives would be much higher. Even more striking, if we assume a cost of $1000 per test, the cost per true positive would be in excess of $300,000 in the first group and $2500 in the second group!

The basic principle of this example is that genetic screening, at least for *BRCA1* mutations, will be most efficiently performed in a high-risk (high prevalence) population. In practice however, a combination of lower cost and lower sensitivity mutation detection approaches may be combined with more expensive strategies of higher specificity and sensitivity (e.g., direct sequencing, functional assays). The mix of these assays will determine an overall sensitivity, specificity, and predictive value, which will define the validity of the approach.

NEGATIVE PREDICTIVE VALUE   Unaffected family members will be as interested in the negative predictive value of a test as they will be in the positive predictive value. Bayesian derivations can be used to address the "conditioning" of risk after genetic testing. For example, a Jewish individual with an extensive family history of breast and ovarian cancer wants to know what it means if she tests negative for the three mutations of *BRCA1* or *BRCA2* that are observed in the Ashkenazi population. What are the chances, given a negative test, that she will still carry a predisposing mutation? Although very few mutations of *BRCA1* or *BRCA2* other than the three founding ones have been observed in the Ashkenazim, some hereditary breast-ovarian cancer families do carry other mutations (see Chapter 4 and Tonin et al., 1996). For example, in a family with two or more cases of breast cancer and two or more cases of ovarian cancer, about 90% will segregate a *BRCA* founder mutation (see Table 4-4). In the example just given, if we approximate p(O|NG) as one, the probabilities for an unaffected daughter in such a family being a gene carrier are:

	Being a Gene Carrier	Not Being a Gene Carrier
Prior probability	0.5	0.5
Conditional probability	.10	1.0
Joint probability	0.05	0.5

The posterior probability of being a gene carrier is equal to 0.5/0.55 = 9%. Thus, a negative three-mutation screen for the unaffected daughter will reduce her risk from 50% to 9%. To reduce it further, it would be necessary to establish the particular mutation (or mutations) segregating in the family and then to offer testing to the daughter.

REFERENCES

Ahlbom A, Lichtenstein P, Malmstrom H, Feychting M, Hemminki K, Pedersen NL. 1997. Cancer in twins: genetic and nongenetic familial risk factors. J Natl Cancer Inst 89:287–93.

American Cancer Society. 1997. Cancer Facts and Figures.

Amos CI, Shaw GL, Tucker MA, Hartge P. 1992. Age at onset for familial epithelial ovarian cancer. JAMA 268:1986–9.

Anderson DE, Badzioch MD. 1993. Familial breast cancer risks: Effects of prostate and other cancers. Cancer 72:114–9.

Benichou J, Gail MH, Mulvhill JJ. 1996. Graphs to estimate an individualized risk of breast cancer. J Clin Oncol 14:103–10.

Claus B, Risch NJ, Thompson WD. 1990. Age at onset as an indicator of familial risk of breast cancer. Am J Epidemiol 131:961–72.

Claus ED, Risch N, Thompson WD. 1991. Genetic analysis of breast cancer in the cancer and steroid hormone study. Am J Hum Genet 48:232–42.

Claus EB, Risch N, Thompson WD. 1994. Autosomal dominant inheritance of early-onset breast cancer. Cancer 73:643–51.

Colditz GA, Willet WC, Hunter DJ et al. 1993. Family history, age, and risk of breast cancer: Prospective data from the Nurses Health Study. JAMA 270:338–43.

Desonie D. 1996. Table: Chances of dying from selected causes. In: Cosmic Collisions. New York: Henry Holt, p. 105.

Dupont WD, Plummer WD Jr. 1996. Understanding the relationship between relative and absolute risk. Cancer 77:2193–9.

Fitzgerald MG, MacDonald DJ, Krainer M et al. 1996. Germ-line *BRCA1* mutations in Jewish and non-Jewish women with early-onset breast cancer. New Engl J Med 334:143–9.

Gail MH, Brinton LA, Byar DP, et al. 1989. Projecting individualized probabilities of developing breast cancer for white females who are being examined annually. J Natl Cancer Inst 81:1879–86.

Gail MH, Benichou J. 1992. Assessing the risk of breast cancer in individuals. In DeVita VT Jr, Hellman S, Rosenberg SA (eds), Cancer Prevention. Philadelphia, PA: J.B. Lippincott, pp. 1–15.

Gayther SA, Warren W, Mazoyer S et al. 1995. Germline mutations of the *BRCA1* gene in breast and ovarian cancer families provide evidence for a genotype-phenotype correlation. Nature Genet 11:428–33.

Grady D, Rubin SM, Petitti DB et al. 1992. Hormone therapy to prevent disease and prolong life in postmenopausal women. Ann Intern Med 117:1016–37.

Offit K, Brown K. 1994. Quantitative risk counseling for familial cancer: a resource for clinical oncologists. J Clin Oncol 12:1724–36.

Offit K. 1996. Breast cancer and *BRCA1* mutations (letter). New Engl J Med 334:1197–8.

Schatzkin A, Goldstein A, Freedman LS. 1995. What does it mean to be a cancer gene carrier? Problems in establishing causality from the molecular genetics of cancer. J Natl Cancer Inst 87:1126–30.

Shattuck-Eidens D, McClure M, Simard J et al. 1995. A collaborative survey of 80 mutations in the *BRCA1* breast and ovarian cancer susceptibility gene. Implications for presymptomatic testing and screening. JAMA 273:535–41.

Shattuck-Eidens D, Oliphant A, McClure M et al. 1997. Complete DNA sequence analysis of *BRCA1* in 798 women at high risk for susceptibility mutations. JAMA (in press).

St. John DJB, McDermott FT, Hopper JL et al. 1993. Cancer risk in relatives of patients with colorectal cancer. Ann Intern Med 118:785–90.

Weinstein MC, Feinberg HV. 1980. Clinical Decision Analysis. Philadelphia: W. B. Saunders.

Willett WC, Hunter DJ, Stampfer MJ et al. 1992. Dietary fat and fiber in relation to risk of breast cancer. JAMA 268:2037–44.

Winawer SJ, Zauber AG, Gerdes H et al. 1996. Risk of colorectal cancer in families of people with adenomatous polyps. New Engl J Med 334:82–7.

Young ID. 1991. Introduction to Risk Calculation in Genetic Counseling. Oxford University Press.

7

Laboratory Methods of Cancer Genetic Testing

Common techniques of genetic testing have been applied to diagnostic, prognostic, and presymptomatic analysis of clinical samples. A familiarity with these methodologies provides the clinician with a better understanding of their strengths and limitations. The commonly employed methods of chromosome or nucleic acid analysis that have been utilized in clinical cancer genetics are summarized in this section.

LABORATORY METHODS OF CHROMOSOME ANALYSIS

Cytogenetic Analysis

Cytogenetic analysis remains one of the few methodologies that provides a bird's eye view of the human genome. Cytogenetic analyses continue to identify sites for novel oncogenes and are also an established diagnostic test in the evaluation of newly diagnosed patients with cancer as well as individuals with congenital abnormalities and cancer predisposition.

The technique of karyotypic analysis has continued to improve over the past decade, as refinements have made possible extremely high resolution studies. Metaphase cells must be harvested in short-term culture, which limits cytogenetic analysis to freshly obtained, or live frozen material. Metaphase chromosomes are visualized after paralysis of the mitotic spindle with colchicine, isotonic expansion, staining, and imaging. The normal human karyotype consists of 22 pairs of autosomes and two sex chromosomes. It is represented as 46,XY (male) or 46,XX (female). Details of chromosome structure are identified by banding. The arm above the centromere, which is usually shorter, is called the p arm, and the lower arm is called the q arm.

Each arm is divided into regions and bands, numbered differently for each chromosome. Chromosome abnormalities in cancer may be numerical or structural. Many cancer karyotypes are *aneuploid*, meaning that the chromosome number is not 46. Rarely, karyotypes are *haploid* (23 chromosomes) or some multiple of the haploid number (e.g., tetraploid = 92 chromosomes). Other common numerical abnormalities are *trisomies* (an extra copy of a chromosome) or *monosomies* (a missing copy of a chromosome). Structural abnormalities include *deletions* (del), *insertions* (ins), *inversions* (inv), or *duplications* (dup) of chromosomal segments. Sometimes an entire arm is duplicated, and the other arm deleted, an *isochromosome*. Chromosome arms can also be involved in *reciprocal translocations* (Figure 3-8).

In 1991, the International System for Cytogenetic Nomenclature was modified for cancer cytogenetics. Karyotypes are now written in ascending order by each chromosome, listing first the numerical and then the structural abnormalities of each chromosome. Thus,

$$49,XY,dup(1)(q22q44),del(6)(q21),+7,+12,t(14;18)(q21;q32),+18$$

signifies a karyotype with extra copies of chromosomes 7, 12, and 18, hence the chromosome number of $46 + 3 = 49$. There is also a duplication of the long arm of chromosome 1 including bands 22 and 44, a deletion of all of the long arm of chromosome 6 beyond band 21, and a reciprocal translocation between the long arms of chromosomes 14 and 18. (From the data listed in Table 8-2, one can deduce that this tumor was a lymphoid neoplasm.)

In general, translocations tend to be more common in leukemias, lymphomas, and sarcomas, whereas complex structural abnormalities are more common in solid tumors. Catalogs have been published listing chromosomal abnormalities associated with human tumors (Mitelman, 1994). Certain chromosomal abnormalities may be seen in the circulating blood cells, representing *constitutional abnormalities*. These may be associated with congenital and other inborn abnormalities (e.g., trisomy 21), or may not be associated with disease (e.g., some translocations).

Fluorescence In Situ Hybridization (FISH)

Hybridization refers to the specificity of binding between DNA basepairs. When a preset sequence of base pairs is tagged with a label and then hybridized with a section of a tumor specimen, or a spread of chromosomes, this is termed *in situ hybridization*. The labels utilized in these studies may be radioisotopes or reagents containing a fluorescent tag that can be visualized under the microscope (*fluorescence in situ hybridization* or *FISH*). FISH can be utilized to visualize hybridization signals on chromosomes in order to localize a gene.

FISH has been applied to mapping of new genes, where a resolution of 1–2 mb can be achieved. It is also used as a diagnostic reagent to detect translocations of known genes, or to detect numerical chromosome abnormalities. Although FISH can be performed on anaphase as well as metaphase cells, preparations still require short-term culture.

LABORATORY METHODS OF ANALYSIS OF GENE STRUCTURE AND EXPRESSION

Southern Blotting

Southern blotting, named after its inventor some 20 years ago, remains one of the standard methods for analyzing DNA structure. It can detect the presence of a gene and can demonstrate whether that gene is grossly intact. It detects rearrangements, deletions, or insertions that may be missed by cytogenetic analysis (Grompe, 1993). However, it does not detect point mutations or small insertions or deletions unless these occur at restriction sites (see next paragraph). In cancer diagnostics, Southern blotting is most commonly utilized to detect alterations of oncogenes associated with hematologic and some solid tumors and to determine clonality of lymphoid cancers.

The technique of Southern blotting is standardized in clinical laboratories. DNA is isolated from blood lymphocytes or tissue and digested by restriction enzymes, which cut the DNA at a specified DNA sequence. These DNA fragments are subjected to agarose gel electrophoresis, which allows the smaller fragments to move more rapidly through the gel. The fragments, which are double-stranded DNA, are denatured with a strong base to separate the strands. At this point the strands are transferred onto filter paper (the blotting process described by Dr. Southern). A cloned DNA probe for the gene of interest is tagged with a radioisotope and allowed to hybridize, i.e., anneal to its complimentary segment. This process is recorded on film. Depending on the particular enzymes used, there will be a band signifying the presence of the gene of interest. An extra or "rearranged" band (compared to a placental control) signifies a structural alteration of the gene in question.

Southern blotting can be performed on fresh or frozen tissues, but not from paraffin-embedded tissues, in which the DNA is already fragmented. It is the standard method of detection of immunoglobulin gene and oncogene rearrangements, and has also been utilized to detect structural alterations of some tumor suppressor genes.

Northern Blotting

Northern blotting is a method to measure size and amount of mRNA for a specific gene. It is performed in a similar fashion to Southern blotting, except that a probe is hybridized to blots with mRNA. There is no restriction enzyme digestion because the various RNA transcripts are of different lengths. This technique has application for determination of the level of gene expression and is used for some prognostic genetic assays.

Northern blotting generally requires fresh tissue or cells from culture in order to isolate RNA. Relatively large amounts of tumor tissue are required. *RNAse protection assays* allow the quantitation of smaller amounts of RNA. In this technique the mRNA is protected by a DNA probe prior to the addition of nucleases that degrade single-stranded DNA or RNA. This technique can detect one RNA molecule in 100 cells. It is a standard technique in the detection of increased expression of oncogenes in malignant tumors.

Polymerase Chain Reaction

Cited as one of the most significant technical advances in modern molecular genetics, the *polymerase chain reaction* (PCR) makes possible the amplification up to 10^5-fold any DNA fragment for which 20 base pair flanking primers can be made (Grompe, 1993; Cohen, 1994). The primers are complementary to the opposite DNA strand flanking the particular region of interest. After repeated cycles of denaturation, annealing of the primers to opposite strands, and extension of the new DNA with DNA polymerase and nucleotides, the amplified fragment is amenable to detection (see Figure 7-1). In the setting of mutation analysis for cancer predisposition genes, PCR has many applications. It is used to amplify particular exons of large genes (e.g., *BRCA1*) so that each exon can be sequenced. Modifications of PCR are also used to screen for mutations by detection of conformational shifts due to mutations in cancer predisposition genes (see following section).

A great advantage of PCR is that, in theory, it can be performed from DNA of a single cell. Thus, DNA from paraffin-stored tissues, if not degraded, is amenable to some methods of PCR-based mutational analysis.

LABORATORY METHODS FOR DETECTION OF KNOWN MUTATIONS

Allele-Specific Oligonucleotide Analysis (ASO)

ASO analysis is a modification of Southern blotting. Small segments of DNA containing the mutated segment of the gene are amplified using PCR, dot-blotted onto filters, and then hybridized with probes specific for known mutation sequences (Saiki et al., 1989). ASO analysis offers a sensitive means to detect a known small deletion, or single base pair substitutions, which would be missed on a routine Southern blot with a full-length cloned DNA probe. ASO screening only detects one specific mutation; thus, panels of ASO probes for the most common mutations of cancer susceptibility genes are commonly utilized. As a two-step PCR/hybridization reaction, ASO is sensitive enough to detect mutations of DNA from paraffin-embedded tissues. ASO is a common technique to detect recurring mutations, e.g., the 185delAG mutation of *BRCA1*, and is used by a number of commercial laboratories offering this test.

Acrylamide Gel Electrophoresis (Band Shift Assays)

In this simple method of detection of a known mutation, the PCR technique is utilized to amplify a small segment of a gene, including the mutated region. The mutation is detected by a shifted band, due to the different mobility of the mutated fragment, utilizing polyacrylamide gel electrophoresis (PAGE). This technique can detect differences of 1 or 2 base pairs, and can be performed using radioisotopes, or by staining the DNA with a dye (ethidium bromide). Such assays have been utilized to detect known *BRCA1* or *BRCA2* mutations (Neuhausen et al., 1996).

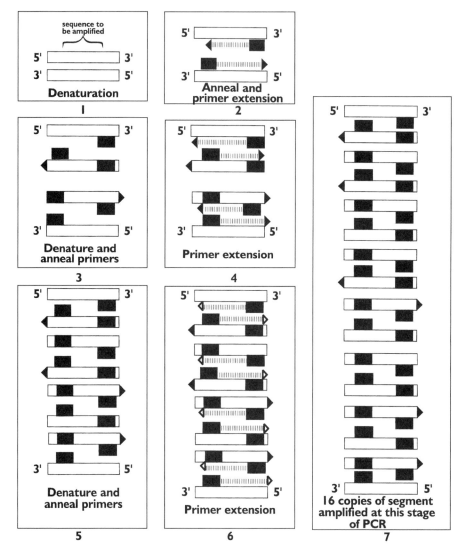

FIGURE 7-1 *The polymerase chain reaction.*

Restriction Site Analysis

In restriction site analysis, the PCR primer is constructed to introduce a restriction site next to the mutant sequence, or the mutation itself creates or destroys a restriction site. Thus, when a specific restriction enzyme is added, the digestion of the mutant sequence results in a fragment of different size than the normal sequence. This technique is ideal for mutation detection tailored to unique mutations in large families, and has been used, for example, to detect a specific *APC* mutation in a large Utah family. It has also been utilized to detect five specific mutations in *BRCA1* (Rohlfs et al., 1997). An advantage of this technique, referred to as "PCR-mediated site directed mutagenesis," is that it does not require radioactivity.

LABORATORY METHODS FOR DETECTION OF UNKNOWN MUTATIONS

Single Strand Conformational Polymorphism (SSCP)

In single strand conformation analysis, double-stranded PCR products from the specimen to be analyzed and a control are denatured into single strands (by heat) and electrophoresed. The mobility in the electrophoresis gel of the conformations of each of the strands will differ, depending on the base pair differences present in the test specimen (see Figure 7-2). The DNA is visualized by using a radionucleotide or fluorescent

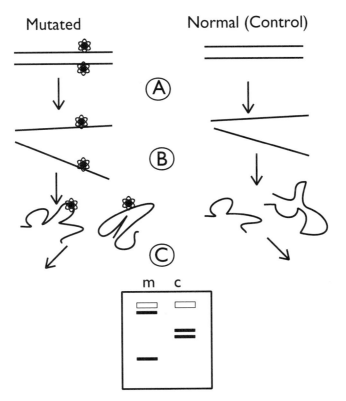

FIGURE 7-2 *Single stranded conformational polymorphism analysis. A. Double-stranded PCR products from the specimen to be analyzed and a control are denatured into single strands (by heat). Stars mark mutations. B. Single strands are allowed to fold under nondenaturing conditions. C. Single strands are electrophoresed. The mobility in the electrophoresis gel of the conformations of each of the strands will differ, depending on the base pair differences present in the test specimen.*

label or by ethidium bromide or silver staining. SSCP detects 70–95% of mutations in PCR products of 200 bp or less. It will easily detect insertions or deletions of four bases or more, but may not detect smaller mutations of one or two bases, especially missense mutations that do not alter the length of the fragment (Grompe, 1993; Sheffield et al., 1993). Abnormal fragments that have shifted mobility on an SSCP gel can then be sequenced to determine the mutation.

SSCP is the most common technique utilized by research laboratories to screen for mutations in specific exons of *BRCA1*, the HNPCC genes, *p53, RET*, and other genes. It is easier to carry out, but somewhat less sensitive than, for example, DGGE or CDGE (see below).

In *heteroduplex analysis*, the denatured samples are allowed to cool so that some will anneal with complementary strands (homoduplexes) and some with mutant strands (heteroduplexes). These double-stranded products can be detected by gel electrophoresis (Grompe, 1993; Ganguly et al., 1993).

Denaturing Gradient Gel Electrophoresis (DGGE)

DGGE is an alternative to SSCP. Single-stranded regions of partially denatured double-stranded DNA fragments have reduced mobility in the electrophoresis gel. In DGGE, fragments from a PCR reaction are run on gels that contain an increasing gradient of urea and formaldehyde. Even a single base pair change may alter the temperature or denaturant concentration at which the DNA strands uncoil or melt (see Figure 7-3). Any method to ensure that the sequence being tested lies within a relatively low melting point region enhances the sensitivity of the reaction. One technique is the attachment of a 30–50 bp high temperature melting point *GC clamp* to one of the PCR primers, thus ensuring that the amplified sequence has a low disassociation temperature. A positive DGGE result, like SSCP, indicates that a mutation exists, but requires sequencing to characterize the specific mutation. DGGE products can also be visualized utilizing nonradioactive dyes (Grompe, 1993; Sheffield, 1989). A modification of DGGE is *constant denaturant gel electrophoresis* (CDGE).

DGGE and CDGE have been utilized to improve the sensitivity of detection of mutations of a number of cancer predisposition genes including *BRCA1* and *BRCA2*. A combination of heteroduplexing and DGGE as a two step, two dimensional DNA electrophoresis reaction has been applied to the detection of mutations of the "HNPCC" genes *hMSH2* and *hMLH1* (Wu et al., 1997).

Chemical Mismatch Cleavage (CMC) Methods

Chemical mismatch cleavage techniques utilize the principle that heteroduplexes will form between mutant and wild-type sequences being analyzed. The CMC technique combines PCR and chemical compounds that modify unhybridized nucleotides so that the fragment can then be cleaved at the modified nucleotide by another chemical compound. Primer extension of these fragments is terminated by the blocked nucleotides. In one CMC technique, the PCR fragment and labeled probe are treated by osmium tetroxide or hyoxylamine in order to modify the unhybridized T or C residues, which

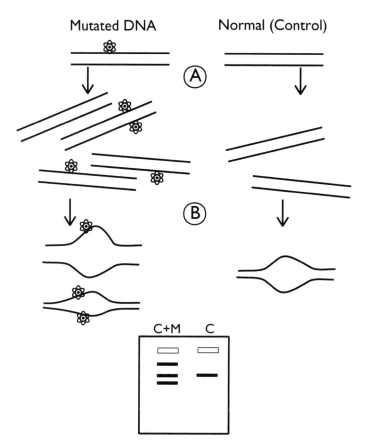

FIGURE 7-3 *Denaturing gradient gel electrophoresis. A. Mutant and normal DNA is denatured into single strands and mixed and allowed to reanneal, making four types of homo- and heteroduplexes. B. These species are subjected to electrophoreses in a gradient of denaturing agents, with different melting of heteroduplexes shown as abnormal bands compared to normal homoduplexes.*

are then cleaved by piperidine. The fragments are analyzed by electrophoresis and autoradiography (Grompe, 1993; Condie et al., 1993).

CMC techniques can analyze PCR products up to 1.7 kb in length and also provide information on the size and location of the change. Because it is a complex technique involving use of hazardous chemicals, CMC is not widely utilized in clinical genetic testing.

Sequencing

Manual methods for determining the nucleotide sequence of DNA fragments have not changed significantly from the protocols that led to a Nobel Prize in 1980. The process is based on analogues of nucleotides (dideoxynucleotides) that halt a DNA polymerase reaction as it generates a complementary fragment of the template stand under analysis. Depending on the concentration of the natural (radiolabeled) analogue nucleotide that is introduced, the reaction will be halted at various points, depending on the location of the nucleotide in the sequence being analyzed. After electrophoresis, the result is a series of radioactive bands on the sequencing gel, corresponding to the locations of the various residues. By running four such reactions for the four nucleotides in four adjoining lanes, it is possible to simply read off the sequence in the order that each band occurs (see Figure 7-4) (Sanger, 1977).

In automated techniques, fluorescently labeled dideoxy terminators, with a different dye coupled to each of the four dideoxynucleotides are utilized (Chadwick et al., 1995). Cycle sequencing is performed, which both amplifies the fragment being sequenced and labels it for sequencing (see Figure 7-5). An advantage of this procedure is that no special primers are needed other than those for the PCR and sequencing. Whether done manually utilizing isotopic detection or by automated sequencers utiliz-

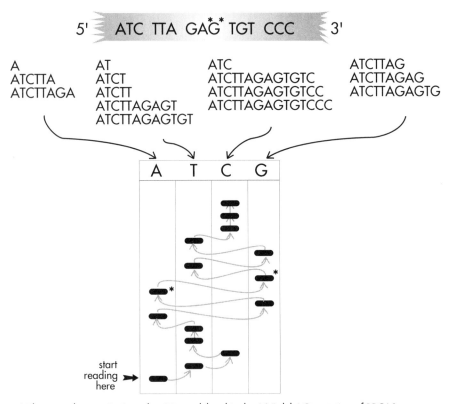

* These two base pairs in codon 23 are deleted in the 185 del AG mutation of BRCA1

FIGURE 7-4 *Direct sequencing of the 185delAG BRCA1 mutation.*

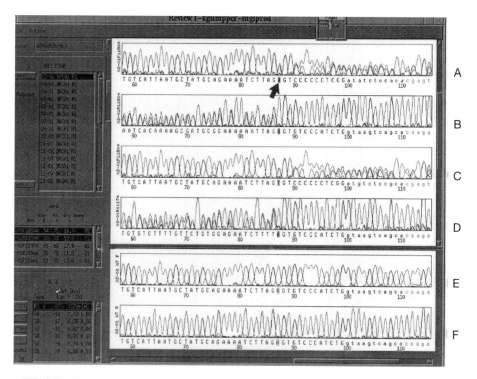

FIGURE 7-5 *Automated fluorescent DNA sequence of a portion of exon 2 of the BRCA1 gene. The cursor in Frame A signifies the location of the first of two deleted bases. From this point downstream (to the right) there is a difference in sequence between the DNA strands as seen by lower peak heights and multiple signals at each base. Frame B is the sequence read in the reverse direction. Frames C and D are repeat experiments of lanes A and B. Frames E and F depict the consensus ("normal") sequence; note the consistent peak heights and single signals at each position [Courtesy of Dr. Brian Ward, Myriad Genetic Laboratories, Inc.].*

ing fluorescence detection technology, direct sequencing is slow and cumbersome. In practice, all the coding regions of a gene and the intron/exon boundaries are amplified by PCR and sequenced in 250–400 base pair segments. Attempts to robotize the process have transformed a tool of basic science into a workhorse of the diagnostic laboratory.

Direct sequencing remains the gold standard for mutation detection for the most common cancer predisposition genes and is required for confirmation of mutations detected by SSCP or band shift methods. Some commercial laboratories rely on SSCP or DGGE methods to identify fragments to be sequenced, whereas other laboratories have committed themselves to sequencing all exons and splice sites. The latter approach is the more sensitive, because single base pair changes may escape detection on SSCP, heteroduplex, or DGGE-based assays. However, even sequencing is not perfectly sensitive, because promotor region or other significant intronic mutations can be missed. In addition, the specificity of sequencing (see Chapter 6) may be decreased by the detection of numerous missense mutations that may be harmless polymorphisms.

A recent innovation in sequencing technologies has been the introduction of the sequencing chip. Using computer-based technologies, microchips that are 1.6 cm^2 in size are constructed containing hundreds of thousands of oligonucleotides of predetermined sequence. These oligonucleotides then interrogate a DNA sample for sequence information. For *BRCA1* screening, families of up to 100,000 oligonucleotides have been designed to detect all possible single base substitutions, single base insertions, and 1–5 base deletions on both strands. Results are read as the relative hybridization to wild-type or mutant targets, labeled with different colored fluorescent tags (Hacia et al., 1996). Although currently limited to research settings, these chip technologies offer the promise of increasing through-put and decreasing cost of future sequence-based analysis.

Monoallelic Mutation Analysis (MAMA)

The *monoallelic mutation analysis* (MAMA) technique utilizes the method of isolating a single allele in a rodent somatic cell hybrid. In this way single alleles can be analyzed to detect heterozygous mutations that would be missed by conventional analysis. It has been applied to detect the 20% of familial adenomatous polyposis (FAP) and 30% of hereditary nonpolyposis colon cancer (HNPCC) cases that do not show mutations by standard techniques (Papadopoulous et al., 1996).

In Vitro Synthesized Protein Assay

In an attempt to screen for mutations and avoid direct sequencing, it was noted that, at least for the majority of mutations of APC and the various HNPCC genes, truncation of the protein results. This holds true for frameshifts causing premature truncation, nonsense mutations, and splice site mutations. In the *in vitro synthesized protein assay* (IVSP), mRNA from lymphocytes is converted to cDNA, amplified by PCR, then converted back to RNA, and translated into a radiolabeled protein. Truncated proteins can be detected when electrophoresed against normal controls on an agarose gel (Powell et al., 1993; Luce et al., 1995).

Because it requires RNA, IVSP assays utilize live lymphocytes. In many of the research studies published, the assay was run from lymphocytes immortalized after exposure to the Epstein-Barr virus. IVSP for mutations of *hHMLH1* and *hMSH2* are commercially available, and truncated protein assays for *BRCA1* and *NFI* have also been developed (Plummer et al., 1995). The technical specifications for these assays have been adapted for clinical laboratory use by Luce and coworkers. For the practicing clinician, obtaining of samples for RNA means that blood specimens have to be processed as soon as possible, unlike methods of DNA analysis, which can be performed on samples stored for several days.

Functional Assays

Functional assays are invaluable to determine whether missense mutations are innocuous polymorphisms or important predisposing mutations. A novel method of assay for the detection of *p53* mutations is based on its function as a transcriptional activator. In this assay, the presence of an inactivating mutation is scored by its ability to interfere with the transcriptional function of *p53*, as measured by binding to the known *p53* binding sites. The patient's *p53* RNA is reverse transcribed to cDNA and amplified by PCR. It is cotransformed into yeast with an expression vector and, through gap repair cloning techniques, put into a plasmid, and the resulting transformants selected by their ability to grow on medium lacking leucine. In this assay, the wild-type *p53* colonies (that bind the receptor) are white and the mutants are red.

These assays appear to be superbly sensitive for missense mutations that affect function, and hence overcome one of the important technical limitations of simpler DNA structure-based techniques such as SSCP, RNAse mismatch cleavage, and chemical mismatch cleavage. They do not detect large deletions or mutant alleles that are poorly expressed due to promotor defects or splicing defects (Ishioka et al., 1993). An assay in which the ability of *BRCA1* mutations to abrogate inhibition of yeast (*S. Cerevesiae*) has been proposed as a functional test for C-terminal *BRCA1* mutations (Humphrey et al., 1997). Functional assays for the DNA replication repair genes are also under development, and similar assays for other genes can be anticipated as their function becomes known.

Choice of Methodologies

Surprisingly few data are available to inform practitioners as to the relative analytic sensitivity and specificity (see Chapter 6) of various methods of mutation detection in cancer-prone families. In addition, no uniform national regulatory program of proficiency testing is in place to guide the consumer of these services. In the absence of these data, the clinician must evaluate the options for molecular diagnosis on a case-by-case and gene-by-gene basis. Mutation-specific hybridization techniques (e.g., ASO, gel shift assays) are cheap and rapid, but unable to detect previously unknown mutations. Sequencing-based techniques are highly sensitive, time-consuming, and expensive. They also suffer due to decreased specificity resulting from detection of missense variants. Functional assays are technically complex and not available for most cancer predisposing genes. Mutation-specific hybridization methodologies (e.g., ASO, gel shift) are best utilized in families in which specific mutations have been identified by SSCP/sequencing or other sequencing-based techniques.

In those instances where specific recurring mutations have been noted in ethnically homogeneous groups (e.g., *BRCA* mutations in Ashkenazi Jews, *hMLH1* mutations in Finland) mutation-specific hybridization techniques may prove useful as initial low-cost screens, but will not detect other mutations that may also occur. For genes that are relatively small or for which mutations occur in a limited region (e.g., *CDKN2/p16*), sequencing can be limited to specific exons. For the most part, however, molecular detection of mutations in cancer predisposition genes involves complex technologies still in the process of clinical translation. An up-to-date list of clinical laboratories providing specific tests is available from the HELIX on-line database. The e-mail address for HELIX and a list of selected laboratories providing these assays is included in Appendix B.

Regulatory Aspects

As highlighted in an interim report by the Task Force on Genetic Testing of the National Institutes of Health, there does not exist an accreditation or proficiency testing program to guarantee the quality of genetic testing services (Task Force on Genetic Testing of the National Institutes of Health, 1997). There does exist a voluntary proficiency testing program run by the College of American Pathologists and the American College of Medical Genetics (CAP/ACMG). At present, laboratories certified under the Clinical Laboratory Improvement Amendments of 1988 (i.e., CLIA-approved labs) are not required to participate in proficiency testing programs for cancer molecular genetic testing. The U.S. Food and Drug Administration oversees genetic reagents marketed as testing kits, but does not regulate laboratories utilizing "home brew" reagents to provide testing services. Health-care providers are well served to inquire if a particular testing laboratory is CLIA-approved and a participant in the CAP/ACMG inspection and survey program and if the lab director is credentialed and holds appropriate state licenses.

For laboratories providing molecular testing for cancer diagnosis, The Association for Molecular Pathology (AMP) has been formed. A list of AMP-member laboratories offering molecular diagnostic testing for cancer, as well as the address of the AMP, is included in Appendix B.

REFERENCES

Chadwick RB, Conrad MP, McGuinnis MD et al. 1996. Heterozygote and mutation detection by direct automated fluorescent DNA sequencing using mutant Taq DNA polymerase. Bio Techniques 20:676–83.

Cohen J. 1994. 'Long PCR' leaps into larger DNA sequences. Science 263:1564–5.

Condie A, Eeles R, Borresen AL et al. 1993. Detection of point mutations in the p53 gene: comparison of single strand conformation polymorphism, constant denaturant gel electrophoresis, and hydroxylamine and osmium tetroxide techniques. Hum Mutation 2:58–66.

Ganguly A, Rock MJ, Prockop DJ. 1993. Conformation-sensitive gel electrophoresis for rapid detection of single base differences in double stranded PCR products and DNA fragments: evidence for solvent-induced bends in DNA heteroduplexes. Proc Natl Acad Sci (USA) 90:10325–9.

Grompe M. 1993. The rapid detection of unknown mutations in nucleic acids. Nature Genet 5:111–6.

Hacia JG, Brody LC, Chee MS, Fodor SPA, Collins FS. 1996. Detection of heterozygous mutations in *BRCA1* using high density oligonucleotide arrays and two-color fluorescence analysis. Nature Genet 14:441–9.

Humphrey JS, Salim A, Erdos MR, Collins FS, Brody LC, Klausner RD. 1997. Human *BRCA1* inhibits growth in yeast: potential use in diagnostic testing. Proc Natl Acad Sci 94:5820–25.

Ishioka C, Frebourg T, Yan Y-X, Vidal M, Friend SH, Schmidt S, Iggo R. 1993. Screening patients for heterozygous p53 mutations using a functional assay in yeast. Nature Genet 5:124–9.

Luce MC, Marra G, Chauhan DP et al. 1995. In vitro transcription/translation assay for the screening of hMLH1 and hMSH2 mutations in familial colon cancer. Gastroenterology 109:1368–74.

Mitelman F. 1994. Catalog of Chromosome Aberrations in Cancer. Ed 5. New York: Wiley-Liss.

Neuhausen S, Gilewski T, Norton L et al. 1996. Recurrent *BRCA2* 6174delT mutations in Ashkenazi Jewish women affected by breast cancer. Nature Genet 13:126–8.

Papadapoulous N, Vogelstein B, Kinzler K. 1996. MAMA: a sensitive strategy for mutation detection. Second plenary meeting of principal investigators. Frederick, Maryland.

Plummer SJ, Anton-Culver H, Webster L et al. 1995. Detection of *BRCA1* mutations by the protein truncation test. Hum Molec Genet 4:1989–91.

Powell SM, Petersen GM, Krush AJ, Booker S, Jen J, Giardiello FM, Hamilton SR, Vogelstein B, Kinzler KW. 1993. Molecular diagnosis of familial adenomatous polyposis. N Engl J Med 329:1982–7.

Rohlfs EM, Learning W, Friedman KJ, Couch FJ, Weber B, Silverman LM. 1997. Direct detection of mutations in the breast and ovarian susceptibility gene *BRCA1* by PCR-mediated site-directed mutagenesis. Clin Chem 43:24–29.

Saiki RK, Walsh PS, Levenson CH, Erlich HA. 1989. Genetic analysis of amplified DNA with immobilized sequence-specific oligonucleotide probes. Proc Natl Acad Sci (USA) 86:6230–4.

Sanger F, Nicklen S, Coulson AR. 1977. DNA sequencing with chain terminating inhibitors. Proc Natl Acad Sci (USA) 74:5463–7.

Sheffield VC, Cox DR, Lerman LS, Myers RM. 1989. Attachment of a 40 base pair G + C rich sequence (GC-clamp) to genomic DNA fragments by the polymerase chain reaction results in improved detection of single base changes. Proc Natl Acad Sci (USA) 86:232–6.

Sheffield VC, Beck JS, Kwitek AE et al. 1993. The sensitivity of single strand conformation polymorphism analysis for the detection of single base substitutions. Genomics 16:325–32.

Task Force on Genetic Testing of the National Institutes of Health. 1997. Proposed Recommendations of the Task Force on Genetic Testing: Notice of Meeting and Request for Comment. Federal Register 62(20):4539–47.

Wu Y, Nystrom-Lahti M, Osinga J et al. 1997. *MSH2* and *MLH1* mutations in sporadic replication error-positive colorectal carcinoma as assessed by two-dimensional DNA electrophoresis. Genes, Chrom, Cancer 18:269–78.

8

Genetic Testing in the Management of Patients with Cancer

Genetic analysis of tumor tissue can provide information that may guide decision making. The use of genetic reagents as diagnostic or prognostic markers has provided a new clinical role for cancer genetics. Since genetic alterations represent causative events of malignant change, they represent ideal tumor markers. This has proved the case for a number of tumor types, as molecular diagnosis has begun to have an impact on clinical pathology and oncology.

Novel methods of detecting alterations in oncogenes and tumor suppressor genes have been applied to the analysis of a broad spectrum of human malignancies. Although some abnormalities are specific for individual types of cancer, other abnormalities are shared among a variety of tumors. Some of the tumor-associated abnormalities have been correlated with progression or clinical outcome. As predicted by the multistep model of tumorigenesis (Chapter 3), some of the tumor-associated abnormalities occur in the same genes that are altered in families with cancer predisposition. The methods of detecting mutations and, in some cases, the regions of the gene mutated, are the same for both inherited and acquired (tumor-associated) genetic alterations. As discussed in Chapter 1, the counseling implications of inherited mutations are distinct from the implications of genetic changes detected in tumors. Increasingly healthcare professionals involved in the management of cancer patients will be called upon to make treatment decisions based upon combinations of both tumor-associated and inherited genetic markers. Genetic information will be combined with other clinical and pathologic data to shape management decisions for patients with cancer.

It is beyond the scope of this chapter to catalogue all genetic alterations associated with human malignancies. Instead, an outline of those genetic tests of tumor cells that are being incorporated into the clinical evaluation of patients is presented. Genetic markers with established diagnostic or prognostic significance are highlighted. Often considered as "additional studies" in the present state of clinical practice, genetic tests will play an expanding role in future cancer diagnosis and treatment.

GENETICS IN CANCER DIAGNOSIS

Genetic Markers of Clinically Distinct Subsets of Malignancy

Table 8-1 highlights selected associations of specific tumor types and recurring cytogenetic or molecular genetic alterations. More complete listings of cytogenetic alterations observed in specific tumor types have been published (Heim and Mitelman, 1995; Mitelman, 1994; Sandberg, 1990). In the examples chosen, the development of genetic markers has led to improvements in pathologic diagnosis or tailoring of therapeutic interventions.

Genetic Alterations in Hematologic Malignancies   As in other aspects of hematologic practice (e.g., hemoglobin disorders), molecular genetics has become central to the diagnosis of hematologic malignancies and premalignancies. Perhaps more than any other aspect of medicine, genetic and molecular diagnosis has been incorporated into the routine management of patients with leukemias and lymphomas. In patients with elevated white blood cell counts, for example, a genetic test is required to secure the diagnosis of chronic myelogenous leukemia. Early detection of the Philadelphia chromosome and other genetic changes, whether by cytogenetic analysis, FISH, Southern blot, or other techniques, may lead to consideration of treatments ranging from chemotherapy and interferon, to bone marrow transplantation. Help may come, too, to the patient with inexplicably low blood counts who is found to have a mono-

TABLE 8-1   Examples of Genetic Aids in Diagnosis of Malignancy

Genetic Marker	Tumor Type	Clinical Utility
Monosomy 7, monosomy 5 deletion of 5q, 7q	Myeloid leukemias and myelodysplastic syndrome	Diagnosis of leukemia or myelodysplastic syndrome
Philadelphia chromosome *BCR* rearrangement	Chronic myeloid leukemia	Diagnosis of leukemia
Specific recurring chromosomal translocations	Histologic subtypes of hematologic malignancies	Confirmation and refinement of histologic diagnoses
Immunoglobulin gene rearrangement	Lymphoproliferative disorders	Diagnosis of malignancy in borderline cases
T-cell receptor gene rearrangement	Lymphoproliferative disorders	Diagnosis of malignancy in borderline cases
iso(12p)	Germ cell tumors	Diagnosis of germ cell neoplasms in small round cell tumors
t(11;22)(q24;q12) *EWS* rearrangement	Ewing's sarcoma/PNET	Confirmation and refinement of histologic diagnosis

somy of chromosomes 5 or 7, or deletion of the long arms of these chromosomes. The diagnosis of myelodysplastic syndrome is made by examination of bone marrow morphology and by documentation, through cytogenetics or FISH, of one of these pathognomonic genetic abnormalities.

Numerous recurring translocations have been associated with specific subtypes of leukemia (Table 8-2), and these careful observations led to discovery of many oncogenes (Chapter 3). The identification of translocations and rearrangements of oncogenes by cytogenetic or molecular analysis can confirm a diagnosis as well as add prognostic information for patients with both myeloid and lymphoid leukemias (Hirsch-Ginsberg et al., 1993; Raimondi, 1993). In the clinical practice guidelines for pediatric acute lymphoblastic leukemia developed for the National Comprehensive Cancer Network, cytogenetic studies were included in the diagnostic studies to be performed on each newly diagnosed patient (Pui et al., 1996). In some cases, genetic markers were proposed as key factors in treatment planning. For example, the detection of t(9;22)(q34;q11), t(4;11)(q21;q23) or rearrangements of *HRX* (also called *MLL, ALL1, HTRX*) identified children as "high-risk" and made them candidates for allogeneic hematopoietic stem cell transplantation protocols (Pui et al., 1996).

Lymphoid Malignancies The molecular genetics of lymphoid differentiation and the immune response were described by several research teams during the 1980s. Their discoveries were rapidly translated into the practice of hematology. By the 1990s, commercial laboratories routinely offered molecular detection of rearrangement of the genes encoding the immunoglobulin light and heavy chains and the T-cell receptor. These assays are utilized in the assessment of the *clonality* of suspicious lesions, i.e., their origin from a single progenitor cell. The identification of an immunoglobulin or T-cell receptor gene rearrangement in a suspicious lesion (e.g., in the skin, or in a lymph node) supports the diagnosis of malignancy. Since not all clonal proliferations

---

Case Example 8.1. A 50-year-old woman presented with axillary lymphadenopathy, fever, and weight loss. Her peripheral blood counts were normal, but her serum lactate dehydrogenase was elevated. A biopsy of the lymph node was interpreted as "reactive hyperplasia." However, immunoglobulin gene rearrangement studies showed a clonal pattern, and karyotype revealed a t(8;14)(q24;q32). The patient was initially told that she should be watched closely, but sought a second opinion. At time of second opinion, biopsy of the bone marrow revealed clusters of both small as well as large, cleaved lymphocytes. Gene rearrangement studies of the marrow showed a clonal proliferation.

This case posed a diagnostic dilemma because of the lack of histologic diagnosis at the time of the initial lymph node biopsy. However, the documentation of the clonal immunoglobulin gene rearrangement and the t(8;14) established a diagnosis of an intermediate-grade B cell neoplasm. This was confirmed by the bone marrow histology. The patient was started on an anthracycline-containing chemotherapy regimen, with a complete remission documented by repeat marrow biopsy, as well as diminution of her symptoms. She ultimately relapsed five years later, with a population of smaller malignant cells detected in the marrow.

TABLE 8-2 Selected Genetic Abnormalities in Cancer

	Chromosomal Alteration	Involved Gene(s)
Malignancy		
Acute Myelogenous	−5, −7, +8	
Leukemia	del(5q)	
	t(6;9)(p23;q24)	*DEK; CAN*
M2	t(8;21)(q22;q22)	*ETO; AML1*
M3	t(15;17)(q22;q21)	*PML; RARα*
M4 with eosinophils	inv(16)(p13;q22)	*MYH11;CBFB*
	inv(3)(q21;q26)	*?EVI-1*
	t(11;19)(q23;p13)	*HRX;AF17*
	t(9;11)(p22;q23)	*HRX;ENL*
	t(11q23)	*HRX*
	t(16;21)(p11;q22)	*FUS;ERG*
	t(7;11)(p15;p15)	*HOXA9;NUP98*
	t(1;22)(p13;q13)	
M5	t(8;16)(p11;p13)	
Acute Lymphoblastic	t(8;14)(q24;q32)	*MYC;IGH*
Leukemia (B lineage)	t(9;22)(q34;q11)	*ABL;BCR*
	t(12;21)(p13;q22)	*TEL;AML1*
	t(4;11)(q21;q23)	*AF4;HRX*
	t(11;19)(q23;p13.3)	*HRX;ENL*
	t(1;11)(p32;q23)	*?HRX*
	t(10;11)(p14-p15;q23)	
	t(1;19)(q23;p13)	*PBX1;E2A*
	t(17;19)(q21-22;p13)	*HLF;E2A*
	t(5;14)(q31;q32)	*IL3;IGH*
Acute Lymphoblastic	t(8;14)(q24;q11)	*c-MYC;TCRδ*
Leukemia (T Lineage)	t(1;14)(p32;q11)	*TAL1;TCRδ*
	t(1;7)(p32;q35)	*TAL1;TCRβ*
	t(7;9)(q35;q32)	*TAL2;TCRβ*
	t(11;14)(p15;q11)	*RBTN1;TCRδ*
	t(11;14)(p13;q11)	*RBTN2;TCRδ*
	t(7;11)(q35;p13)	*RBTN2;TCRβ*
	t(10;14)(q24;q11)	*HOX11;TCRδ*
	t(7;10)(q35;q24)	*TCRβ;HOX11*
	t(7;9)(q35;q34)	*TCRβ;TAN1*
	t(1;7)(p34;q35)	*LCK;TCRβ*
	t(7;19)(q35;p13)	*TCRβ;LYL1*
Chronic Myelogenous	t(9;22)(q34;q11) and variants	*ABL;BCR*
Leukemia	+8,+19,+Ph, abn 17	
	t(3;21)(q26.2;q22)	*EVI1;AML1*

(continued)

TABLE 8-2 continued

	Chromosomal Alteration	Involved Gene(s)
Tumor Type		
Polycythemia vera	del(20)(q11) +8,+9 del(1)(p11) del(3)(p11p14) t(1;6)(q11;p21) t(1;9)(q10;p10) del(13)(q12q14)	
Myeloid Metaplasia	del(13)(q12q14) del(20)(q11) +21, -7,+8,+9	
Lymphoma [F = follicular lymphoma; DLC= diffuse large cell lymphoma; ALC= ana-plastic large cell lym-phoma; MCL= mantle cell lymphoma; BL= Burkitt lymphomas; PL= plasmacytoid lym-phoma]	t(14;18)(q32;q21) (F) t(8;14)(q24;q32) (BL) t(11;14)(q13;q32) (MCL) t(2;5)(p23;q35) (ALC) t(9;14)(p13;q32) (PL) t(3;22)(q27:q11) (DLC) t(3;14)(q27:q32) (DLC) t(10;14)(q24;q32) del(6)(q21-25) +7,+12	*BCL2* *MYC* *BCL1* *ALK;NPM* *PAX5* *BCL6* *BCL6* *LYT10/NFk-B*
Multiple Myeloma		*MUM1*
Breast Cancer	6q24-27 7q 8q24 10q22-23 11q13 13q12-3 13q14 17p13 17q21	*ER* *c-MET; WNT2* *c-MYC* *PTEN* *INT2, cyclin D1* *BRCA2* *RB1* *p53* *BRCA1, c-ERBB2*
Colorectal Cancer	2p16 2q31-33 3p21 5q21 5q21 7p22	*hMSH2* *hPMS1* *hMLH1* *APC* *MCC* *hPMS2*

TABLE 8-2 *continued*

	Chromosomal Alteration	Involved Gene(s)
Tumor Type		
Colorectal Cancer	12p	*K-RAS*
(continued)	17p13	*p53*
	17q22	*NM23*
	18q21	*DCC*
Desmoplastic small round cell tumor	t(11;22)(p13;q11.2)	*EWS; WT1*
Lipogenic tumors	t(12)(q13→14)	*CHOP*
Melanoma	del(9p), del(1)(p12-22), t/del(6q),i(6p), 10q11	*CDKN2/p16*
Neuroblastoma	del(1)(p31→32)	*NMYC*
	1p36	*p73*
Ovarian adenocarcinoma	t(6;14)(q21;q24), +12, chromosome 1 abnormality	
Pleomorphic adenomas of the salivary gland	t(3;8)(p21;q12) t(9:12)(p13-22;q13-15)	
Renal cell carcinoma	t/del(3)(p11→p21)	*VHL*
Retinoblastoma	del(13)(q14), -13	*RB1*
Sarcomas		
Ewing's sarcoma; peripheral neuroepithelial tumors	t(11;22)(q24;q12)	*EWSR1,EWSR2* *(FLI1; EWS)*
Myxoid liposarcoma	t(12;16)(q13;p11)	*CHOP; FUS*
Rhabdomyosarcoma (alveolar)	t(2;13)(q37;q14)	*PAX3; FKHR*
Synovial sarcoma	t(1;13)(p36;q14)	*PAX7; FKHR*
	t(X;18)(p11;q11)	*SSX; SYT*
Clear cell sarcoma	t(12;22)(q13;q12)	*ATF; EWS*
Small-cell lung cancer	del(3)(p14p23)	
	13q14	*RB1*
Testicular germ cell tumors	i(12p)	

(continued)

TABLE 8-2 continued

	Chromosomal Abnormality	Involved Gene(s)
Tumor Type		
Transitional cell bladder carcinoma	i(5p), +7, del(8p)	
Wilms' tumor	t/del(11)(p13)	*WT1*

Key: M2 = AML with maturation; M3 = acute promyelocytic leukemia; M4 = acute myelomonocytic leukemia; M5 = acute monocytic leukemia.

are malignant (e.g., monoclonal gammopathies in the elderly), it may be necessary to demonstrate additional genetic changes. The identification of rearrangements of specific oncogenes in lymphoma can assist in the diagnosis of different subtypes of the disease (see Table 8-2 and review by Gaidano and Dalla-Favera, 1995).

Specific genetic abnormalities in lymphomas may also suggest different treatment strategies. For example the identification of *BCL1* rearrangement denoting mantle cell lymphomas may lead to treatment with purine analogues. Identification of 18q21 (*BCL2*) rearrangement in the elderly patient with recurrent large cell lymphoma may suggest palliative treatment to gain extended survival with disease (Offit, 1992). *BCL2* overexpression and *p53* mutation have been correlated with an adverse prognosis (Gascoyne et al., 1997; Ichikawa et al., 1997). At present, however, the identification of specific oncogene rearrangements in T- and B-cell lymphomas have supplemented, rather than supplanted, such histopathologic nosologies as the Revised European-American Lymphoma classification system. Cytogenetic markers also have been documented to be independent prognostic indicators in multiple myeloma (Tricot et al., 1997) and other well-differentiated lymphoid neoplasms (Juliusson et al., 1990).

Isochromosome 12p in Poorly Differentiated Carcinomas of Unknown Primary Site The identification of an extra copy of the long arm of chromosome 12 [isochromosome 12p or i(12p)] has proved pathognomonic for germ cell tumors. Of 101 germ cell tumors with an abnormal karyotype, an i(12p) was found in 80% (Bosl et al., 1994). Detection of i(12)p has also provided clinically relevant diagnostic information in patients with undifferentiated neoplasms of unknown primary site. Of 40 such patients analyzed by Motzer and coworkers, 17 demonstrated i(12)p by cytogenetic or FISH analysis, or increased 12p copy number by Southern analysis. In 5 cases, characteristic cytogenetic abnormalities suggested the diagnoses of neuroepithelioma, lymphoma, or desmoplastic small round cell tumors (Table 8-2). Of the 17 cases with i(12)p or equivalent abnormalities, 75% demonstrated a response to platinum-based chemotherapy, compared to 18% of cases with no diagnosis suggested by cytogenetic analysis (Motzer et al., 1995). Because platinum-based chemotherapy can be curative for germ cell malignancies at any stage, these results demonstrate the clinical utility of cytogenetic or molecular analysis in this subset of patients.

t(11;22)* in *Peripheral Neuroepithelioma Peripheral neuroepithelial tumors (PNET) generally arise in peripheral nerves, but can metastasize to bone, bone marrow, lung, and other sites. The disease poses diagnostic as well as therapeutic challenges in managing the children affected by these tumors. The observation of a cytogenetic abnormality in almost all of these tumors has aided diagnosis. The t(11;22)(q24;q12) seen in cases of PNET was identical to the abnormality in Ewing's sarcoma. Rearrangement of the oncogene *ESW* was noted in both tumor types. This observation was clinically relevant because the PNET patients responded to the same combination chemotherapy regimens designed for patients with Ewing's sarcoma, and because the histologic distinction between the various entities of small round cell tumors in children was a challenge for pathologists (Fletcher et al., 1991; Delattre et al., 1994). Thus, molecular diagnosis of these entities can assist in clinical diagnosis of these diseases.

Table 8-2 lists selected genetic-pathologic associations of human neoplasias. The identification of recurring chromosomal abnormalities in the hematologic malignancies has led to the incorporation of genetic analysis in the diagnostic evaluation of patients with leukemia and lymphoma. The recent characterization of many of the genes involved in chromosomal rearrangements in the hematologic malignancies has offered the potential for molecular diagnosis of these lesions. With the possible exception of

---

Case Example 8.2. A 30-year-old man came to the emergency room complaining of difficulty breathing. A chest radiograph revealed a large mediastinal mass, with retroperitoneal adenopathy later noted on CT scan. There was no other adenopathy, and the rest of the physical exam, including examination of the testes, was normal. Serum lactate dehydrogenase was elevated. Blood indices were normal. A biopsy of the mass revealed a poorly differentiated neoplasm of unknown primary site. Serum alpha-fetoprotein (AFP) and human chorionic gonadotropin (HCG) levels were normal. Karyotypic analysis of the tumor revealed an isochromosome 12. On the basis of the genetic studies, platinum-based chemotherapy was instituted for presumed extragonadal germ cell cancer syndrome. The patient remained in complete remission five years after cessation of therapy.

The recent genetic identification of the extragonadal germ cell cancer syndrome in men with poorly differentiated midline tumors (Motzer et al., 1995) is now a recognized aspect of oncologic management. It is important, however, to remember that AFP will be positive in only 60–80% and HCG in 30–50% of non-seminomatous germ cell tumors, while AFP is absent in seminomas and HCG may be low. These markers may thus be non-diagnostic in some cases of poorly differentiated neoplasms. In addition, immunoglobulin gene rearrangement studies can rule out the diagnosis of lymphoid malignancy in difficult cases, although immunohistochemical stains can also serve this purpose.

the sarcomas, the diagnostic genetics of the solid tumors is still in a formative stage. As discussed in Chapter 3, for the most part, the "primary" or early genetic events associated with the common human malignancies remain to be elucidated.

Although the tumor specificity of the molecular markers listed in Table 8-2 is quite high, factors limiting their clinical use are their relative complexity and expense. At present, the proportion of human cancers that pose diagnostic dilemmas to pathologists is limited, and the costs of additional genetic assays can be considerable. As genetic reagents become standardized and more readily available, the use of these assays in cancer diagnosis will increase.

GENETICS IN CANCER DETECTION

In addition to their specificity, the very high sensitivity of some molecular assays poses remarkable clinical opportunities. By combining knowledge of specific cancer genetic associations (Table 8-2) with the power of the polymerase chain reaction (Chapter 7), powerful methods of detection of tumor cells have been devised. These techniques have the potential to detect as few as one tumor cell mixed with a million normal cells. Table 8-3 lists several PCR-based applications of molecular detection of residual cancer cells. These methodologies have already had clinical application in the treatment of certain hematologic malignancies; PCR assays have been utilized to measure the effectiveness of treatments aimed to purge bone marrows of tumor cells prior to transplantation (Gribben et al., 1993). For solid tumors, PCR-based assays have been used as supersensitive tests for tumor cells in body fluids (urine, sputum, etc.), and these same techniques may be utilized to assist surgeons in determining operative margins free of tumor cells. Although most of the assays listed in Table 8-3 are not part of clinical practice, they represent potential tools for future cancer management and many are being tested in clinical trials.

GENETICS IN CANCER PROGNOSIS

The published literature relating to genetic markers of clinical prognosis has grown rapidly over the past decade. With the exception of the hematologic malignancies, where cytogenetic prognostic markers were first described, there have been few prospective trials to validate the utility of the markers tested. Thus, small sample sizes, different treatment regimens, and different methods of genetic analysis have limited the clinical impact of the studies thus far published. Nonetheless, molecular medicine sections of leading journals continue to communicate novel observations, some of which have considerable potential to influence current therapeutic strategies. Table 8-4 highlights selected genetic prognostic markers that are in the process of being integrated into the clinical management of patients with cancer. Table 8-5 provides a broader survey of candidate markers that have been proposed as prognostic indicators in patients treated for a variety of malignancies.

TABLE 8-3 Polymerase Chain Reaction-Based Applications of Genetic Diagnosis in the Detection of Small Populations of Tumor Cells

Tumor Type	PCR Target	Tissue Site Studied
Colon	*RAS* mutations	Stool
Pancreatic	*RAS* mutations	Stool
Bladder	*p53* mutations	Urine
Lung	*RAS* mutations	Sputum
Lymphoma	*IGH-BCL2* rearrangement	Blood
Leukemias	Specific rearrangements (see Table 7-1)	Blood
B-cell leukemia	*IGH* rearrangement	Blood
T-cell leukemia	*TCR* rearrangement	Blood
Sarcomas	Specific rearrangements (see Table 8-2)	Tumor margin
Melanoma	Tyrosinase	Circulating cells
Prostate cancer	Prostate specific antigen	Pelvic lymph nodes, bone marrow, blood
Breast cancer	Keratin 19	Bone marrow
Gastrointestinal malignancies	Carcinoembryonic antigen	Bone marrow
Hepatoma	Alpha-fetoprotein albumin	Circulating cells
Neuroblastoma	Tyrosine hydroxylase PGP 9.5	Circulating cells
Small cell lung cancer	Microsatellite instability	Circulating cells
Head and neck cancer	Microsatellite instability	Circulating cells
	p53 mutations	Surgical margins

Sources: From Tables 12-1 and 12-3 in Seiden M, Sklar JL. PCR and RT-PCR based methods of tumor detection: potential applications and clinical applications. In Devita VT, Hellman S, Rosenberg SA. *Important Advances in Oncology 1996.* Philadelphia: Lippincott-Raven, 1997, pp. 191–204. Also Sidransky D, Frost P, von Eschenbach A et al. Identification of *p53* mutations in bladder cancers and urine samples. Science 1991; 252:706–9; Sidransky D, Tokino T, Hamilton SR et al. Identification of ras oncogene mutations in the stools of patients with curable colorectal tumors. Science 1992; 256:102–5; Gribben JG, Neuberg D, Freedman AS et al. Detection by polymerase chain reaction of residual cells with the BCL-2 translocation is associated with increased risk of relapse after autologous bone marrow transplantation for B-cell lymphoma. Blood 1993; 81:3449–57; Caldas C, Hahn SA, Hruban RH, Redston MS, Yeo CJ, Kern SE. Detection of k-ras mutations in the stool of patients with pancreatic cancer and pancreatic ductal hyperplasia. Cancer Res 1994; 54:3568–73; Mao L, Hruban RH, Boyle JO et al. Detection of oncogene mutations in sputum precedes diagnosis of lung cancer. Cancer Res 1994; 54:1634–37; Chen XQ, Stroun M, Magnenat J-L, et al. Microsatellite alterations in plasma DNA of small cell lung cancer patients. Nat Med 1996; 2:1033–4; Nawroz H, Koch W, Anker P, Stroun M, Sidransky D. Microsatellite alterations in serum DNA of head and neck cancer patients. Nat Med 1996; 2:1035–7; Brennan JA, Mao L, Hruban RH et al. Molecular assessment of histopathologic staging in squamous-cell carcinoma of the head and neck. New Engl J Med 1995; 332:429–35.

p53 Mutation and Overexpression as a Prognostic Marker

As introduced in Chapter 3, the *p53* tumor suppressor gene plays an important role in programmed cell death (*apoptosis*), as well as binding tumor-transforming proteins such as the SV40 large T antigen, and inducing p21, a protein inhibitor of the cyclin-

TABLE 8-4 Selected Genetic Prognostic Markers in Cancer Management

Marker	Tumor Type	Significance
t(15;17) *PML/RARα* rearrangement	Promyelocytic leukemia	Signifies response to retinoic acid therapy
NMYC amplification	Neuroblastoma	Amplification identifies poor prognosis group
HER2/neu/*ERBB2* overexpression	Breast cancer	Overexpression in stage II disease is one of many known prognostic factors
p53 mutation or overexpression	Breast cancer Bladder cancer Colon cancer Leukemia Lung cancer Lymphoma Prostate cancer Uterine cancer	Associated with shortened patient survival or aggressive features
18q loss of heterozygosity/ absence of *DCC* expression	Colon cancer	May signify need for adjuvant treatment in stage II disease

dependent kinases that regulate the cell cycle. These actions result in the tumor-suppressing and growth-controlling function of the gene. It has also been observed that the vulnerability of tumor cells to irradiation or chemotherapy is greatly decreased by mutations that inactivate *p53* and interfere with its role in apoptosis (Lowe et al., 1993). This later observation has formed the central hypothesis for the numerous correlations of *p53* mutations with "tumor aggressiveness" or poor clinical outcome. In breast cancer, for example, specific *p53* mutations have been correlated with resistance to doxorubicin-containing chemotherapy (Aas et al., 1996).

Mutations of the tumor suppressor gene *p53* are among the most common genetic alterations found in tumors (Greenblatt et al., 1994), observed in about half of cases studied. However, *p53* mutations are not observed in all tumor types. They are rare in testicular and Wilms' tumors. However, *p53* mutations commonly occur in histologies in transition from premalignant to frankly malignant type. For example, *p53* mutations are common in *in situ* breast and bladder cancers, and in the transition from colon polyps to frank malignancy. They are also commonly observed in cancers caused by environmental exposures, including sun-damage-induced skin cancers, head and neck cancers due to tobacco use, and colon cancers associated with Barrett's esophagus (Ruley, 1996; Harris, 1993; Chang et al, 1995).

Despite differing treatment strategies, different methods of detecting *p53* alterations, and a variety of clinical settings, numerous studies have demonstrated the association of *p53* alterations with adverse clinical outcome or aggressiveness of tumors. Table 8-5 summarizes studies documenting the prognostic utility of assessing *p53* mu-

TABLE 8-5 Examples of Genetic Prognostic Markers in Cancer Management

Malignancy	Genetic Marker	Method of Detection	Prognostic Significance	Representative References or Reviews
Acute myelogenous leukemia	t(8;21)(q22;q22), inv(16)	CG	+	Hirsch-Ginsberg, 1993
	t(15;17)(q22;q11), *RAR*α rearrangement	CG/SB	Responsive to retinoids	Warrell et al., 1993
	p53 mutation	SS	−	Wattel et al., 1994
	WT1 overexpression	RTPCR	−	Inoue et al., 1994
	RB underexpression	IHC	−	Kornbleau et al., 1994
Acute lymphocytic leukemia	11q23 (*HRX*) rearrangements	CG/SB	−	Chen et al., 1993
	t(9;22)(q34;q11)	CG/FISH	−	Rubnitz et al., 1994
	Hyperdiploidy	CG	+	Raimondi, 1993
Myelodysplastic syndrome	del(5q) or del(7q)	CG	−	Verhoef and Boogaerts, 1996
	p53 mutations	SS	−	Wattel et al., 1994
	BCL2 expression	IHC	+	Lepelley et al., 1995
	MPL expression	mRNA	−	Bouscary et al., 1995
Chronic myelogenous leukemia	+8, i(17q), +19	CG	Progression	Kantarjian et al., 1993
	p53 mutations	SS	Progression	Nakai et al., 1992
Chronic lymphocytic leukemia	+12, del(6q)	CG	−	Juliusson et al., 1990
	p53 mutations	SS	−	Dohner et al., 1995
Non-Hodgkin's lymphoma	*BCL2* rearrangement	SB	−	Yunis et al., 1989
	+7, del(6q), 17p, 1q abnormalities	CG	−	Offit, 1992
				Whang-Peng et al., 1995
	BCL6 rearrangement	SB	+	Tilly et al., 1994
	p53 overexpression	IHC	−	Offit et al., 1994
	p53 mutation	SS	−	Piris et al., 1994
				Louie et al., 1995;
				Lo Coco et al., 1993
	BCL2 expression	IHC	−	Gascoyne et al., 1997

(continued)

TABLE 8-5 continued

Malignancy	Genetic Marker	Method of Detection	Prognostic Significance	Representative References or Reviews
Bladder cancer	p53 expression	IHC	—	Dalbagni et al., 1995
	RB underexpression	IHC	—	Tetu et al., 1996
Breast cancer	HER2/neu/ERBB2 expression	mRNA, SB, IHC	– in stage II	Ravdin e al., 1995
	p53 overexpression	IHC	– in stage I	Allred et al., 1993
				Gasparini et al., 1994
	p53 mutation	SS	—	Kovach et al., 1996; Aas et al., 1996; Bergh et al., 1996
				Henry et al., 1993
	INT2 amplification	SB	—	Tan et al., 1997
	p27 underexpression	IHC	—	Kihana al., 1994
Cervical cancer	HER2/neu/ERBB2 expression	IHC	No correlation	Costa et al., 1995
Colon cancer	LOH at 18q	SB/PCR	– in stage II	Jen et al., 1994
	p53 overexpression	IHC	– in stage III	Pricolo et al., 1996
		IHC	– in node positive	Zeng et al., 1994
	BCL2 expression	IHC	– in stage II	Sinicrope et al., 1995
	p27 underexpression	IHC	—	Loda et al., 1997
	DCC underexpression	IHC	– in stage II	Shibata et al., 1996
Gastric and Esophageal carcinoma	HER2/neu/ERBB2 expression	IHC	Little or no significance	Miller et al., 1994
				Nakamura et al., 1994
				Duhaylongsod et al., 1995
				Hilton et al., 1992
	p53 overexpression	IHC	Little or no significance	Sarbia et al., 1994

Non-small cell lung cancer	p53 overexpression	IHC	In esophagus – (gastric)	Fonseca et al., 1994
	K-RAS mutations	SS	– 5 studies of >200 patients	Slebos et al., 1990
				Sugio et al., 1990
				Mitsudomi et al., 1991
				Rosell et al., 1993
	HER2/neu/ERBB2 expression	IHC	—	Giaccone et al., 1996
	EGFR level	IHC	—	Tateishi et al., 1991
	Cyclin D1 expression	IHC	—	Veale et al., 1993
	BCL2 expression	IHC	—	Betticher et al., 1996
	p53 mutation	SS	—	Passlick et al., 1995
	RB underexpression	IHC	—	Mitsudomi et al., 1993
Melanoma	NM23 expression	mRNA	– time to relapse	Xu et al., 1994
	p53 overexpression	IHC	No prognostic role in thin lesions	Xerri et al., 1994
				Sparrow et al., 1995
Neuroblastoma	p53 overexpression	IHC	Histologic progression	McGregor et al., 1993
	tyrosinase	mRNA	—	Kunter et al., 1996
	NM23 expression	mRNA	+	Florenes et al., 1992
	NMYC expression	SB	—	Seeger et al., 1985
	NMYC, 1p LOH, extra 17q	SB	—	Caron et al., 1996
	BCL2 expression	IHC	—	Castle et al., 1993
	NMYC expression	SB	No prognostic role in localized tumors	Cohn et al., 1995

(continued)

TABLE 8-5 continued

Malignancy	Genetic Marker	Method of Detection	Prognostic Significance	Representative References or Reviews
Ovarian cancer	*NM23* expression	mRNA	–	Scambia et al., 1996
	BCL2 expression	IHC	+	Herod et al., 1996
	EGFR expression	IHC	–	Berchuk et al., 1991
	HER2/neu/*ERBB2* expression	IHC	Minimal or no prognostic role	Rubin et al., 1993
				Fajac et al., 1995
	p53 overexpression	IHC	Minimal or no prognostic role	Niwa et al., 1994
Pancreatic cancer	*BRCA1* mutation	SS	+	Rubin et al., 1996
	CDKN2 mutations	SS	–	Bartsch et al., 1996
	HER2/neu/*ERBB2* expression	IHC	–	Lei et al., 1995
	p53 overexpression	IHC	Little or no prognostic role	DiGiuseppe et al., 1994
Prostate cancer	*HER2*/neu/*ERBB2* expression	IHC	–	Sadasivan et al., 1993
	p53 overexpression	IHC	–	Stricker et al., 1996
Thyroid (medullary)	*RET* codon 918	SS	–	Zedenius et al., 1995
Thyroid (papillary)	*p21* RAS	SS	–	Bosolo et al., 1994
Uterine	*p53* overexpression	IHC	–	Ito et al., 1994
Wilms' Tumor	*p53* mutation	SS	–	Bardeesy et al., 1994

Key: Method of Detection: CG = cytogenetic; SB = Southern blot; SS = SSCP (or variant) and sequencing; IHC = immunohistochemistry; mRNA = Northern blot; RTPCR = reverse transcriptase PCR; FISH = fluorescence in situ hybridization.

Prognostic Significance: – means correlated with poor clinical outcome with regard to survival or disease-free survival.
+ means correlated with a more favorable clinical outcome.

tation or overexpression in patients with cancers of the bladder, breast, colon, lung, prostate, as well as leukemias and lymphomas. These studies represent initial reports and require confirmation in prospective trials including other known genetic and clinical prognostic markers.

HER2/neu/*ERBB2* Expression and Prognosis in Breast and Other Cancers

The *HER2/neu* gene encodes a protein tyrosine kinase that is homologous with the human epidermal growth factor receptor. For this reason, it is also referred to as *C-ERBB2* (or *C-erbB-2*). The gene is located at 17q21 and is transcribed to a 4.5-kb mRNA which is translated to a 185-kd glycoprotein.

Initial studies of expression of *C-ERBB2* in breast cancer utilized measures of gene amplification. These included gene copy number (by Southern blot) and amount of mRNA transcript (by Northern blot). Later studies utilized measurements of the amount of protein (Western blot) or histologic location and expression on paraffin-fixed material (immunohistochemical analysis). Although most overexpression of the protein is associated with amplification of the gene, this is not always the case. Thus, methods of measurement of protein level may sometimes be preferable.

Starting with the initial report by Slamon in 1987, there have been dozens of studies addressing the issue of the prognostic significance of genetic markers in early stage breast cancer. In stage II (lymph node positive) disease, overexpression of the *ERBB2* oncogene has been correlated with increased chance for relapse and decreased survival. In a number of studies (reviewed by Ravdin et al., 1995), the prognostic power of *ERBB2* amplification was independent of other known factors, including number of lymph nodes involved. In node-negative breast cancer, there have been conflicting, mostly negative, reports of the ability of *ERBB2* assays to add prognostic power to known prognostic markers.

At present, the prognostic role for *ERBB2* is limited to the setting of node-positive disease, suggesting that *ERBB2* gene amplification or protein expression represent markers for chemotherapy resistance. This hypothesis has been supported by some studies (Tetu and Brisson, 1994) in which this genetic prognostic factor was only useful in patients treated with chemotherapy. Other studies, however, have found that tumors overexpressing *HER2*/neu can still demonstrate a significant dose-response to chemotherapy (Muss et al., 1994). Larger, prospective trials will be needed to resolve these issues. Until these trials are completed, *ERBB2* gene amplification or protein expression constitute one of a number of prognostic markers utilized by clinicians in planning treatment strategies.

In addition to patients with breast cancer, overexpression of *ERBB2* has been associated with poor prognosis in a variety of other tumors, including prostate (Sadasivan et al., 1993; Veltri et al., 1994) and lung cancer (Harpole et al., 1995).

NMYC, MRP Amplification and 1p Loss in Neuroblastoma

Neuroblastoma is one of the five most common cancers of childhood, with an incidence of 10 cases per million. Patients with localized disease are generally cured by surgery. However, patients with disseminated disease often fare poorly, despite intensive therapies. Because of the need for prognostic indicators, neuroblastoma is a cancer in which molecular genetic tests have become accepted as part of the routine clinical assessment of the newly diagnosed child (Cheung NK et al., 1996).

Two decades of genetic analysis of neuroblastoma tumors and cell lines in the laboratories of Biedler, Brodeur, and Alt led to the discovery of homogeneously staining regions and double minutes in the karyotypes of neuroblastoma tumors, the observation that these structures contained regions of gene amplification, and the discovery that the gene amplified was *NMYC* (Biedler and Spengler, 1976; Kohl et al., 1984). *NMYC* amplification, noted in about a third of children with advanced disease, was associated with a shorter time to relapse (Seeger et al., 1985). Southern blot analysis of amplification of *NMYC* is now considered part of the standard diagnostic workup for children with this disease (Cheung et al., 1996). Increased copy number of *NMYC* correlates with prognosis and is independent of other factors including stage.

In the neuroblastoma practice guidelines developed for the National Comprehensive Cancer Center Network, amplification of *NMYC* resulted in high risk classification for all stage II–IV patients regardless of age or other prognostic features (Cheung et al., 1996). In up to 80% of sporadic cases, a tumor suppressor gene at 1p36 has been implicated because of allelic loss or cytogenetic deletion at this locus. A study of 89 patients revealed that molecular detection of 1p deletion or 17p duplication identified a high-risk subset of patients with both limited and disseminated disease who would not otherwise have been detected by virtue of stage, age, or other clinical factors. In this analysis, 1p deletion actually provided more prognostic power than all the other variables (Caron et al., 1996). A candidate tumor suppressor gene, *p73,* has been mapped to 1p36 (Kaghad et al., 1997).

In a separate study of 60 patients, overexpression of the gene for multidrug resistance protein (*MRP*) was also a more powerful prognostic marker than *NMYC* amplification alone (Norris et al., 1996). These later results are of practical interest because *MRP*, like p-glycoprotein, mediates resistance to drugs including vinca alkaloids, anthracyclines, and epipodophyllotoxins. The measurement of expression of drug resistance genes may eventually assist in treatment planning for these patients.

PML, RARα and Promyelocytic Leukemia

Acute promyelocytic leukemia (APL) comprises about 10% of acute myelocytic leukemia in adults. Its characteristic clinical hallmark is disseminated intravascular coagulation, caused by the release of procoagulants from the malignant cells. This process often leads to fatal complications of hyperfibrinolysis and hemorrhage. Conventional chemotherapy for the disease results in 5-year survivals of 35–45%.

In the 1970's and 1980's a number of observations about the genetics and clinical course of APL established this disease as a model for the prognostic relevance of molecular markers in cancer treatment. First was the observation by Rowley and co-workers of a chromosomal translocation t(15;17)(q22;q11) that could be utilized as a diagnostic marker for the disease. In 1987, the gene encoding the retinoic acid receptor-alpha (*RARα*) was mapped to the chromosomal breakpoint 17q21, and found to be rearranged in all cases of APL. The breakpoints on chromosome 15 were in a region termed *PML*. The *PML/RARα* fusion protein was found in all patients with APL, and the *RARα/PML* fusion was found in about two thirds of APL patients (reviewed in Warrell et al., 1993; Pandolfi et al., 1991). Molecular detection of *PML/RARα* rearrangement by PCR analysis became available as a diagnostic assay for the disease (Miller et al., 1993).

Subsequently, it was discovered by clinicians in Shanghai, and confirmed in New York, that about 85% of APL patients treated with all-*trans*-retinoic acid (ATRA) achieved a complete clinical remission. While it seemed surprising that a defect that caused a mutation in a receptor would result in a remarkable sensitivity of that receptor to one of its ligands, the initial clinical response to ATRA correlated precisely with the presence of t(15;17). Several models were proposed to account for this observation (reviewed in Warrell et al., 1993). More recent clinical follow-up utilizing a combination of ATRA and conventional chemotherapy have documented a sustained 80% 5-year survival, with the prospect of decreasing the relapse rate further by ablating residual disease with monoclonal antibody-based experimental protocols (reviewed in Soignet et al., 1997).

Loss of Heterozygosity at Chromosome 18q or Underexpression of *DCC* and Prognosis in Colorectal Cancer

Of the 15,000 new cases of colorectal cancer diagnosed each year, about a third will be stage II (B2) disease (tumor extending through the muscularis propria, but not involv-

---

Case Example 8.3. A 49-year-old man presented with a recent history of thrombophlebitis of the lower extremities, and bleeding after a minor injury. Laboratory analysis revealed a total leukocyte count of 2000 cells/mm^3; hemoglobin of 11 gm/dl, platelets of 90,000 cells/mm^3, prothrombin time of 15.0 seconds, partial thromboplastin time of 28 seconds, fibrinogen of 150 g/dl, and fibrin degradation products of 100 (normal less than 10). Bone marrow aspirate revealed a large number of granulated promyelocytes, and cytogenetic analysis revealed a reciprocal translocation involving the long arms of chromosome 15 and 17.

The diagnosis of acute promyelocytic leukemia led to initiation of treatment with all-*trans*-retinoic acid, and entry into a protocol that involved consolidation with a humanized anti-CD33 monoclonal antibody followed by cycles of cytosine arabinoside and idarubicin. The patient achieved a complete remission after induction treatment, and was followed by a PCR assay for the *PML/RARα* fusion mRNA.

This case illustrates the diagnostic and prognostic utility of detection of the t(15;17) in a newly diagnosed leukemic patient, and the availability of sensitive PCR-based techniques to monitor remission after therapy. In contrast to patients with chronic myeloid leukemia, where similar molecular markers for the t(9;22) are available, APL patients do not appear to harbor residual clonal populations of leukemic cells while in remission. Long-term follow up of APL patients will document the predictive utility of the PCR-based assays.

ing lymph nodes). While surgery can result in long-term remission in 80% of these cases, the remainder fare poorly. Some studies have suggested a role for adjuvant chemotherapy for stage II disease.

Two reports have demonstrated the prognostic importance of molecular markers on chromosome 18q in patients with stage II colorectal cancer. An initial study of 144 consecutive colon cancer patients analyzed paraffin-embedded tumor specimens for loss of heterozygosity at chromosome 18q. Five-year survival reached 93% among those patients with stage II disease and no evidence of allele loss, compared to 54% in those who had allele loss (P = 0.005). Allele loss at 18q was a strong predictor for death, even when adjusted for other known prognostic factors, including tumor differentiation, vein invasion, and TNM stage (Jen et al., 1994).

A second study involved 132 patients with stage II or III colorectal cancers. Expression of DCC protein, measured by immunohistochemical analysis from routine pathology sections, was inversely correlated with survival for patients with stage II or stage III disease. For patients with stage II disease whose tumors expressed DCC, survival was 94% at five years, compared to 62% for patients whose tumors were DCC negative. Corresponding survival rates for stage III patients were 59% and 33%, respectively. Multivariate analysis confirmed the independent prognostic significance of *DCC* expression when compared to age, sex, and tumor site (Shibata et al., 1996).

Taken together, these results hold the promise to identify patients with stage II disease whose survival may significantly be impacted by adjuvant therapies. These observations will be tested in the setting of prospective intergroup trials.

REFERENCES

Aas T, Borresen AL, Geisler S et al. 1996. Specific p53 mutations are associated with de novo resistance to doxorubicin in breast cancer patients. Nature Medicine 2:811–14.

Allred DC, Clark GM, Elledge R et al. 1993. Association of *p53* protein expression with tumor cell proliferation rate and clinical outcome in node-negative breast cancer. J Natl Cancer Inst 85:200–6.

Bardeesy N, Falkoff D, Petruzzi MJ et al. 1994. Anaplastic Wilms' tumor, a subtype displaying poor prognosis, harbours *p53* gene mutations. Nature Genet 7:91–7.

Bartsch D, Shevlin DW, Callery MP, Norton JA, Wells SA, Jr., Goodfellow PJ. 1996. Reduced survival in patients with ductal pancreatic adenocarcinoma associated with CDKN2 mutation. J Natl Cancer Inst 88(10):680–2.

Basolo F, Pinchera A, Fugazzola L, Fontanini G, Elisei R, Romei C, Pacini F. 1994. Expression of p21 ras protein as a prognostic factor in papillary thyroid cancer. Eur J Cancer 30A:171–4.

Bell SM, Scott N, Cross D et al. 1993. Prognostic value of *p53* overexpression and c-Ki-ras gene mutation in colorectal cancer. Gastroenterol 104:57–64.

Berchuck A, Rodriguez GC, Kamel A et al. 1991. Epidermal growth factor receptor expression in normal ovarian epithelium and ovarian cancer. I. Correlation of receptor expression with prognostic factors in patients with ovarian cancer. Am J Obstet Gynecol 164:669–74.

Bergh J, Norberg T, Sjogren S, Lindgren A, Holmberg L. 1996. Complete sequencing of the p53 gene provides prognostic information in breast cancer patients, particularly in relation to adjuvant systemic therapy and radiotherapy. Nature Medicine 1:1029–34.

Betticher DC, Heighway J, Hasleton PS et al. 1996. Prognostic significance of CCND1 (Cyclin D1) overexpression in primary resected non-small-cell lung cancer. Br J Cancer 73:294–300.

Biedler JL, Spengler BAA. 1976. A Novel chromosome abnormality on human neuroblastoma and anti-folate resistant Chinese hamster cell lines in culture. J Natl Cancer Inst 57:683–95.

Bosl GJ, Ilson DH, Rodriguez E, Motzer RJ, Reuter VE, Chaganti RSK. 1994. Clinical relevance of the i(12p) marker chromosome in germ cell tumors. J Natl Cancer Inst 86: 349–55.

Bouscary D, Preudhomme C, Ribrag V, Melle J, Viguie F, Picard F et al. 1995. Prognostic value of c-mpl expression in myelodysplastic syndromes. Leukemia 9:783–8.

Caldas C, Hahn SA, Hruban RH, Redston MS, Yeo CJ, Kern SE. 1994. Detection of k-ras mutations in the stool of patients with pancreatic adenocarcinoma and pancreatic ductal hyperplasia. Cancer Res 54:3568–73.

Caron H, van Sluis P, de Kraker J et al. 1996. Allelic loss of chromosome 1p as a predictor of unfavorable outcome in patients with neuroblastoma. New Engl J Med 334:225–30.

Castle VP, Heidelberger KP, Bromberg J et al. 1993. Expression of the apoptosis-suppressing protein bcl-2 in neuroblastoma is associated with unfavorable histology and N-myc amplification 3-5. Am J Path 143:1543–50.

Chang F, Syrjanen S, Syrjanen K. 1995. Implications of the *p53* tumor-suppressor gene in clinical oncology. J Clin Oncol 13:1009–20.

Chen CS, Sorenson, PHB, Domer PH et al. 1993. Molecular rearrangements on chromosome 11q23 predominate in infant acute lymphoblastic leukemia and are associated with specific biologic variables and poor outcome. Blood 81:2386–93.

Cheung NK, Bowman L, Castle V et al. 1996. NCCN pediatric neuroblastoma practice guidelines. The Nation Comprehensive Cancer Network. Oncology 10:1813–22.

Cohn SL, Look AT, Joshi VV, Holbrook T, Salwen H, Chagnovich D et al. 1995. Lack of correlation of N-myc gene amplification with prognosis in localized neuroblastoma: a pediatric oncology group study. Cancer Res 55:721–6.

Costa MJ, Walls J, Trelford JD. 1995. c-erbB-2 oncoprotein overexpression in uterine cervix carcinoma with glandular differentiation: a frequent event but not an independent prognostic marker because it occurs late in the disease. Amer J Clin Pathol 104:634–642.

Dalbagni G, Cordon-Cardo C, Reuter V, Fair WR. 1995. Tumor suppressor gene alterations in bladder cancer: translational correlates to clinical practice. Surg Oncol Clin N Amer 4:231–40.

Delattre O, Zucman J, Melot T et al. 1994. The Ewing Family of tumors—a subgroup of small-round-cell tumors defined by specific chimeric transcripts. New Engl J Med 331:294–9.

DiGiuseppe JA, Hruban RH, Goodman SN, Polak M, van den Berg FM, Allison DC et al. 1994. Overexpression of *p53* protein in adenocarcinoma of the pancreas. Amer J Clin Pathol 101:684–8.

Dohner H, Fischer K, Bentz M et al. 1995. *p53* gene deletion predicts for poor survival and non-response to therapy with purine analogs in chronic B-cell leukemia. Blood 85:1580–9.

Duhaylongsod FG, Gottfried MR, Iglehart JD, Vaughn AL, Wolfe WG. 1995. The significance of c-erb B-2 and *p53* immunoreactivity in patients with adenocarcinoma of the esophagus. Ann Surg 221:677–83.

Fajac A, Benard J, Lhomme C et al. 1995. c-erb B2 gene amplification and protein expression in ovarian epithelial tumors: evaluation of their respective prognostic significance by multivariate analysis. Int J Cancer 64:146–51.

Fletcher JA, Kozakewich HP, Hoffer FA et al. 1991. Diagnostic relevance of clonal cytogenetic aberrations in malignant soft-tissue tumors. New Eng J Med 324:436–40.

Florenes VA, Aamdal S, Mykebost O et al. 1992. Levels of *NM23* mRNA in metastatic malignant melanomas: inverse correlation to disease progression. Cancer Res 52:6088–91.

Fonseca L, Yonemura Y, De Aretxabaia X et al. 1994. *p53* detection as a prognostic factor in early gastric cancer. Oncology 51:485–90.

Gaidano G, Dalla Favera R. 1995. Molecular biology of lymphoid neoplasms. In Mendelsohn J, Howley PM, Israel MA, Liotta LA (eds), The Molecular Basis of Cancer. Philadelphia: W. B. Saunders, pp. 251–80.

Gascoyne RD, Adomat SA, Krajewski S et al. 1997. Prognostic significance of Bcl-2 protein expression and Bcl-2 gene rearrangement in diffuse aggressive non-Hodgkin's lymphoma. Blood 90:244–51.

Gasparini G, Weidner N, Bevilacqua P et al. 1994. Tumor microvessel density, *p53* expression, tumor size, and peritumoral lymphatic vessel invasion are relevant prognostic markers in node-negative breast carcinoma. J Clin Oncol 12:454–66.

Giaccone G. 1996. Oncogenes and anti-oncogenes in lung tumorigenesis. Chest 109:130S–4S.

Glick SH, Howell LP, White RW. 1996. Relationship of *p53* and bcl-2 to prognosis in muscle invasive transitional cell carcinoma of the bladder. J Urol 155:1754–7.

Gribben JG, Neuberg D, Freedman AS et al. 1993. Detection by polymerase chain reaction of residual cells with the BCL-2 translocation is associated with increased risk of relapse after autologous bone marrow transplantation for B-cell lymphoma. Blood 81:3449–57.

Harpole DH Jr., Herndon JE 2nd, Wolfe WG, Iglehart JD, Marks JR. 1995. A prognostic model of recurrence and death in stage I non-small cell lung cancer utilizing presentation, histopathology, and oncoprotein expression. Cancer Res 55:51–6.

Harris CC, Hollstein M. 1993. Clinical implications of the *p53* tumor suppressor gene. New Engl J Med 329:1318–27.

Heim S, Mitelman F. 1995. Cancer Cytogenetics. New York: Wiley-Liss.

Henry JA, Hennessy C, Levett DL, Lennard TW, Westley BR, May FE. 1993. int-2 amplification in breast cancer: association with decreased survival and relationship to amplification of c-erbB-2 and c-myc. Int J Cancer 53:774–80.

Herod JJ, Elipoulos AG, Warwick J et al. 1996. The prognostic significance of BCL-2 and *p53* expression in ovarian cancer. Cancer Res 56:2178–84.

Hilton DA, West KP. 1992. C-ErbB2 oncogene product expression and prognosis in gastric carcinoma. J Clin Pathol 45:454–6.

Hirsch-Ginsberg C, Huh YO, Kagan J et al. 1993. Advances in the diagnosis of acute leukemia. Hem Onc Clin N Amer 7:1–46.

Ichikawa A, Kinoshita T, Watanabe T et al. 1997. Mutations of the p53 gene as a prognostic factor in agressive B-cell lymphoma. New Eng J Med 337:529–34.

Inoue K, Sugiyama H, Ogawa H et al. 1994. *WT1* as a new prognostic factor and a new marker for the detection of minimal residual disease in acute leukemia. Blood 84:3071–9.

Ito K, Watanabe K, Nasim S, Sasano H, Sato S, Yajima A et al. 1994. Prognostic significance of *p53* overexpression in endometrial cancer. Cancer Res 54:4667–70.

Jaros E, Lunec J, Perry RH et al. 1993. *p53* protein overexpression identifies a group of central primitive neuroectodermal tumours with poor prognosis. Br J Cancer 68:801–7.

Jen J, Kim H, Piantadosi S et al. 1994. Allelic loss of chromosome 18q and prognosis in colorectal cancer. New Eng J Med 331:213–21.

Juliusson G, Oscier DG, Fitchett M et al. 1990. Prognostic subgroups in B-cell chronic lymphocytic leukemia defined by specific chromosomal abnormalities. New Eng J Med 323:720–4.

Kaghad M, Bonnet H, Yang A et al. 1997. Monoallelically expressed gene related to p53 at 1p36, a region frequently deleted in neuroblastoma and other human tumors. Cell 90: 809–19.

Kantarjian HM, Deisseroth A, Kurzrock R et al. 1993. Chronic myelogenous leukemia: a concise update. Blood 82:691–703.

Kern JA, Schwartz DA, Nordberg JE et al. 1990. p185 neu expression in human lung adenocarcinomas predicts shortened survival. Cancer Res 50:5184–7.

Kihana T, Tsuda H, Teshima S, Nomoto K, Tsugane S, Sonoda T et al. 1994. Prognostic significance of the overexpression of c-erbB-2 protein in adenocarcinoma of the uterine cervix. Cancer 73:148–53.

Kohl NE, Gee CE, Alt FW. 1984. Activated expression of the N-myc gene in human neuroblastomas and related tumors. Science 226:1335–7.

Kornblau SM, Xu HJ, Zhang W et al. 1994. Levels of retinoblastoma protein expression in newly diagnosed acute myelogenous leukemia. Blood 84:256–61.

Kovach JS, Hartmann A, Blaszyk H, Cunningham J, Schaid D, Sommer SS. 1996. Mutation detection by highly sensitive methods indicates that *p53* gene mutations in breast cancer can have important prognostic value. Proc Natl Acad Sci (USA) 93:1093–6.

Kunter U, Buer J, Probst M et al. 1996. Peripheral blood tyrosinase message RNA detection and survival in malignant melanoma. J Natl Cancer Inst 88:590–4.

Lassam NJ, From L, Kahn HJ. 1993. Overexpression of *p53* is a late event in the development of malignant melanoma. Cancer Res 53:2235–8.

Lei S, Appert HE, Nakata B, Domenico DR, Kim K, Howard JM. 1995. Overexpression of the *HER2*/neu oncogene in pancreatic cancer correlates with shortened survival. Int J Pancreatol 17:5–21.

Lepelley P, Soenen V, Preudhomme C et al. 1995. Bcl-2 expression in myelodysplastic syndrome and its correlation with hematologic features, *p53* mutations, and prognosis. Leukemia 9:726–30.

Levine, MN, Andrulis, I. 1992. The Her-2/neu oncogene in breast cancer: so what is new? J Clin Oncol 10: 1034–6.

Lo Coco F, Gaidano G, Louie DC, Offit K, Chaganti RSK, Dalla-Favera R. 1993. *p53* mutations are associated with histologic transformation of follicular lymphoma. Blood 82:2289–95.

Loda M, Cukor B, Tam P et al. 1997. Increased proteasome-dependent degradation of the cyclin-dependent kinase inhibitor p27 in aggressive colorectal carcinomas. Nature Medicine 3:231–4.

Louie DC, Offit K, Jaslow R, et al. 1995. *p53* overexpression as a marker of poor prognosis in mantle cell lymphoma with t(11;14)(q13;q32). Blood 86:2892–99.

Lowe SW, Ruley HE, Jacks T, Housman DE. 1993. *p53*-dependent apoptosis modulates the cytotoxicity of anticancer agents. Cell 74:957–67.

Mao L, Hruban RH, Boyle JO et al. 1994. Detection of oncogene mutations in sputum precedes diagnosis of lung cancer. Cancer Res 54:1634–7.

McGregor JM, Yu CC, Dublin EA et al. 1993. *p53* immunoreactivity in human malignant melanoma and dysplastic nevi. Br J Dermatol 128:606–11.

Miller TA. 1994. ErbB-2 Expression: A useful prognostic indicator in gastric carcinoma? Gastroenterology 107:1209–10.

Miller WH Jr., Levine K, DeBlasio A, Frankel SR, Dmitrovsky E, Warrell RP Jr. 1993. Detection of minimal residual disease in acute promyelocytic leukemia by reverse transcriptase polymerase chain reaction assay for the PML/RAR-α fusion mRNA. Blood 82:1689–94.

Mitelman F. 1994. Catalog of Chromosome Aberrations in Cancer, ed 5. New York: Wiley-Liss.

Mitsudomi T, Oyama T, Kusano T, Osaki T, Nakanishi R, Shirakusa T. 1993. Mutations of the *p53* gene as a predictor of poor prognosis in patients with non-small-cell lung cancer. J Natl Cancer Inst 85:2018–23.

Mitsudomi T, Steinberg SM, Oie HK et al. 1991. Ras gene mutations in non-small cell lung cancers are associated with shortened survival irrespective of treatment intent. Cancer Res 51:4999–5002.

Motzer RJ, Rodriguez E, Reuter VE, Bosl GJ, Mazumdar M, Chaganti RS. 1995. Molecular and cytogenetic studies in the diagnosis of patients with poorly differentiated carcinomas of unknown primary site. J Clin Oncol 13:274–82.

Muss HB, Thor AD, Berry DA et al. 1994. c-erbB-2 expression and response to adjuvant therapy in women with node-positive early breast cancer. New Eng J Med 330:1260–6.

Nakai H, Misawa S, Toguchida J et al. 1992. Frequent *p53* gene mutations in blast crisis of chronic myelogenous leukemia, especially in myeloid crisis harboring loss of a chromosome 17p. Cancer Res 52:6588–93.

Nakamori S, Yashima K, Murakami Y et al. 1995. Association of *p53* gene mutations with short survival in pancreatic adenocarcinoma. Jpn J Cancer Res 86:174–81.

Nakamura T, Nekarda H, Hoelscher AH et al. 1994. Prognostic value of DNA ploidy and c-erbB-2 oncoprotein overexpression in adenocarcinoma of Barrett's esophagus. Cancer 73:1785–94.

Niwa K, Itoh M, Murase T et al. 1994. Alteration of *p53* gene in ovarian carcinoma: clinicopathological correlation and prognostic significance. Br J Cancer 70:1191–7.

Offit K. 1992. Chromosome analysis in the management of patients with non-Hodgkin's lymphoma. Leukemia and Lymphoma 7:275–82.

Offit K, Parsa NZ, Lo Coco F et al. 1994. Rearrangement of the bcl-6 gene as a prognostic marker in diffuse large-cell lymphoma. New Engl J Med 331:74–80.

Pandolfi PP, Grignani F, Alcalay M et al. 1991. Structure and origin of the acute promyelocytic leukemia myl/RARα cDNA and characterization of its retinoid-binding and transactivation properties. Oncogene 6:1285–92.

Passlick B, Izbicki JR, Häussinger K, Thetter O, Pantel K. 1995. Immunohistochemical detection of *p53* protein is not associated with a poor prognosis in non-small-cell lung cancer. J Thorac Cardiovasc Surg 109:1205–11.

Piris MA, Pezzella F, Martinez-Montero JC et al. 1994. *p53* and bcl-2 expression in high grade B-cell lymphomas: correlation with survival time. Br J Cancer 69:337–41.

Pricolo VE, Finkelstein SD, Wu TT et al. 1996. Prognostic value of T*p53* and k-ras-2 mutational analysis in stage III carcinoma of the colon. Am J Surg 171:41–6.

Pui CH, Kernan N, Sallan S, Sanders J, Steinherz P, Wharam M, Zipf T. 1996. NCCN pediatric acute lymphoblastic leukemia practice guidelines. The National Comprehensive Cancer Network. Oncology 10:1787–94.

Raimondi SC. 1993. Current status of cytogenetic research in childhood acute lymphoblastic leukemia. Blood 81:2237–51.

Ravdin PM, Chamnes GC. 1995. The c-erbB-2 proto-oncogene as a prognostic and predictive marker in breast cancer: a paradigm for the development of other macromolecular markers. Gene 159:19–27.

Rosell R, Li S, Skacel Z et al. 1993. Prognostic impact of mutated k-ras gene in surgically resected non-small cell lung cancer patients. Oncogene 8:2407–12.

Rubin SC, Finstad CL, Wong GY et al. 1993. Prognostic significance of HER-2/neu expression in advanced epithelial ovarian cancer: a multivariate analysis. Am J Obstet Gynecol 168:162–9.

Rubin SC, Benjamin I, Behbakht K et al. 1996. Clinical and pathological features of ovarian cancer in women with germ-line mutations of *BRCA1*. New Engl J Med 335:1413–6.

Rubnitz JE, Link MP, Shuster JL et al. 1994. Frequency and prognostic significance of HRX rearrangements in infant acute lymphoblastic leukemia: a Pediatric Oncology Group study. Blood 84:570–3.

Ruley HE. 1996. p53 and Response to chemotherapy and radiotherapy. In DeVita VT, Hellman SH, Rosenberg SA (eds), Important Advances in Oncology 1996. Philadelphia: Lippincott-Raven, pp. 37–56.

Sadasivan R, Morgan R, Jennings S et al. 1993. Overexpression of her-2/neu may be an indicator of poor prognosis in prostate cancer. J Urol 150:126–31.

Sandberg AA. 1990. The Chromosomes in Human Cancer and Leukemia, ed 2. New York: Elsevier.

Sarbia M, Porschen R, Borchard F, Horstmann O, Willers R, Gabbert HE. 1994. *p53* protein expression and prognosis in squamous cell carcinoma of the esophagus. Cancer 74:2218–23.

Scambia G, Ferrandina G, Marone M et al. 1996. *NM23* in ovarian cancer: correlation with clinical outcome and other clinicopathologic and biochemical prognostic parameters. J Clin Oncol 14:334–42.

Seeger RC, Brodeur GM, Sather H et al. 1985. Association of multiple copies of the N-Myc oncogene with rapid progression of neuroblastomas. New Eng J Med 313:1111–6.

Shibata D, Reale MA, Lavin P et al. 1996. The DCC protein and prognosis in colorectal cancer. New Engl J Med 335:1727–32.

Sidransky D, Frost P, Von Eschenbach A et al. 1991. Identification of *p53* mutations in bladder cancers and urine samples. Science 252:706–9.

Sidransky D, Tokino T, Hamilton SR et al. 1992. Identification of ras oncogene mutations in the stool of patients with curable colorectal tumors. Science 256:102–5.

Sinicrope FA, Hart J, Michelassi F, Lee JJ. 1995. Prognostic value of bcl-2 oncoprotein expression in stage II colon cancer. Clin Cancer Res 1:1103.

Slebos RJ, Kibbelaar RE, Dalesio O et al. 1990. K-ras oncogene activation as a prognostic marker in adenocarcinoma of the lung. New Eng J Med 323:561–5.

Soignet S, Fleischauer A, Polyak T, Heller G, Warrell RP Jr. 1997. All-*trans*-retinoic acid significantly increases 5-year survival in acute promyelocytic leukemia: an updated analysis of the New York study. Cancer Chemother Pharmacol (in press).

Sozzi G, Veronese ML, Negrini M et al. 1996. The FHIT gene at 3p14.2 is abnormal in lung cancer. Cell 85:17–26.

Sparrow LE, English DR, Heenan PJ et al. 1995. Prognostic significance of *p53* overexpression in thin melanomas. Melanoma Res 5:387–92.

Stock C, Ambros IM, Mann G et al. 1993. Detection of 1p36 deletions in paraffin sections of neuroblastoma tissues. Genes Chrom Cancer 6:1–9.

Stricker HJ, Jay JK, Linden MD, Tamboli P, Amin MB. 1996. Determining prognosis of clinically localized prostate cancer by immunohistochemical detection of mutant *p53*. Urology 47:366–9.

Sugio K, Ishida T, Yokoyama H et al. 1990. Ras gene mutations as a prognostic marker in adenocarcinoma of the human lung without lymph node metastasis. Cancer Res 52:2903–6.

Tan P, Cady B, Wanner M et al. 1997. The cell cycle inhibitor p27 is an independent prognostic marker in small (T1a, b) invasive breast carcinomas. Cancer Res 57:1259–63.

Tateishi M, Ishida T, Mitsudomi T, Kaneko S, Sugimachi K. 1990. Immunohistochemical evidence of autocrine growth factors in adenocarcinoma of the lung. Cancer Res 50:7077–80.

Tateishi M, Ishida T, Mitsudomi T, Kaneko S, Sugimachi K. 1991. Prognostic value of c-erbB-2 protein expression in human lung adenocarcinoma and squamous cell carcinoma. Eur J Cancer 27:1372–5.

Tetu B, Brisson J. 1994. Prognostic significance of HER2/neu oncoprotein expression in node-positive breast cancer. Cancer 73:2359–65.

Tetu B, Fradet Y, Allard P et al. 1996. Prevalence and clinical significance of *her2*/neu, *p53* and Rb expression in primary superficial bladder cancer. J Urol 155:1784–8.

Tilly H, Rossi A, Stamatoullas A et al. 1994. Prognostic value of chromosomal abnormalities in follicular lymphoma. Blood 84:1043–9.

Tricot G, Sawyer JR, Jagannath S et al. 1997. Unique role of cytogenetics in the prognosis of patients with myeloma receiving high-dose therapy and autotransplants. J Clin Oncol 15:2659–66.

Veale D, Kerr N, Gibson GJ, Kelly PJ, Harris AL. 1993. The relationship of quantitative epidermal growth factor receptor expression in non-small cell lung cancer to long term survival. Br J Cancer 68:162–5.

Veltri RW, Partin AW, Epstein JE et al. 1994. Quantitative nuclear morphometry, Markovian texture descriptors, and DNA content captured on a CAS-200 Image analysis system, combined with PCNA and HER-2/neu immunohistochemistry for prediction of prostate cancer progression. J Cell Biochem 19:249–58.

Verhoef GE, Boogaerts MA. 1996. Cytogenetics and its prognostic value in myelodysplastic syndrome. Acta Haematol 95:95–101.

Warrell RP, Jr., De Thé H, Wang ZY, Degos L. 1993. Acute promyelocytic leukemia. New Engl J Med 329:177–89.

Wattel E, Preudhomme C, Hecquet B et al. 1994. *p53* mutations are associated with resistance to chemotherapy and short survival in hematologic malignancies. Blood 84:3148–57.

Whang-Peng J, Knutsen T, Jaffe ES et al. 1995. Sequential analysis of 43 patients with non-Hodgkin's lymphoma: clinical correlations with cytogenetic, histologic, immunophenotyping, and molecular studies. Blood 85:203–16.

Xerri L, Grob JJ, Battyani Z et al. 1994. *NM23* expression in metastasis of malignant melanoma is a predictive prognostic parameter correlated with survival. Br J Cancer 70:1224–8.

Xu H J, Quinlan DC, Davidson AG et al. 1994. Altered retinoblastoma protein expression and prognosis in early-stage non-small-cell lung carcinoma. J Natl Cancer Inst 86:695–9.

Yunis JJ, Mayer MG, Arnesen MA et al. 1989. *bcl*-2 and other genomic alterations in the prognosis of large-cell lymphoma. N Engl J Med 320:1047–54.

Zedenius J, Larsson C, Bergholm U, Bovee J, Svensson A, Hallengren B et al. 1995. Mutations of codon 918 in the RET proto-oncogene correlate to poor prognosis in sporadic medullary thyroid carcinomas. J Clin Endocrinol Metab 80:3088–90.

Zeng ZS, Sarkis AS, Zhang ZF et al. 1994. *p53* nuclear overexpression: an independent predictor of survival in lymph node-positive colorectal cancer patients. J Clin Oncol 12:2043–50.

9

Reproductive Counseling for Cancer Patients and Familes

An important aspect of risk counseling for individuals affected by cancer relates to reproductive choices after successful completion of therapy. Counseling regarding the potential gonadal toxicities of cancer therapies has been part of the practice of clinical oncology, and detailed discussions are available in cancer medicine texts (Meistrich et al., 1997). Treatment planning for some patients, for example those with Hodgkin's disease or seminoma, may be modified based on these concerns.

Discussions of posttreatment reproductive choices has been limited by the databases available to guide decisions. Prenatal genetic testing for cancer predisposition has not yet emerged as a clinical need, although this may change as technologies become more widely available to medical geneticists and genetic counselors. This aspect of clinical cancer genetics needs to be responsive to considerations of the ethical and medical appropriateness of reproductive options that technology has now made possible. The scope of genetic counseling for reproductive risks in cancer patients is outlined in Table 9-1.

PRETREATMENT REPRODUCTIVE COUNSELING FOR THE CANCER PATIENT

All three modalities of cancer treatment—surgery, chemotherapy, and radiation therapy—have potential toxicities affecting the reproductive organs.

The risk for ovarian failure in women being treated for cancer varies with age, dose and type of chemotherapy, and duration of treatment. For example, in patients being treated with cyclophosphamide-based therapies for breast cancer, women younger than 40 experienced amenorrhea after twice the dose of drug compared to older women

TABLE 9-1   Scope of Counseling for Reproductive Risks in Cancer Patients

1. Risks of infertility due to treatment.
2. Risks for genetic diseases, including cancer, in offspring of cancer patients. This component may include germline DNA testing or constitutional karyotype analysis, if appropriate.
3. Risks of, and contraindications for, attempts at conception during and after treatment.
4. Pretreatment evaluation of sperm count and function in males.
5. Consideration of pretreatment sperm banking, oophoropexy, or embryo harvesting and cryopreservation.
6. Discussion of risks of mutation-causing effects of chemotherapy and radiation therapy.
7. Referral or liaison counseling with obstetrician for fetal imaging, monitoring, or prenatal genetic counseling and analysis, as appropriate, for level of risk.

(Dnistrian et al., 1983). More than half of women treated with MOPP (nitrogen mustard, vincristine, procarbazine, prednisone) chemotherapy for Hodgkin's disease experienced ovarian dysfunction, but the risk for persistent amenorrhea was much greater in women older than 35–40. Gonadal toxicity of the MOPP regimen has been one factor in the greater acceptability of the ABVD (doxorubicin, bleomycin, vinblastine, DTIC) regimen for younger patients with this disease (Horning et al., 1981; Bonnadonna et al., 1984).

Young girls appear to be resistant to the gonadal toxicities of even the most intensive chemotherapy regimens, with radiation therapy noted as the most significant agent to impact on fertility in survivors of a range of childhood cancers (Byrne et al., 1987). This testifies to the resilience of the immature ovary to chemotherapy-induced toxicities. Effects of radiation therapy to the ovaries are dependent on age and dose, with exposures over 500–600 cGy producing permanent loss of ovarian function (Sanders et al., 1988).

It was originally thought that prepubertal males tolerated high doses of alkylating agents in treatment protocols for leukemia without testicular damage. However long-term follow-up has noted that there is a dose-dependent decrease in male gonadal function in long-term survivors of childhood cancer (Dhabhar et al., 1993). In postpubertal males, the testes is susceptible to damage, particularly by alkylating drugs, which produce azoospermia. In general, there is increased incidence of azoospermia as dose increases, although dose-toxicity data for most drugs are not available. The ABVD regimen is less toxic to the male gonads, producing azoospermia in only 0–35% of males, while it is observed in up to 100% of men treated with MOPP (da Cunha et al., 1984; Viviani et al., 1985). About half of young males treated with platinum-based regimens for germ cell tumors will recover sperm count and function. It should be noted that a significant proportion of male Hodgkin's disease patients and males with germ cell cancer have abnormal sperm motility before treatment.

Effects of radiation therapy to the testes are dose dependent. Exposures over 600 cGy produce sterility, with compromise in function noted at lower doses. Despite efforts to preserve neurologic function in patients receiving radical prostatectomy, cystoprostatectomy, and retroperitoneal lymph node dissection, compromise of sexual function may occur in a significant proportion of cases.

Techniques standardly employed to preserve gonadal function in patients undergoing radiation therapy include testicular shielding and surgical repositioning of the ovaries behind the uterus (oophoropexy). In this latter procedure, radiation dose to the ovaries can be diminished to 4 to 5 Gy, with good preservation of gonadal function in younger women (Sy Ortin et al., 1990). Cryopreservation of sperm samples is part of the routine prechemotherapy workup of patients with lymphoma or germ cell cancer, although, as noted, compromised sperm function may limit the effectiveness of this procedure. Newer techniques such as intracytoplasmic sperm injection may be successful with sperm samples of 0% motility, as long as viability is documented (Palmero et al., 1995). Cryopreservation of eggs has recently become feasible. Banking of *in vitro* fertilized embryos is an option available for couples (Buster et al., 1985), as long as there is sufficient time available prior to initiation of treatment. Electrical stimulation to produce semen has been applied to males post lymph node dissection.

POSTTREATMENT REPRODUCTIVE COUNSELING

Numerous studies have addressed the outcomes of pregnancies in over 3000 cancer survivors. Because most cancer therapies cause mutations in DNA, it is conceivable that germ cell mutations could also be induced, especially in the female where the total complement of oocytes has completed the first phase of meiosis by birth. Significantly, there was no increase in congenital abnormalities or other chromosome abnormalities noted in survivors of the atomic detonations over Japan in 1945. The same findings have been noted among survivors of cancer treatment regimens. A literature review of over 1000 live births from cancer survivors revealed a 4% rate of birth defects, a rate comparable to the general population (Mulvihill and Byrne, 1985). Analysis of over 4000 offspring of survivors of childhood cancer showed no increase in cancer rates when families with cancers associated with known hereditary predisposition syndromes were taken into account (e.g., retinoblastoma) (Mulvihill et al., 1987; Hawkins et al., 1989).

An increasingly frequent issue in cancer care relates to requests for reproductive counseling for young survivors of breast cancer. From 10 to 20% of breast cancer occurs in women of child-bearing age. The question of risk is not so much for the fetus as for the patient. Two large retrospective Scandinavian studies involving 324 women who became pregnant after breast cancer failed to show any evidence of a worse prognosis compared to a control group of 7,465 breast cancer patients (von Schoultz et al., 1995; Kroman et al., 1997). The need for prospective data remains (Petrek, 1994). Conventional advice pending definitive data has been to postpone childbearing until at least two years after completion of treatment for breast cancer.

The evaluation for infertility in young cancer patients in long-term remission should involve the same level of scrutiny (including constitutional karyotype, infectious, endocrinologic and other evaluation) as patients without cancer.

Case Example 9.1. A 32-year-old woman diagnosed with Hodgkin's disease of mediastinal lymph nodes desired to preserve her childbearing options after treatment. The planned treatment was to include both radiation and chemotherapy, with a possibility for stem cell bone marrow transplantation, depending on the treatment arm assigned in the protocol. The patient opted to delay treatment so as to arrange for harvesting of ova and cryopreservation of *in vitro* fertilized embryos. Treatment was successful, resulting in a complete remission, and the stem cell transplant was not administered. The patient sought counseling regarding options for reproduction. Menstrual function resumed posttreatment and hormonal evaluation was unremarkable. Reassurances were provided regarding the minimal increase in risk for low birth weight or congenital abnormalities in offspring of survivors of Hodgkin's disease. Nonetheless, the patient opted for implantation of the cryopreserved embryos. Healthy twins were delivered after an uncomplicated pregnancy.

This case indicates the range of reproductive options now available to young individuals considering curative treatments for hematopoietic malignancies and some solid tumors. Because of the need for rapid initiation of treatment, banking of *in vitro* fertilized embryos is often not practical. As indicated in the text, cryopreservation of harvested eggs is now feasible, and sperm samples from affected males are routinely cryopreserved prior to cytotoxic therapies.

COUNSELING FOR EXPOSURE TO ANTINEOPLASTIC AGENTS DURING PREGNANCY

Pregnancy is contraindicated during cancer therapies. In those circumstances where drugs or radiation have been administered inadvertently or on a life-saving basis, counseling must be provided. The literature relating to the pharmacology of antineoplastic agents during pregnancy and reports of pregnancy outcomes have been reviewed (Aviles et al., 1991; Dodds et al., 1993; Hawkins et al., 1989; Wiebe and Sipila, 1994; Zemlickis et al., 1992). In addition, a registry of pregnancies exposed to cancer therapy is maintained by J. Mulvihill at the University of Pittsburgh.

In general, exposure of the 8–15 week fetus to even low levels of radiation (10 cGy) may result in diminished IQ. Microcephaly and short stature result from higher radiation doses. Exposure to chemotherapy agents in the first trimester results in an increased teratogenic risk, in the range of 10–15% in some series. Remarkably, the older fetus is quite resistant to the teratogenic effects of even combination chemotherapy regimens. There are numerous reports in the literature of successful pregnancy outcomes when treatments were commenced after the first trimester.

Treatment of lymphoma, leukemia, and breast cancer in the pregnant patient poses a special challenge to the oncologist. In some circumstances, an understanding of the pharmacology of antineoplastic agents can lead to the fashioning of temporizing strategies. Consultation with available registries and toxicologic databases are critical resources for clinical cancer genetics counselors. One such telephone consultation service for assessing chemotherapy risk for pregnant patients is the "Motherisk" program in Toronto, Canada (described in Koren et al., 1996).

Case Example 9.2. In the course of a genetic analysis for engraftment after bone marrow transplantation for acute leukemia, a patient was found to be a full chimera (i.e., the hematopoietic cells were of 100% donor origin). However, karyotypic analysis revealed a balanced translocation that was not known to be associated with malignancy. A second sample from the patient's HLA-matched donor was requested. The translocation was confirmed to be a constitutional abnormality. After consultation with the institutional ethics committee, it was decided that the donor should be offered counseling regarding the results because the consent for marrow donation did not preclude such notification and because this abnormality could aid in reproductive planning. The donor was a 36-year-old woman who had experienced multiple miscarriages and who had gone on to adopt two children. Counseling was provided regarding the association of constitutional chromosomal abnormalities and the donor's reproductive history. The donor had consulted a fertility specialist in the past and chromosomal studies had been recommended but not performed. Further counseling was provided, including reassurance about the benign nature of abnormality detected and its presumed role in the pregnancy outcomes.

This case indicates one indication for reproductive counseling in the setting of a cancer genetics laboratory. Chromosome abnormalities, usually sex chromosome mosaicism or structural chromosome abnormalities, are observed in about 5% of couples with two consecutive miscarriages. Reciprocal translocations are relatively common and have been observed in up to 1 in 500 newborns. They are usually innocuous for the carrier. However, as in this case, spontaneous abortions can result from the generation of unbalanced gametes at meiosis with large duplications or deficiencies in the unbalanced products leading to a failure in implantation or development. In some circumstances, viable conceptuses may result, although the generation of unbalanced gametes may lead to dysmorphism and altered mental development. Pregnancy outcomes depend on the relative frequencies of gametes produced, which are determined by the specific type of translocation present.

PREIMPLANTATION GENETICS FOR HEREDITARY CANCER SYNDROMES

Preimplantation genetics is a modification of in vitro fertilization (IVF) in which embryos unaffected for a genetic disease are selectively implanted. Because of the extremely early stage at which genetic diagnosis is performed, this technique may be viewed differently than selective termination of pregnancy after chorionic villous sampling or amniocentesis. As in IVF, the woman is treated with a hormonal regimen to cause ovulation of multiple eggs, which are collected by aspirating ovarian follicles through a needle inserted transvaginally. The eggs are fertilized *in vitro* with the husband's sperm. One or two cells are then biopsied from the developing embryo at the eight-cell stage, at about the third day after insemination. Embryos found to be unaffected for the genotype in question are then transferred to (implanted in) the uterus (Gullick and Handyside, 1994).

Preimplantation genetic diagnosis was initially utilized for X-linked recessive disorders. In these circumstances, only female embryos were selected for transfer. Successful application of this technique has now been reported for cystic fibrosis, Lesch-Nyhan syndrome, Tay-Sachs disease, hemophilia A, and Duchenne muscular dystrophy. To date, there have been no published attempts to use these techniques for dominant cancer predisposition syndromes, although, in theory, this is feasible (Gullick and Handyside, 1994).

The technical limitation of the procedure is the determination of genotype at the single-cell level. These considerations are critical, as rare technical errors of diagnosis have been reported in preimplantation diagnosis of recessive disorders. In these circumstances, the probability of transferring an affected embryo should be far less than in a dominant disorder, since failure to amplify one allele would not affect the ability to exclude homozygotes, but could result in accidental implantation of a heterozygote. For families with known mutations (e.g., 185delAG mutations of *BRCA1*), PCR-based techniques could be applied, using sensitive techniques of detection of specific mutations. For breast and ovarian cancer predisposition, sex-specific selection could also be performed, although there may also be an increased cancer risk in male carriers of mutations of *BRCA1* or *BRCA2*.

Clearly, ethical and social factors in addition to technical feasibility will determine the availability of preimplantation genetics for late onset disorders for which early detection and prevention options of presumed benefit exist. Because of limited insurance reimbursement for IVF procedures, it is unlikely that the demand for preimplantation cancer genetic diagnosis will be substantial. IVF can cost $40,000–50,000 per pregnancy. Cancer genetic counselors should stay apprised of public policy debates that are sure to emerge regarding the potential applications and limitations on these technologies.

REFERENCES

Aviles A, Diaz-Maqueo JC, Talavera A, Guzman R, Garcia E. 1991. Growth and development of children of mothers treated with chemotherapy during pregnancy: current status of 43 children. Amer J Hem 36:243–8.

Bonadonna G, Santoro A, Viviani S et al. 1984. Gonadal damage in Hodgkin's disease from cancer chemotherapy regimens. Arch Toxicol 7(suppl):140–5.

Buster JE, Bustillo M, Rodi IA et al. 1985. Biologic and morphologic development of donated human ova recovered by nonsurgical uterine lavage. Am J Obstet Gynecol 153:211–7.

Byrne J, Mulvihill JJ, Myers MH et al. 1987. Effects of treatment on fertility in long-term survivors of childhood or adolescent cancer. New Engl J Med 317:1315–21.

da Cunha MF, Meistrich ML, Fuller LM et al. 1984. Recovery of spermatogenesis after treatment for Hodgkin's disease: limiting dose of MOPP chemotherapy. J Clin Oncol 2:571–7.

Dhabhar BN, Malhotra H, Joseph R et al. 1993. Gonadal function in prepubertal boys following treatment for Hodgkin's disease. Am J Pediatr Hematol Oncol 15:306–10.

Dnistrian AM, Schwartz MK, Fraccia AA et al. 1983. Endocrine consequences of CMF adjuvant chemotherapy in premenopausal and postmenopausal breast cancer patients. Cancer 51:803–7.

Dodds L, Marrett LD, Tomkins DJ, Green B, Sherman G. 1993. Case-control study of congenital anomalies in children of cancer patients. Br Med J 307:164–8.

Gullick WJ, Handyside AH. 1994. Pre-implantation diagnosis of inherited predisposition to cancer. Eur J Cancer 30A:2030–2.

Hawkins MM, Draper GJ, Smith RA. 1989. Cancer among 1,348 offspring of survivors of childhood cancer. Int J Cancer 43:975–8.

Horning SJ, Hoppe RT, Kaplan HS et al. 1981. Female reproductive potential after treatment for Hodgkin's disease. New Engl J Med 304:1377–82.

Koren G, Lishner M, Farine D (eds), 1996. Cancer in pregnancy. Cambridge: Cambridge University Press.

Kroman N, Jensen MB, Melbye M, Wohlfahrt J, Mouridsen HT. 1997. Should women be advised against pregnancy after breast-cancer treatment? Lancet 350:310–22.

Meistrich ML, Vassilopoulou-Sellin RV, Lipshultz LI. 1997. "Gonadal Dysfunction" in: DeVita VT, Jr, Hellman S, Rosenberg SA (eds). Cancer: Principles and Practice of Oncology. Lippincott-Raven, Philadelphia. pp. 2758–72.

Mulvihill JJ, Byrne J. 1985. Offspring of long-time survivors of childhood cancers. Clin Oncol 4:333–43.

Mulvihill JJ, Myers MH, Connelly RR et al. 1987. Cancer in offspring of long-term survivors of childhood and adolescent cancer. Lancet 2:813–7.

Palmero GD, Cohen J, Alikani M et al. 1995. Intracytoplasmic sperm injection: a novel treatment for all forms of male factor infertility. Fertil Steril 63:1231–40.

Petrek JA. 1994. Pregnancy safety after breast cancer. Cancer 74:528–31.

Sanders JE, Buckner CD, Amos D et al. 1988. Ovarian function following marrow transplantation for aplastic anemia or leukemia. J Clin Oncol 6:813–8.

Sy Ortin TT, Shostak CA, Donaldson SS. 1990. Gonadal status and reproductive function following treatment for Hodgkin's disease in childhood: the Stanford experience. Int J Radiat Oncol Biol Phys 19:873–80.

Viviani S, Santoro A, Ragni G et al. 1985. Gonadal toxicity after combination chemotherapy for Hodgkin's disease. Comparative results of MOPP vs. ABVD. Eur J Cancer Clin Oncol 21:601–5.

von Schoultz E, Johansson H, Wilking N, Rutqvist LE. 1995. Influence of prior and subsequent pregnancy on breast cancer prognosis. J Clin Oncol 13:430–34.

Wiebe VJ, Sipila PEH. 1994. Pharmacology of antineoplastic agents in pregnancy. Crit Rev Oncol/Hematol 16:75–112.

Zemlickis D, Lishner M, Degendorfer P, Panzarella T, Sutcliffe SB, Koren G. 1992. Fetal outcome after *in utero* exposure to cancer chemotherapy. Arch Intern Med 152:573–6.

10

Psychological, Ethical, and Legal Issues in Cancer Risk Counseling

The clinician, though well versed in the technical and statistical aspects of genetic testing summarized in the preceding chapters, may be unprepared for the psychological challenges and ethical complexities of communicating hereditary cancer risk information to families. In this chapter, the psychological principles that underlie counseling interactions are presented, along with the special vulnerabilities and untoward reactions to genetic information that may occur. The extraordinary scope of the ethical implications of genetic testing and counseling is also explored. The organization of this latter discussion follows the classical elements of biomedical ethics, with an emphasis on autonomy, nonmaleficence (do no harm), and privacy. The evolving federal and local legal statutes that bear on genetic testing are reviewed. The concept of informed consent is presented as the unifying process that sets the stage for the discussion of both the medical and nonmedical risks and benefits of cancer genetic testing.

PSYCHOLOGICAL ISSUES IN CANCER GENETIC COUNSELING

Seymour Kessler has defined two broad schools of genetic counseling: content-oriented and person-oriented (Kessler, 1979). In content-oriented genetic counseling, there is a strong emphasis on risk assessment, facts, and figures. In person-oriented counseling, the timing of when and how information is delivered and the psychologic characteristics of the client are emphasized. Advocates of person-centered approaches argue, quite convincingly, that studies indicate that 21–75% of counselees do not remember, or do not understand, the information they have received (Sorenson, 1974). Studies of individuals seeking counseling for cancer risk reveal that an individual's perception of cancer risk may be completely unrelated to actual risk. Even more significantly, a persons' desire for genetic testing may stem from profound psychologic stresses and "intrusive thoughts" about the dangers of cancer. The most accurate genetic test that molecular biology can produce must ultimately be translated into a behavioral endpoint: the ability of an individual to take positive actions following testing. Clearly, recognition of the psychological forces that define preventive and other behaviors are critical components of cancer risk counseling.

Psychological Principles

Borrowing from Rogerian theory, four features are particularly relevant to effective counseling: empathy, respect, positive regard, and genuineness (Kessler, 1979). Derived over 40 years ago, these therapeutic goals still serve as useful guideposts for clinicians. Carl Rogers defined *empathy* as the ability to sense "the client's private world as if it were your own, but without ever losing the 'as if' quality" (Rogers, 1951). *Positive regard* represents the counselor's ability to express respect and care for the counselee. According to Rogers, this must be without condition. *Genuineness* refers to the counselor's ability to "freely and deeply" break down the facade with the counselee, to communicate a sense of personal sincerity and conviction.

The ability to empathetically project these qualities is clearly dependent on the personality of the individual counselor. In some regards, the specific knowledge of the cancer specialist (e.g., oncologist or oncology nurse) can be an enormous asset. In the taking of the personal and family history, the cancer specialist can demonstrate understanding of the specific features of a chemotherapeutic regimen or surgical procedure. She or he can convey a sense of first-hand knowledge, and appreciation, of the way in which the proband or family member coped with their treatment travails. As familiarity with cancer treatments and experiences grows, genetic counselors, primary care physicians, and other health professionals can project this same empathetic understanding of the family's cancer care experiences. On occasion, an admission, by the counselor, of a similar experience with another patient, friend, or colleague can do much to break down the formality of the physician–patient relationship. Such gestures, while good-intentioned, must be broached carefully. The "as if" clause in the Rogerian definition of empathy is a critical one. In members of families where hereditary disease is characterized by multiple cancers and very early age of onset, the magnitude of grief and suffering can be extraordinary and unique.

In addition to Rogerian sensitivities, a number of powerful constructs are particularly useful in cancer risk counseling. Emphasis on the notion of empowerment, an ability to change the future, can provide a positive focus to most cancer risk counseling interactions. It is almost always helpful, both to the counselor and the consultand, to pause during a session to take stock of the special nature of the encounter and the rapid progress in research that has made accurate risk prediction possible. The ability to predict the future brings with it a burden, but also extraordinary opportunities new to the practice of preventive medicine. In the context of a positive genetic test, it should be emphasized that risk for inheriting a mutation is very different from risk for developing the cancer. And both of these risks are very different from the risk of dying of a cancer, which will be significantly lower.

Psychological Barriers to Counseling: The Individual Unaffected by Cancer

Psychological barriers may impact both the tendency to seek counseling and the effectiveness of the counseling that is offered. When an individual comes to seek guidance regarding cancer risk, it is often in the setting of a recent personal experience with cancer in a close family member. Doubts about the patient's ability to receive the results of a genetic test should serve as a contraindication to DNA evaluation for this individual. In a situation where the grieving survivor seeks prophylactic surgery after witnessing the death of a relative, it is prudent to defer testing and to seek time to put into perspective urgent requests for surgery. A recognition of, and sensitivity to, the especially trying circumstances of the grieving relative should influence the approach to counseling.

Numerous authors have attached different labels to the phases of coping that follow a stress-evoking event; those used here are from Horowitz as modified by Kessler (Horowitz, 1976; Kessler, 1979). They include: outcry, denial, intrusion, working through, and completion. Although the first two stages are straightforward, the intrusion phase is complex. It includes a fear of repetition, shame over one's helplessness, rage and fault-finding, and survivor guilt.

The concept of *survivor guilt* has generally been applied to family members of cancer survivors. It has emerged from studies of the psychological aspects of late-onset diseases. Renewed interest in survivor guilt has grown from observations of the stress reactions of individuals who test negative for cancer susceptibility mutations, particularly when siblings test positive. It can come as a surprise to the clinician that the individual requiring acute psychiatric intervention is the one who tests negative, not the individual who is told he or she carries a predisposing mutation. A lack of awareness of this phenomenon is common among oncologists and other physicians, who feel they are experienced in the communication to patients of "bad news."

In the working through phase, the acceptance of reality gradually emerges. The completion phase is characterized by a termination of stress due to cognitive factors. These may even occur in the dying patient, as explored by Kubler-Ross. According to some psychologists, the completion phase rarely occurs, and cycles of grief, denial, and intrusion may be recurrent (Kubler-Ross, 1969).

It might appear that cancer genetic counseling would best be reserved for the later phases in the cycle of reactions to a stress-evoking event. However, a basic tenet of genetic counseling is that it is effective at any stage in the coping process, and may serve as a critical opportunity for emotional support and guidance. Different mixes of information and support will be appropriate for the family member at different stages in the coping process.

Beyond severe stress reactions to the sickness or death of family members, additional psychological barriers to cancer risk counseling are specific to the familial syndromes themselves. Most studies have been directed toward the fears of disfigurement and loss of body image in women at risk for breast cancer. These same concerns are relevant to the child undergoing prophylactic thyroid surgery or the adolescent with adenomatous polyposis. For some individuals, pervasive fear of cancer can color life choices or become disabling. In other circumstances the pervasive fear of cancer repre-

---

Case Example 10.1. A 50-year-old woman was diagnosed with a 3-cm infiltrating intraductal breast cancer at age 45. She had five positive lymph nodes, which were estrogen receptor negative, and expressed high levels of HER2/neu protein. She received six cycles of anthracycline-containing chemotherapy. Liver metastases was documented 2 months after completion of chemotherapy. After induction therapy with taxotere, a stem-cell transplant was successfully performed. Four years posttransplant, the patient developed abdominal symptoms, which gradually emerged over 6 months. An evaluation ultimately revealed ovarian cancer. An intensive chemotherapy protocol was initiated.

The patient had a limited family history. Her relatives were lost in the Holocaust. She had no sisters or children. She sought genetic testing for *BRCA1* and *BRCA2*.

On first appearance, there seemed little indication for genetic testing in this case. There were no therapeutic benefits and no relatives at risk. However, in the course of counseling, the patient expressed a desire to better understand the origins of her disease. She had followed a "healthy" lifestyle and had adhered to the dietary and exercise recommendations of her physicians. She articulated a need to know if she was "fated" by inherited predisposition to cancer despite her best efforts. She said that this would provide her with meaningful information.

This case serves as an example of the nonmedical or psychological considerations surrounding cancer genetic counseling. The individual was offered genetic testing.

---

sents a symptom of a larger set of character or personality disorders. These issues are particularly relevant in the preoperative evaluation of patients seeking prophylactic mastectomy. In this context, formal psychological evaluation can be of enormous benefit both to the individual considering the procedure and the health-care providers seeking to counsel her about the emotional risks and benefits entailed.

Psychological Barriers to Counseling: The Individual Affected by Cancer

It must be recognized that some elements of cancer genetic counseling are unsettling and create an additional burden for the patient. This is no more evident than in the individual already affected by cancer. Often such individuals participate in genetic testing to allow their children to better estimate their risk. In the process, individuals with cancer may be confronted with unexpected information about their own risk for secondary cancers, or new primary cancers. These individuals are at the greatest risk for serious psychological compromise, including suicidal thoughts. At least one suicide attempt has occurred in an affected individual given results of *BRCA1* mutation status. Such vulnerabilities should be identified in the pretest phase of counseling and appropriate consultations organized. Ethical commitments to the autonomy of the patient and attention to possibly coercive elements within the family must be recognized. In some research settings, it may be possible for the affected proband to elect not to be told the results of genetic testing. In routine medical practice, such an option is fraught with concerns about responsibility and liability.

Because of the unique medical circumstances of each cancer survivor, it is essential that risk notification for these individuals be coordinated with the patient's oncologist. In keeping with the Rogerian model, the oncologist is in a favorable position to integrate new genetic information into the context of the patient's life, values, and experiences. In some situations, the identification of a genetic predisposing mutation can even provide an intellectual explanation for the seemingly random course of events that afflicted the patient and the family.

Behavioral Research in the Risk Counseling Clinic

There is a rich tradition of research on the psychological aspects of genetic counseling and testing (reviewed in Kessler, 1989). Psychological research on aspects of cancer genetic counseling has focused on three broad areas: factors predicting interest in cancer genetic testing, the psychological impact of genetic testing and counseling for inherited cancer risk, and the relationship between genetic risk and preventive behaviors. In each of these areas, preliminary conclusions have implications for the management of at-risk families.

Early reports of heightened interest in genetic testing for cancer susceptibility mirrored the initial findings for cystic fibrosis, Duchenne muscular dystrophy, and Huntington disease. In some studies, more than 90% of individuals expressed their desire to undergo genetic testing for breast cancer susceptibility (Struewing et al., 1995; Botkin et al., 1996), and a majority of individuals expressed interest in colon cancer testing (Croyle and Lerman, 1993). The most common shared motivation was a desire to learn of children's risks. In Huntington disease, a similar level of interest was documented, but the uptake fell to 16% once testing was actually made available (Craufurd et al., 1989). It was not clear if the proportion of individuals seeking genetic testing for cancer risk would also drop once testing became available. A study of 279 women in hereditary breast-ovarian cancer families showed that the proportion opting to receive test results fell to 60% (Lerman et al., 1996). The factors predicting the decision to receive test results were: having health insurance, knowledge about *BRCA1* testing, and number of first degree relatives affected with breast cancer.

A number of studies (Table 10-1) have addressed the impact of cancer genetic counseling and/or testing for breast cancer susceptibility. Research is underway for other syndromes. Because of cultural differences in populations studied, the complexity of the instruments used in research studies, and the varying levels of resources for support offered to participants, it may be difficult for the clinician to select from these data for everyday practice. However, some of these research findings are clinically relevant. Counseling must be tailored to the individual, with respect to education, life experience, and level of anxiety. To many health professionals not involved in risk counseling, the conventional wisdom has been that the more a person is made aware of an increased personal risk of developing cancer, the more motivated that individual should be to comply with medical recommendations. A paradoxical conclusion of psychosocial research in this area is that heightened levels of anxiety actually interfere with regular clinical exams and a woman's ability to perform breast self-examination or follow through with preventive services such as mammography (Kash et al., 1992 Alagna et al., 1987; Lerman et al., 1990). One of the tenets of cancer risk counseling is

Table 10-1 Studies of Psychological Impact of Breast Cancer Genetic Counseling and/or Testing

Author	Type of Study	Size	Findings
Lynch et al., 1993	Prospective descriptive interview	32 relatives in one family offered *BRCA1* testing	• No emotional trauma following genetic testing • Some depression, but no interventions needed • *BRCA1* positive patients better able to plan interventions
Lerman et al., 1995	Prospective randomized comparative study	200 women with family history of breast cancer	• Individualized counseling improved risk comprehension • African-American women more likely to sense benefit • Anxious preoccupation with risk interfered with efficacy of counseling
Lerman et al., 1996	Prospective cohort with follow-up after counseling	279 women in *BRCA1*-linked families	• 60% requested test results • In *BRCA1* negative: significant reduction in depressive symptoms and functional impairment • In *BRCA1* positive: no increase in depression or functional impairment
Lynch et al., 1997	Prospective descriptive interview	181 relatives in 14 families offered *BRCA1* testing	• In *BRCA1* positive group: 35% considered mastectomy, 76% considered oophorectomy • 80% who tested negative had emotional relief • 33% who tested positive had sadness, anger, guilt
Lerman et al., 1997	Prospective randomized comparative study of counseling methods	400 women at low to intermediate risk for breast cancer	• Counseling significantly increased perceived limitations and decreased perceived benefit of *BRCA1* testing • Neither counseling or educational approach altered intention to have genetic testing
Croyle et al., 1997	Prospective interview	60 individuals from one kindred	• Carriers with no history of cancer had greatest stress • Gene carriers had higher general distress (state anxiety) compared to non-carriers

that, to the extent that anxiety is based on misperceptions, the educational component of counseling will reduce these misperceptions. Thus, effective risk assessment and counseling can provide a potent psychotherapeutic effect.

Research studies have shown that counseling can have a significant role in reducing personal risk estimation in some cancer families. It is common for unaffected individuals in these families to overestimate their cancer risk, mostly from a lack of understanding of Mendelian mechanisms. In addition, individuals tend to think in an anti-Bayesian manner. An individual whose grandmother and aunt died of breast cancer and whose mother and sister have not been affected was convinced that she would be the unlucky one, although Bayesian inference would argue that her risks were lower than 50%. In addition, the classical observations of Pearn have identified the broad spectrum of variation in attitude to risk as "varying from extreme cautiousness to recklessness" (Pearn, 1973). Characteristics such as pessimism ("just my luck"), optimism ("it can't happen to me"), and achievement-oriented versus failure-threatened personalities have been shown to impact on both risk perception and willingness to take risks. These patterns of risk-taking personalities are as recognizable in the counseling clinic as in the gambling parlor.

Preliminary psychological research studies in clinical cancer genetics have largely been performed in the setting of counseling and testing for hereditary breast cancer. Comparing the psychological outcome after counseling and testing in mutation carriers, noncarriers, and decliners of testing, there was a greater reduction in depression and role impairment in noncarriers compared to the other groups. This latter category was measured utilizing questionnaires about impairment in daily, functional activities, as well as other measures. Thus, these results document psychological benefits of counseling in noncarriers, and no seriously adverse sequelae in carriers (Lerman et al., 1996). Another study of 60 women tested for *BRCA1* showed a sustained increase in general distress 1–2 weeks after counseling for genetic test results. These findings were more severe in women without a history of cancer or cancer-related surgery (Croyle et al., 1996).

A special psychological concern in cancer genetic counseling is the possibility of ambiguous results. Experience from Huntington disease has shown that ambiguous results can be more stressful than positive results (Wiggins et al., 1992). The possibility that results may be of unclear significance (e.g., missense mutations) should be included in pre-test counseling.

Ongoing psychological studies based on such models as the decision-balance and stages of change theories (Prochaska, 1994) will explore both the psychological characteristics in families seeking and receiving genetic testing and counseling.

ETHICAL AND LEGAL ASPECTS OF CANCER RISK COUNSELING

Careful attention to ethical considerations is a prerequisite for the humane translation of the new genetic technologies to clinical cancer medicine. Without anticipation and careful framing of the ethical and legal issues surrounding predictive genetic testing and counseling, the clinician may be overwhelmed by the unexpected dilemmas that emerge.

For example, the children of a mother who died of colon cancer at age 40 wanted to know if they were carrying the same genetic predisposition. In order to be tested with the best chance of meaningful results, it was first necessary for their aunt, who had a successful resection of colon cancer, to be screened for an identifiable mutation in one of the five genes associated with this syndrome. She, however, was tired of doctors and hospitals and was unwilling to participate. The family asked the physicians to help "convince" her to cooperate. In another case, a parent and survivor of colon cancer wanted his 10-year-old son tested for a colon cancer predisposition gene. He promised not to tell the boy, but felt it was his right as a parent to know his son's health risks. He was concerned, however, about his child's ability to get insurance and asked that the results of the genetic tests be kept out of the medical chart.

In these and other cases, ethical dilemmas may have legal or economic repercussions. It is the central premise of this chapter that open discussion, planning, involvement of the family, and a shared approach to decision making, grounded in ethical theory, is the best strategy to confront these issues. Although this approach will not diminish the difficulty or intensity of the decision process, it allows the family member and the health-care professional to face obstacles together, and under a shared set of values. A client-centered decision-making strategy is in keeping with the nondirective tenets of genetic counseling. It also offers a framework to address complex moral conflicts which are in many ways unavoidable consequences of a technology growing so rapidly that it has outpaced the social and medical infrastructure that spawned it. In such an environment, in which rules and guidelines may change rapidly, unusual diligence is necessary to provide up-to-date counseling and guidance.

There is a sound and well-established framework of biomedical ethics that can be called upon to aid decisions framed in genetic counseling sessions. Hospital ethics committees and institutional review boards (IRBs) include individuals with experience and perspective that can be drawn upon to guide these deliberations. In this section, the basic tenets of biomedical ethics and existing legal guidelines that pertain to genetic testing are outlined. At present these concerns relate primarily to *germline* genetic testing, because of social implications as well as implications to others. As genetic tests of tumor (*somatic*) cells improve in predictive accuracy (see Chapter 8), additional concerns about consent and ethical implications may emerge.

The Grounding of Biomedical Ethics in Moral Theory

Codes and Guidelines   The relatively young discipline of biomedical ethics has sought to examine the moral implications of medical decisions and new technologies. "Normative" ethics tries to set norms for the guidance of medical conduct that meet with established notions of what is right and wrong. The distinction of moral correctness (right and wrong), at least from a theoretical perspective, may vary according to the ethical model adopted. The models include a number of ethical theories, some of which predate Hippocrates. They range from the moral theory of utilitarianism, in which an individual acts to provide the greatest good (utility) for the greatest number, to Kantian theory, in which one acts only in a way that the actions may be generalized to become universal law (the categorical imperative), to more complex theories based on assumptions of basic rights that protect individuals within a society. Although discussions of how one arrives at a "right" decision utilizing each of these models makes for lively graduate seminars and meetings of hospital ethics committees, the translation and generalization of these norms to clinical situations can be daunting. Professional societies have sought to aid in this dialectic by formulating various uniform "codes" of professional ethics.

Codes of ethics, however, must be utilized carefully, since they may vary in their grounding in moral theory. The early American Medical Association (AMA) codes of ethics, starting with the 1847 ban on criticism of another physician in charge of a case and mandatory full professional courtesy, were cynically compared to the Pirates Creed of Ethics. (In the 1640 version of the ethical code of the Brothers of the Coast, detailed formulas were laid down for the distribution of the spoils and "courts of honour" to resolve disputes among the pirates.) The example of these historical codes only serves to underscore the importance of principle-driven normative ethics, firmly grounded in moral theory (Beauchamp and Childress, 1994).

Recent codes, including those of the AMA and the *Office for Protection from Research Risks (OPRR)*, reflect the impact of modern ethical theory in the area of human genetic information (NIH Office for Protection from Research Risks, 1993). Guidelines for the ethical application of genetic testing of human subjects are discussed on pages 5-42 through 5-63 of the 1993 edition of the OPRR recommendations. The OPRR recommendations have become a critical resource for institutional IRBs, and constitute basic reading for the cancer risk counselor. On important issues (e.g., the duty to warn family members at risk), the OPRR recommendations offer guidelines rather than prescriptions. To resolve individual issues, clinicians and IRBs are expected to reach decisions based on the fundamental tenets of biomedical ethics as applied to genetic testing.

Grounding in Ethical Theory: Autonomy

In their scholarly discussion of biomedical ethics, Beauchamp and Childress define the principles central to the current notion of ethical conduct in medicine. These concepts include: respect for individual autonomy of the patient, the imperative to do no harm (nonmaleficence), the concept of beneficence and justice, and certain obligations of the health professional relating to truth telling, privacy, confidentiality, and morally correct behavior. Each of these principles has special application to cancer genetics, but the principle of autonomy is perhaps the most fundamental.

Strictly defined, *autonomy* refers to self-rule, but in bioethical parlance this concept is more broadly defined. It refers to the right of the individual to act freely, with adequate information, and without coercion or interference. The concept of autonomy has also been invoked to justify the individual's right not to know medical information. This later imperative is not universally applicable, however, because in some circumstances the moral obligation to know is driven by a risk to others (e.g., in the case of an HIV test). For most cancer genetic susceptibilities tested in the context of research, the balance is tipped in favor of the individual's autonomous right not to know the results of a genetic test, or to have the test at all.

Thus, as in the case of the aunt who does not want to be tested despite the family's desire to know if there is a mutation in the family, the autonomy of the aunt may be viewed as the prevailing opinion. In this analysis, the coercive influences of the family should be avoided. One potential resolution, which can be built into IRB-sponsored research protocols for genetic testing, utilizes the option to be tested but not to know the results [OPRR 5-53]. This option can provide data needed to interpret genetic data in a family, while sparing the affected individual from what may be perceived as unwanted knowledge. Such individuals should be counseled that the information they are declining to know may relate to their risk of a second neoplasm, and medical screening can

Case Example 10.2. A brother and sister, both in their 20's, desired genetic testing for hereditary colon cancer risk. During counseling, they were informed that according to the research protocol being followed, testing should begin with the father, to establish if a mutation was segregating in the family. Their father, affected by colon cancer in his 30's, did not want to participate. After extensive counseling and discussion, it was clear that he did not feel able to cope with the psychological burden of knowing, beyond a reasonable doubt, that he was responsible for passing "bad genes" on to his children.

This understandable psychological response is encountered in testing for all cancer predisposition syndromes. Education and support about the advantages of early detection and prevention can often overcome the concerns and fears of some family members, but the "autonomy rule" ultimately determines individual participation in testing for inherited cancer risk. In this case, the children were not encouraged to coerce the father to participate. They were offered the opportunity to pursue testing on their own. If they were found to harbor a mutation, it would be possible for them to infer that their genetic susceptibility to colon cancer was inherited from their father. They recognized that without testing their father, a negative genetic test for each of them would not be definitive.

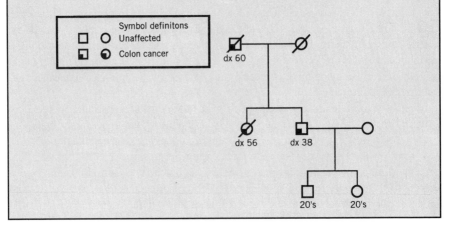

Case Example 10.3. A woman sought help in deriving her familial cancer risk. She was an adopted daughter who was concerned about her family history of multiple cancers. In speaking to her biological mother, she had learned of the extensive history of cancer. She insisted that her biological mother participate in genetic testing so that she could determine her cancer risk.

This case highlights the principle of autonomy. Attempts by the daughter to coerce the natural mother into genetic evaluation were discouraged. It was emphasized that the medical and counseling relationship between the mother and health professionals should be independent and autonomous. After these principles were communicated, the mother agreed to enter into a research protocol that allowed her to participate in genetic testing without receiving the results of the analysis.

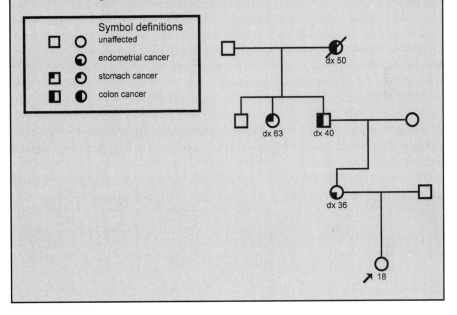

be advised to address these risks regardless of the outcome of testing. Thus, the aunt with colon cancer may desire to undergo colonoscopy and pelvic ultrasound and not be told the results of her genetic test. Even if the individual declines to know the test results, it may be possible to infer this information from the actions of other family members. The family's sensitivity to an affected relative can protect his or her desire for privacy.

A dramatic test of the autonomy principle in genetic testing occurs when an adopted child seeks the involvement of the natural (affected) parent as a participant in the process. The principle of autonomy requires a separate counseling relationship with the natural parent. This means fully informed choice, free from coercion. Genetic counseling, with its emphasis on education and empowerment is fully consistent with the concept of autonomy. However, in some cases, the principles of autonomy and beneficence collide, leading to ethical conundrums of paternalism.

Nonmaleficence

Whether or not Hippocrates actually stated it, the maxim *primum non nocere*—"above all do no harm"—has become a central dogma in medical ethics. This doctrine has been applied to guiding decisions about terminal care and withdrawing of life-sustaining treatments. As related to cancer, the concept of *nonmaleficence* also has major application to genetic testing.

Negative Results One of the most worrisome concerns about a genetic test is that it will do more harm than good. For a negative test, there is the concern that the individual, buoyed by the knowledge that he/she is not a carrier (heterozygote) for a particular genetic mutation, may still be at risk for mutations in other genes. Although false negative tests may be avoided by baseline testing of an affected family member, the negative test for the proband may still be deleterious if the individual abandons cancer screening altogether. For malignancies such as colon or breast cancer, in which the population risk remains quite high in the absence of a known predisposing mutation, continued surveillance may be essential.

As discussed earlier, negative test results may, paradoxically, be more emotionally devastating than positive results. The existence of survivor guilt was dramatically evident in the early families counseled for linkage to breast cancer susceptibility genes. Adverse psychological results of testing must always be anticipated in the process of posttest counseling.

Positive Test Results The damaging effects of positive test results appear self-evident. A widely cited research study followed a highly selected cohort of individuals that agreed to testing and went on to test positive for susceptibility to Huntington disease, a degenerative neurological disorder without effective treatment (Wiggins et al., 1992). Interestingly, the levels of psychological distress peaked post testing, but then declined to values close to those of the test-negative group. In genetic counseling for most adult-onset cancers, interventions of presumed medical benefit will be increased in frequency or intensity if the individual tests positive. However, for some conditions, such as the risk for brain or visceral tumors in Li-Fraumeni syndrome, the harm:benefit ratio may be greater, and the principle of nonmaleficence may be a central consideration.

As discussed earlier, there can be important psychological benefits even for positive results for high-penetrance cancer predisposing mutations. In the case of the affected individual, and in some unaffected individuals with striking family histories, the documentation of a positive DNA result can provide a sense of "closure" following the uncertainty that preceded it.

Even for those circumstances where a genetic test may lead to increased surveillance, hidden dangers may lurk ahead. The surveillance procedures may be risky or may identify an abnormality that may prove to be a benign process after surgery (e.g., ovarian cancer screening). The most troubling negative outcome to result from genetic testing and/or counseling is stigmatization and genetic discrimination.

Genetic Discrimination   *Genetic discrimination* is defined as social stigmatization due to one's hereditary disease risks. It can lead to purely social traumas, such as discrimination against potential spouses based entirely on their risk for disease, a practice sanctioned by certain Greek Orthodox and Jewish Orthodox sects. In other cases, genetic discrimination can create economic hardship, for example, when genetic knowledge is used by potential employers in hiring or promotion decisions, or by insurance carriers to exclude groups from coverage or to charge them higher rates. Perhaps for these reasons, England, France, and the Netherlands declared moratoria on the use of genetic information in insurance.

In the United States, where no such moratoria exist, instances of genetic discrimination have been reported for a number of disorders (e.g., Gaucher's disease, fragile X syndrome, cystic fibrosis, Huntington disease). This concern has largely been a theoretical issue for common adult cancer predisposition syndromes, with very few cases of insurance discrimination thus far documented.

As T. H. Murray has written, "Genetic risk testing is important because it exposes the logic of a system that provides access to health insurance to those least likely to need it." Although the ethical basis for exclusion of at-risk individuals from insurance pools is debatable, the practice of underwriting is the basis of a major American industry. A survey of medical directors of U.S. life insurance companies indicated that over half felt that a strong family history of breast cancer constituted sufficient justification to disallow all life insurance, or to substantially increase the rates (McEwen et al., 1993). From the perspective of "distributive justice," combined with the notion of insurance as a commodity and not a right, the option of excluding high-risk groups to guarantee the lowest possible rates seems logical. Antiselection, the bane of insurers, occurs when those at increased risk more actively seek insurance. This is precisely what some cancer genetic counselors advise consulting families before they obtain genetic testing!

Legislative Approaches   In response to the emerging concerns about genetic discrimination, in 1993 a task force on genetic information and health insurance was organized by the National Institutes of Health. The task force made sweeping recommendations regarding the need to exclude genetic information as a consideration in determining access to, or cost of insurance coverage. The recommendations, which included a moratorium on the use of genetic testing in underwriting, did not have the force of law.

At least three federal initiatives impact on the potential for discrimination by health insurers or employers based on genetic knowledge. Each of these initiatives has yet to be fully tested in a court of law. The *Americans with Disabilities Act* (ADA), a sweeping civil rights legislative initiative enacted in 1990 to protect the disabled, makes illegal discrimination against an employee, or potential employee, based solely on "an impairment which substantially limits a major life activity." In theory, the Americans with Disabilities Act [US Code 12111–12201, 1990] prevents employers from inquiring about health conditions in the course of evaluation for employment. However, unlike life insurance, 90% of which is purchased by the policy holder, most health insurance in America is provided by employers. Issues of genetic discrimination in the workplace are intertwined with those of insurance discrimination, because employers are most likely to have knowledge of individuals medical histories. It was not clear whether discrimination by an employer based on one's genetic background would fall within the ADA regulations. An enforcement guideline, promulgated on March 15, 1995, by the Equal Employment Opportunity Commission [EEOC compliance manual, vol. 2, section 902, order 915.002, 902-45] defined "disability" as including genetic predisposition.

The Kennedy-Kassebaum bill, enacted as the *Health Insurance Portability and Accountability Act*, was signed into law in August of 1996 and took effect in July of 1997. It defined genetic information as a component of the "health status" of the individual, along with obvious manifestations of disease, disability, and medical history. It was the legislation's intent that a health insurance plan could not be designed to exclude any individuals on the basis of their health status. The law was intended to prohibit employers or insurers from excluding employees in a group from coverage or charging them higher rates on the basis of health status, including genetic conditions. The intent of the legislation was to spread risk among insurance pools, while protecting individuals with specific conditions from losing the portability of their insurance when they changed jobs.

The Kennedy-Kassebaum provisions signified an attempt to include those with genetic predisposition to common diseases, including cancer, in insurance plans. However, the act allows insurance plans to exclude benefits or coverage for specific conditions, presumably including genetic predispositions, for *all* members of the group. The plan may also increase rates or provide caps on benefits for specified conditions, as long as *individuals* are not singled out. This would seem to leave the door open to potential hardships for those groups of individuals who will have to pay higher premiums in order to be included in specific plans. Thus, until the composition of the menu of benefits for group health plans is specified, the impact of the 1997 law on individuals with hereditary cancer predisposition will remain unclear. These protections, it should be remembered, apply only to health insurance, and not life insurance. Exclusions and rate discrimination for life insurance applicants are more widely accepted and fall outside the purview of health insurance regulations. The provisions of both the ADA enforcement guideline and the health insurance portability and accountability act will need to be tested in court before their impact is secured. It will be left to the individual to prove that genetic information was misused by an insurer. During this period, and in response to political initiatives in many communities, state legislatures have taken on the issue of the special nature of genetic information.

By mid-1997, 14 states had passed various types of legislation bearing on issues of genetic discrimination, with legislation pending in an additional 10 states, and upgrades of existing laws pending in other states. These state initiatives are summarized in Table 10-2. This table is not intended to describe the specific protections relevant to individual families considering genetic testing, but it should encourage cancer risk counselors to seek updates of the status of existing or pending legislation in their state. The major focus of this legislation is on protecting employees from discrimination by employers based on the results of genetic tests. This legislation was modeled after the

Table 10-2 State Legislation Bearing on Genetic Discrimination and Health Insurance

State	Year Enacted or Introduced	Provision[a]	Pending
Alabama	1982, 1997	D(ss), D	H
Arizona	1997	P, D	
California	1994	P, D, H	
Colorado	1994	P, D	
Connecticut	1997	D, H	
Florida	1978, 1992, 1997	D(ss), P, H, D	
Georgia	1995	P, D	
Hawaii	1996, 1997	D, H	
Illinois	1997	P, D	
Indiana	1997	P, D, H	
Iowa	1992, 1997	P	D
Kansas	1996		P, D, H
Maryland	1986, 1996	H[b], P, D	
Massachusetts	1996		P, D, H
Michigan	1997		D
Minnesota	1995	P, D, H	
Nebraska	1996	(c)	
Nevada	1997	D, H	
New Hampshire	1995	P, D, H	
New Jersey	1996	P, D, H	
New York	1996	P	D, H
North Carolina	1975, 1997	D(ss), H(ss), D, H	
Ohio	1993	P, D	
Oklahoma	1996	(c)	
Oregon	1995	P, D, H	
Rhode Island	1992	P	
Tennessee	1997	P, D, H	
Texas	1997	P, D, H	
Virginia	1996	P, D, H	
Wisconsin	1991	P, D, H	

Sources: Data modified from that compiled by Professor Karen Rothenberg and Barbara Fuller, Esq., University of Maryland School of Law. (Rothenberg KH. Genetic Information and Health Insurance: State Legislative Approaches, Journal of Law, Medicine, and Ethics 23: 312-9, 1995; and Rothenberg K and Fuller B, unpublished data.) For specific provisions and status of legislation, consult records of appropriate state legislatures.

Key: P = Privacy protection for genetic information, generally by prohibiting employers from requiring genetic test or by requiring written release for disclosure of genetic information.

D = Prohibits denial of health insurance based on genetic characteristics.

H = Prohibits higher rates of health insurance based on genetic characteristics.

(ss) = Protections apply to sickle cell testing only.

[a] Anti-discrimination provisions modeled on Kennedy-Kassebaum law ("*Health Insurance Portability and Accountability Act*, 1996"), but include small employers and individuals, not covered in federal legislation. In general, these provisions ban discrimination against individuals, but allow a range of policies relating to groups (see web-site http://gatekeeper.dol.gov/dol/pwba/public/pubs/q&aguide.htm#hipaa). These provisions passed in 49 of 50 states (except Missouri) in 1997.

[b] Allowed to charge high rates if there is actuarial justification.

[c] State legislature created a study commission (Nebraska) or genetic information task force (Oklahoma), but no anti-genetic discrimination passed in 1996 session.

1991 Wisconsin mandate which prohibited employer-access to test results. Similar legislation was enacted in Iowa, Rhode Island, New Hampshire, and New York (Rothenberg et al., 1997). Legislation in New Jersey went even further, including not only genetic testing, but also family history information.

The provisions of the state laws with respect to health insurance vary, but generally parallel the legislation on privacy and employer discrimination. The impact of many of these state laws is limited by the *Employee Retirement Income Security Act (ERISA)*, which preempts self-insured employers from many of the state insurance provisions. From the perspective of the individual with a genetic predisposition to cancer, one of the potential benefits of the 1997 Health Insurance Portability and Accountability Act is that its provisions apply to employers providing health insurance plans, including small employers (with 2-50 employees).

Because of the limitations in this law, however, more definitive federal legislation bearing on genetic discrimination and privacy of information was developed in 1997. A number of bills were introduced in the 1997 legislative session. One bill, the *Genetic Information Nondiscrimination in Health Insurance Act* introduced by Representative Louise M. Slaughter and Senator Olympia Snowe, garnered bipartisan support. It called for a ban on the use of "genetic information" in denying or setting rates for group health insurance. "Genetic information" was defined broadly to include genetic tests as well as "information about inherited characteristics." The bill also called for limits on the collection or disclosure of genetic information without the written consent of the individual. In the summer of 1997, President Clinton endorsed the Slaughter-Snowe bill with some modifications. The passage of such a bill, during the 1997-1998 legislative session will be of enormous value in consolidating other provisions in this area, especially as they relate to self-insured employers, those in individual plans, and those on Medicare supplement policies. The Slaughter-Snowe bill, like the Kennedy-Kassebaum bill that preceded it, called for a year before implementation would go into effect. During the period before its passage, and until its eventual implementation, consumers would need to rely on those protections already in place in some states, and in some research studies.

Impact on counseling   It is evident that, in seeking to counsel the concerned family member, the cancer geneticist must be informed about the scope of numerous state and federal statutes that have been formulated in this area. This information, plus the specific exemptions and provisions of individual group insurance or managed care plans, must be factored into the cost benefit equation for genetic testing. As a potential risk discussed in the context of informed consent, the issue of genetic discrimination has an enormous weight, which can overshadow the medical content of these discussions. In many cases, the medical record may already have documented the family history of cancer. However, the more concrete nature of genetic tests poses a greater perceived danger, and this remains one of the compelling reasons cited to veil this information behind the protective cloak of "research." Indeed, it is possible to protect genetic information gathered during the course of research from the reach of legal discovery. As discussed in the section on confidentiality of genetic information, *Certificates of Con-*

fidentiality can be sought to protect research-associated data. However, when the results of genetic tests are shared with individuals, these individuals may be asked by insurers if they are aware of any conditions that might increase their health risks.

As a practical matter, the potential risk of genetic discrimination based on cancer predisposition has largely remained a theoretical concern. It is true that precedent for discrimination was documented for individuals with or at risk for AIDS, Huntington disease, cystic fibrosis, and a number of other medical conditions. However, each of these conditions had no known or presumed means of definitive medical intervention, which is not the case for the common adult cancers, where early detection can lead to curative intervention. It seems reasonable to anticipate that managed care and health maintenance organizations will take a more progressive stance toward predisposition testing for colon, breast, or prostate cancers. Some networks have been willing to pay for such procedures as prophylactic surgery, and some (e.g., Kaiser-Permanente) are already including some cancer genetic tests as a component in their coverage. Despite these developments, for most individuals the risks due to potential abuse of genetic information must remain a prominent component of the informed consent discussion preceding genetic testing.

Beneficence

Medical interventions based on genetic testing and counseling should not only respect individual autonomy and cause no harm, but they should also be helpful. One of the fundamental benefits of genetic counseling is the psychological benefit of the negative test. As has been discussed, for many fatal genetic disorders with no known treatment, this potential benefit must be weighed against the potentially devastating effect of the positive test. For most common cancer predisposition syndromes, however, even the positive test can be considered "beneficent" if it leads to more effective medical management. Starting in 1995, a task force under the auspices of the Ethical, Legal, and Social Implications (ELSI) Branch of the National Center for Human Genomic Research (NCHGR) undertook to survey the published data relating to management of individuals at hereditary risk for cancer. For many on the task force, the exercise was a sobering experience because it became clear that virtually all of the medical recommendations for high-risk families were based on presumed rather than proven benefit. In many cases, recommendations were simply the personal opinions of scholars or clinicians. The ELSI documents, published in 1997, nonetheless serve as a critical resource in the ethical counseling of families because they indicate the possible limitations as well as presumed benefits of such interventions as mammography, breast self-examination, ovarian screening, colonoscopy, and prophylactic surgery (Burke et al., 1997).

As discussed earlier, the psychological and supportive aspects of genetic counseling, with or without testing, can have important beneficial effects. When an individual's anxiety regarding a cancer risk is very great, that individual may be less able to perform such basic preventive medical practices as monthly breast self-examination. An important benefit of counseling and education, being documented in a number of formal research studies, is their effect in reducing anxiety and increasing acceptance of screening and prevention behaviors.

Paternalism: The Collision of Beneficence and Autonomy In a recent malpractice suit in Florida, *Pate v Threlkel* [661 So.2d 278 (Fla. 1995)], the plaintiff's mother had received treatment for medullary thyroid cancer. Three years later, the daughter learned that she had the condition. The daughter, the plaintiff, sued, claiming that the physician was under a duty to warn the mother that it was necessary to test her daughter for the disease. If the daughter had been tested, preventive measures could have been taken, leading to a better chance for cure. The intermediate appellate court rejected this argument, based on the general rule of privity, but this decision was overturned by the State Supreme Court. The court felt that "prevailing standards of care" created a "duty" to warn the mother of the potential risk to other family members. Expanding on the *Pate* opinion, the New Jersey Superior Court did not agree that "in all circumstances the duty to warn will be satisfied by informing the patient." In this decision, *Safer* v. *Pack* [677 A. 2d 1188 (N.J. 1996)] a plaintiff diagnosed with colon cancer sued the estate of the physician who had treated her father for colon cancer more than forty years earlier. The father had expressed the wish, honored by his physician, that the details of his condition not be shared with his family. The plaintiff claimed that the physician had an overriding duty to inform her of her familial cancer risk.

These decisions, if they establish a precedent in other states, will create special challenges in the counseling and testing of families with hereditary cancer predisposition. They also illustrate the murky area where the principles of autonomy (patient confidentiality) and beneficence (duty to warn relatives) conflict. What of the circumstance when the relative at hereditary risk is present in the waiting room of the health provider's office? Is there a duty to warn? In many of these scenarios neither legal case law nor ethical codes provides definitive guidance. In the example cited, the OPRR guidelines offer some advice, suggesting that "to the extent possible, persons undergoing genetic screening should be asked to consent in advance to the disclosure of genetic information to relatives in the event that such useful information is discovered" [OPRR 5-53]. But what if the individual tested wants the results kept private? What are the potentially at-risk relatives's legitimate claims? The OPRR is silent, stating "whether a legal duty exists to warn relatives of possible genetic defects has not yet been established." Some legal scholars argue that the controlling case in such a claim would be *Tarasoff v Reagents of California*. In this case, a psychiatrist was held to have a duty to have warned the patient's girlfriend that he had threatened to harm her. A number of pending cases will test the applicability of this principle to cancer genetic testing and may redefine the nature of informed consent guarantees of confidentiality that health-care professionals may provide.

As the knowledge of the health risks associated with specific mutations becomes more precise and the proof of efficacy of interventions becomes available, issues of paternalism will be even more frequent. What is a clinician to do when she holds in her hands both the warning of the future risks for an individual and the power to intervene dramatically and effectively? John Stuart Mill gave the example of a person ignorant of the risk starting to cross a dangerous bridge. But what if the individual wants to push ahead, aware of the consequences? Some biomedical ethicists are quite tolerant of what they term "strong paternalism" in selected medical situations. In these instances, one must intervene despite a person's autonomous wishes, choices, and actions in order to protect the individual. Such a view is represented by the conclusions expressed by a recent NIH Task Force on Genetic Testing when it stated that it is appropriate to override autonomy concerns and inform other at-risk family members "when the person tested refuses to communicate information despite reasonable attempts to persuade him or her to do so, and when failure to give that information has a high probability of resulting in . . . harm" (Task Force on Genetic Testing, 1997).

Paternalistic actions may be justified in some circumstances. Surely, the bedrail must be forced up, even if the young postoperative patient doesn't want it to obscure the view out the window. But what of the individual who doesn't want to know the results of a genetic test associated with greater than 90% risk for colon cancer? There are a number of ethical theories to invoke in these situations. They range from Rawls and Dworkin's theories of "justified paternalism," to consent-based theories in which paternalism is viewed as a sort of "social insurance policy" that must always be balanced against autonomy interests. In each of these circumstances it becomes necessary to carefully consider the context of the decision, the probability of an adverse outcome, and the efficacy of the interventions available.

In some circumstances in which autonomy and beneficence come into conflict, there may emerge different orders of legal and ethical responsibility. For example, is it acceptable to conduct a research study on the frequency of a specific mutation, without the informed consent of the participants, utilizing anonymous samples stripped of all personal identifiers? What if the results indicate that a certain percentage of the participants have a genetic mutation with a highly lethal—and preventable—outcome. Such studies on selected racial or ethnic groups have been subject to peer review and published in distinguished journals. Legal opinions, as exemplified by the provisions of New York State's 1996 Civil Rights Law 79-1 relating to genetic testing, specifically exempt "anonymous" genetic testing from the requirements of informed consent. However, an ethicist might argue the participants in such studies should be recontacted and offered the autonomous choice to repeat the test, this time with full knowledge, consent, and counseling. But who will bear the cost of these added services? What about research studies where personal identifiers are removed retrospectively to protect confidentiality and at the same time make future contact impossible? The ethical obligations of investigators to the at-risk but unknowing participants must be weighed against the vital public health significance of these studies.

Numerous policy statements have been issued by professional organizations and researchers who have studied the ethical obligations to obtain consent for research genetic testing of specimens from which personal identifiers have been removed. It is useful to distinguish between truly *anonymous* samples (obtained without identifiers), those which have been *anonymized* (by removing identifiers), samples which are *identifiable* (e.g., coded), and those which are clearly *identified*. Different requirements for informed consent apply to each of these categories (American Society of Human Genetics Report, 1996), and no uniform recommendations have been agreed upon (Clayton et al., 1995). In these circumstances, as in the other ethical conundrums that will emerge in the course of cancer predisposition testing, the clinician is well advised to develop research protocols in concert with ethics committees and local IRBs.

The Professional Obligations of Privacy, Confidentiality, Veracity and Fidelity

Genetic testing by its very nature raises fundamental questions about privacy. Privacy, as has been noted by ethicists, is a relatively recent area of legal scholarship. A series of decisions by the U.S. Supreme Court starting in the 1920s carved out a notion of privacy as arising from the "penumbra" of the first, third, fourth, fifth, ninth, and fourteenth amendments to the Constitution. While not explicitly spelled out in these amendments, an implied notion of privacy was invoked to protect individual choice on birth control and reproductive matters, raising of children, and other areas of family life. Privacy became almost a negative right, i.e., an ability to shield personal information or information of a personal act, or, as Justices Warren and Brandeis put it, "the right to be left alone." Shifting legal decisions regarding the "right to privacy" have sought to apply this doctrine to such personal matters as abortion or termination of life-sustaining equipment. In the setting of these controversies, a major theme in medical ethics has been to define levels of privacy for different components of medical information. Genetic information can be viewed as the most basic aspect of personal information, because a small amount of DNA may serve to fingerprint the individual as well as provide a glimpse into both the medical past and future of the individual's family.

As established earlier, some aspects of access to genetic information can also be linked to the concept of autonomy, because proper information is necessary to act responsibly. Such is the case when the patient requests that information regarding a genetic test not be shared with other family members. Privacy refers to those special situations when the individual seeks to act to limit personal information, when such an action has no effect on the autonomy of other family members or members of society. For example, disclosure of genetic information to an unauthorized party would be considered a serious violation of profession notions of privacy and confidentiality.

Two common scenarios in which privacy and confidentiality considerations can be raised as they relate to cancer predisposition testing are population screening and record keeping. Population screening for common genetic disorders has had a stormy past. In 1970 it was reported that individuals with sickle cell trait, which comprised 7–13% of African-Americans, were at risk for sudden death during exercise. Within 2 years many states enacted mandatory screening laws. Other research reports did not replicate the original findings about risk of sudden death. Unfortunately, the screening programs led to both employment and insurance discrimination against those with sickle cell trait, as well as psychological distress and stigmatization. In considering the conditions that justified widespread screening for a genetic trait, the Institute of Medicine cited certain prerequisites, including the high relative frequency of the disease, the validity of the test, and the ability to mount effective interventions (Institute of Medicine, 1994). The technology for rapid screening of mutations of large genes is not yet available, and the infrastructure to allow access to genetic counseling does not exist. Even if these barriers were to be surmounted, significant economic obstacles remain. The costs for genetic testing will be significant, and such costs may not be reimbursed by some third-party carriers.

Even if costs were routinely covered, at what point would genetic screening be performed. At birth? At marriage? A classic study of screening for cystic fibrosis among high school students in Canada demonstrated that the students actually changed their dating patterns based on knowledge of the gene status of their partner. If such behavioral changes were noted for a recessive condition, how would the prospective spouse view a marriage to a partner in which the offspring had a 50% chance of inheriting a gene that conferred an increased risk of early-onset breast cancer?

The issue of confidentiality of patient records is a pressing concern in cancer genetic testing. In the growing number of circumstances where cancer genetic testing is undertaken with full informed consent but outside of established research protocols, privacy considerations must be perceived as identical to—and no more secure than—any other medically sensitive information. As Earley and Strong (1995) point out, one of the major advantages of providing genetic testing in the context of a research study is the availability of *certificates of confidentiality.* Originally applied to drug-abuse studies, federal protection is available for genetic information which "if released could reasonably be damaging to an individual's . . . employability . . . or which could lead to social stigmatization or discrimination" (Earley and Strong, 1995). The certificate, issued by the Department of Health and Human Services, protects the researcher from being compelled to reveal the identity of a research subject "in any Federal, State, or local civil, criminal, administrative, legislative, or other proceedings." [Note: Investigators interested in applying for a certificate of confidentiality should write or phone the Office of Health Planning and Evaluation, Public Health Service, 737F Humphrey Building, Department of Health and Human Services, Washington, D.C. 20201; phone (202) 690 7100.]

When information derived from a "research" genetic test is utilized to inform a clinical decision, then the protection afforded by the certificate of confidentiality may seem moot. As previously discussed, once the individual is aware of a genetic susceptibility, then this information can be expected to be included in the voluntary disclosure process required by insurers. Verbal communication of this information by the individual to another physician may result in a notation in the medical record.

Thus, if communication of genetic results to the patient and informing of medical decisions based on these results are anticipated benefits of participation in genetic research, certificates of confidentiality may be of limited benefit. The ability of certificates of confidentiality to protect genetic information from subpoena has not been tested in court. Thus, even in the context of research protocols, investigators should include language in the informed consent that explains the procedures that will be taken to guarantee confidentiality, but which do not guarantee a level of confidentiality beyond that afforded other medical information.

The issue of record keeping of genetic test results has brought into conflict two professional obligations: privacy and veracity. Clinicians are left to choose between two bad alternatives: recording genetic data in patient charts (posing insurance risks to patients), or keeping genetic data in separate records (compromising availability of information to be used in making medical decisions). In research centers, the latter option is most often taken, with certificates of confidentiality requested to protect the research charts. In clinical practice, the precedent of "secret psychiatric records" has been invoked to justify the keeping of separate charts, at the same time that critical information is utilized to inform medical decisions (e.g., prophylactic surgery). As has been discussed, in the absence of specific legal protections these "psychiatric charts" are fully discoverable by insurers or other authorized parties. Keeping separate charts for genetic data outside of IRB-approved research studies runs the risk that insurance carriers or other parties may construe this practice as deceptive.

Veracity

The concern with truth telling, as Beauchamp and Childress (1994) point out, is also a relatively recent one in biomedical ethics. It is ignored in the Hippocratic oath, in the Declaration of Geneva, and was not addressed by the AMA Principles of Medical Ethics until the 1980 version. In most medical practice, obligations of disclosure and truth telling are most difficult in the case of a diagnosis of a fatal disease or other potentially damaging medical information in the setting of an elderly or compromised patient. In cancer genetics, in virtually every case, the rules of disclosure should be anticipated in the pretest counseling.

A special, and potentially devastating disclosure unique to genetic testing is the issue of relatedness (i.e., paternity and maternity). Nonpaternity has been a potential concern to medical geneticists since the advent of prenatal testing. Remarkably, greater than 90% of geneticists indicated in a survey that they would not disclose nonpaternity to the father, with about 80% electing first to tell the mother and letting her decide how to handle it. Since cancer predisposition testing is generally performed on families with adult members, the issue of nonrelatedness among family members comes even more unexpectedly, and with even greater emotional and legal consequences. The best solution to these particular dilemmas of veracity is to anticipate the problem at the pretest stage, and to establish if this information is to be disclosed, or is deemed irrelevant to the medical concerns at hand.

The Unifying Concept of Fidelity: Informed Consent

In the absence of the contractual obligations of the marketplace, the concept of fidelity has been invoked to capture the spirit of the trust, commitment, and faithfulness that exists in the doctor-patient relationship. Fidelity is the reason a doctor cannot simply walk away from a family or patient; this is abandonment and a breach of trust. Fidelity concerns can become split into divided loyalties when a physician is given an economic incentive by a capitated health plan to defer certain medical interventions. In the area of biomedical research, divided loyalties can lead to a confusion between the interests of the patient and the interests of the researcher, particularly in the case of randomized placebo-controlled trials. Because of the need to make explicit the agreement between subject and researcher, and in keeping with the principles of autonomous choice, the concept of informed consent was developed. The basic requirements of informed consent are: (1) competence to understand the informed consent discussion; (2) disclosure of procedures, risks, and benefits of the research; (3) understanding of what has been discussed; (4) voluntariness of the decision; and (5) consent by the individual or the appropriate surrogate.

Careful attention to each of these issues is required for biomedical research. In its 1994 report on genetic screening, the Institute of Medicine recommended informed consent as a prerequisite for genetic testing. Informed consent is not a new concept to medical practice. It is required before all surgical or invasive procedures. The concept of informed consent for a diagnostic blood test reached its first widespread application with HIV testing. Similar requirements for informed consent confront the practicing physicians seeking to offer a genetic test. In its elemental form (Table 10-3), pretest genetic counseling is synonymous with informed consent. Informed consent is not simply the signing of a document that absolves the clinician from certain liabilities associated with genetic testing. Instead, informed consent is a process of education and

TABLE 10-3   Basic Elements of Informed Consent for Germline DNA Testing

Autonomy Provisions

1. Information on the specific test being performed
2. Implications of a positive and negative result
3. Possibility that the test will be inconclusive or not informative
4. Options for risk estimation without genetic testing (e.g., population-derived risks)
5. Risk of passing mutation to children
6. Options to withdraw from study

Beneficence Provisions

7. Options and limitations of medical surveillance and screening following testing

Nonmaleficence Provisions

8. Technical accuracy of the test
9. Risks of psychological distress
10. Risks of insurance or employer discrimination

Paternalism Provisions

11. Procedures if relatedness is not as expected
12. Procedures governing notification of family

Privacy-Professional Responsibilities

13. Confidentiality issues
14. Fees involved in testing, counseling, and follow-up care

Special Considerations

15. Banked tissue specimens
16. Ownership of material
17. Anonymous testing provisions for other studies

understanding about the risks and benefits of a procedure. In a research context, informed consent also represents a mutual commitment of subject and investigator to a research endeavor. When cancer genetic testing is offered as part of a research protocol, it requires an incremental level of explanation to the participant (Reilly et al., 1997). Even for genetic testing in clinical practice, the basic elements of informed consent are required.

In its discussion of the special nature of genetic research, the OPRR emphasizes that social and psychological harm, rather than physical injury, are the primary risks to be anticipated. In clinical practice as well as research, care must be taken to avoid coercion or undue influence, for example, by other relatives or the family physician. The disclosure portion of the informed consent process should be as specific as possible. Table 10-3 lists the basic elements of the informed consent for genetic cancer predisposition testing, grouped according to the aspect of ethical theory that they address. These elements are also elaborated below.

The Elements of Informed Consent for Genetic Testing   Discussion of the elements of informed consent should be performed at the time a sample is taken for study, not when a result is available. It should include discussion of:

1. Information on what the test is intended to do, i.e., determine whether a mutation can be detected in a specific cancer susceptibility gene.
2. What can be learned from both a positive and negative test, including the most recent information on the type and magnitude of health risks associated with a positive test, as well as the risks that may remain even after a negative test.
3. The possibility that no additional risk information will be obtained at the completion of the test, or that the test will result in a finding of unknown significance (e.g., a polymorphism) that may require further studies.
4. The options for approximation of risk without genetic testing, e.g., using empiric risk tables for breast cancer given differing family histories.
5. The risk of passing a mutation on to children.
6. The options to withdraw from the study, with mention that samples will be destroyed, identifiers removed, etc.
7. The medical options and limited proof of efficacy for surveillance and cancer prevention for individuals with a positive test, as well as the accepted recommendations for cancer screening even if genetic testing is negative. This discussion is important to avoid false security and inadequate surveillance for those whose genetic test may be negative, but who are still at risk based on different genetic factors, age, environment, or other causes.
8. The technical accuracy of the test.
9. The risks of psychological distress and family disruption, whether a mutation is found or not found.
10. The risk of employment and/or insurance discrimination following disclosure of genetic test results.

11. The risks that nonrelatedness will be discovered, and how this information will be disclosed (or not disclosed).

12. The procedure to be followed regarding notification of results to other family members, including the eventualities in the event of the death or incapacitation of the proband.

13. The level of confidentiality of results compared to other medical tests and procedures.

14. The fees involved for both the laboratory test and the associated consultation by the health professional providing pretest education, results disclosure, and follow-up, and the costs of preventive procedures, which may not be covered by third-party payers.

The informed consent discussion should emphasize that the process of disclosure makes the individual considering testing more fully aware of what is known and what is not known about cancer risk determination and possible means of reducing cancer-associated mortality. Implicit in all discussions of the options for genetic testing is the right of the individual not to be tested.

Justice

Biomedical ethicists formally define "justice" as the notion that equals should be treated equally. Ethicists differ, however, on what the term "equal" refers to. The material principles of how justice is to be distributed can vary according to individual need, merit, free-market resources, and other determinants. Although justice may seem a theoretical consideration, with little evident clinical relevance at present, important concerns exist about the long-term social and ethical implications of genetic screening and testing.

In the current health-care debate, the need-based entitlement theories of the egalitarians have given way to the market-driven theories of the libertarians. Indeed, the molecular biotechnology sector is an important part of the national marketplace. In some measure this is a result of the enormous venture capital that has poured into "gene discovery" and the current need to reward investors with lucrative cancer diagnostic and therapeutic discoveries. The underpinnings for these developments resulted from basic ethical and legal decisions regarding the patenting of human genes.

Ethics of Patenting Genes In 1980, the U.S. Supreme Court ruled 5–4 that a genetically engineered organism that aided in the clean-up of oil spills was a new invention. That case served as the precedent for the patent office's granting of patents to products involving human genes. Such patents provide companies exclusive rights to gene products for 17 years. Since that ruling, the patent office has granted over 12,000 patents for genetically engineered substances. In addition to genetically modified organisms, purified cDNAs have been patented as tools to manufacture protein products. These types of patents are different from recent applications to patent oligonucleotides or cDNAs to be used as tools to detect disease-causing mutations or the actual sequences of the genes themselves. To patent a gene sequence, its function also needs to be known.

Each of these attempts to gain patent protection for genetic research has met with specific objections from religious and lay consumer groups. In May of 1995, 187 religious leaders representing all of the major religious movements in the United States condemned the practice of patenting human genes. In the spring of 1996, a number of prominent feminists circulated a petition condemning the possibility that a genetic testing company might have an exclusive license for testing after the patenting of *BRCA1*. Such an initiative could result in decreased public access to testing and limitation of availability of alternative testing technologies. In response, it has been noted that the millions of dollars of investor capital raised by companies led to the "robotizing" of automated sequencing that allows wider access to this information. The prospect of patenting genes has clearly resulted in a stimulus for basic research. To name but one example, in 1995, a biotechnology company paid a New York academic research institution $20 million for exclusive license to develop products from a gene associated with obesity.

The human genome project, conducted by the National Institutes of Health and the Department of Energy has a budget of approximately $180 million a year. Its goal is to sequence the human genome by the year 2005, at a cost $3 billion for the 50,000–80,000 human genes. It is already ahead of schedule and under budget, and may be finished by 2002. It has been aided by both private charities and for-profit corporations. The rush to identify functions for these genes, necessary to apply for patent rights, is an area of intense competition.

The Ethics of Eugenic Applications of Genetic Technologies At the same time that capital markets for biotechnology are expanding, corporate markets providing managed care are taking control of the health-care delivery system. Whether one recognizes or rejects the notion of a moral right to health care, one is faced with the practical implications of a limited health-care budget and the need to allocate resources. Few argue that expensive medical procedures should be denied those who can afford them. These privileges of the affluent become more troublesome when they extend to eugenics or "selective breeding."

There exist in the U.S. health-care system today powerful forces affecting the practice of clinical cancer genetics that may create a wealth-driven eugenic effect. Contributing factors are: (1) the poor, less able to pay out-of-pocket for "confidential" genetic testing, are more vulnerable to genetic discrimination; (2) the poor have less access to such eugenic technologies as preimplantation genetics, which are not covered by most third-party payers; and (3) many procedures considered following genetic testing (e.g., colonoscopy, prophylactic surgery) are not covered by third-party payers, and must be reimbursed out-of-pocket.

It is useful to remember the strong roots of the eugenic movement in America because they may predict the relative acceptance of eugenic concepts in medical practice today. Coined by Francis Galton in his 1859 book *Hereditary Genius*, eugenics was introduced as the practice of arranged marriages to make a "gifted race." The American Eugenics Society in 1926 called for the sterilization of insane, epileptic, and retarded.

Laws were passed in more than half of the states, with over 100,000 individuals involuntarily sterilized from 1907–1960. Sterilization of this group of individuals was viewed as a public health issue. In a landmark Supreme Court ruling, *Buck vs. Bell*, Justice Holmes wrote that "the principle that is sufficient to justify compulsory vaccination is sufficient to justify cutting the fallopian tube." In the 1960s the Nobel Laureate William Shockley called for voluntary sterilization of all those with an IQ of less than 100. In 1974, a class action suit, *Relf vs Weinberger*, noted that the "dividing line between family planning and eugenics is murky" and state sterilization laws were ended (Mehler, 1994).

Case Example 10.4. A religious leader called the cancer geneticist to seek guidance on whether he should give approval for a proposed courtship. He had the permission of both parties to make these investigations. The religious leader was aware that the young lady's mother and aunt died of breast cancer, and that the young man's mother and sister died of breast cancer. He stated that if marriages between carriers of recessive traits, which have a 25% chance of producing an "affected" child, were not desired, then unions between those with dominant traits should also not be sanctioned. He worried about the possible 75% chance for an affected child given a marriage between heterozygotes for a dominant cancer predisposing mutation. He was also aware of the high frequency of certain *BRCA1* and *BRCA2* mutations in certain ethnic groups. He explained that he usually did not approve testing for dominant traits, since this created stigmas. However he felt compelled in this circumstance because of the higher-than-usual range of potential risks involved. For this reason, he felt that both individuals should have genetic testing, so that he could decide, as he had been entrusted to do, if the individuals were suitable to enter into a relationship that might lead to marriage.

This case illustrates a specific ethical challenge posed by the practices of some members of some religious groups. Questions about basing reproductive decisions on carrier status for adult-onset traits for which effective therapies exist are controversial. Professionals providing cancer genetic testing will need to anticipate the degree to which they should provide genetic information for the purposes of fashioning "passive eugenic" strategies, whether by individuals, religious groups, or social institutions.

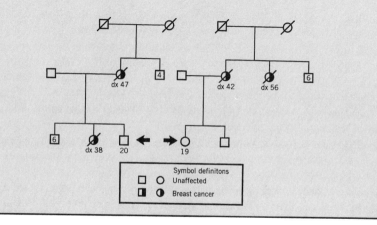

The "genetics revolution" of the 1980s and 1990s led to the identification of genes for muscular dystrophy, cystic fibrosis, Marfan syndrome, fragile X syndrome, and myotonic dystrophy. Over the period of two decades, prenatal selection based on genetic tests has become an accepted component of medical practice. As the technology became available, a natural extension of these efforts has been the attempt to genetically manipulate embryos so they would not bear altered copies of "deleterious" genes, or to select embryos with "normal" genes. While the possibility of cloning an identical copy of a human resulted in an immediate Presidential condemnation in 1997, the availability of options for the genetic selection of embryos resulted in little public attention. As discussed in Chapter 8, preimplantation genetics is currently available for couples at risk for having children with cystic fibrosis and other genetic disorders.

Although the medical and humanitarian justification for these procedures seems evident, certain long-term consequences of germline genetic selection are ominous. Because of the high prevalence of cancer susceptibility genes, clinical cancer geneticists are likely to become involved in this dialogue. The results of the public debate about genetic selection will extend beyond medicine. To some, the fate of our egalitarian society hangs in the balance. The historian Charles Van Doren wrote that the greatest threat to our democracy "comes not from the totalitarianism of the left or the right, but from democracy's oldest foe, which is oligarchy, the rule of the few, who claim to be the best, over the many. Democracy could be eroded by the cunning merchants of genetic superiority." The responsible and humanitarian translation of the genetic revolution in medical practice remains a critical need for patients, their families, and society.

REFERENCES

Alagna SW, Morokoff PJ, Bevett JM et al. 1987. Performance of breast self-examination by women at high risk for breast cancer. Women Health 12:29–46.

American Society of Human Genetics. 1996. Statement on informed consent for genetic research. Am J Hum Genet 59:471–4.

Beauchamp TL, Childress JF. 1994. Principles of Biomedical Ethics. Oxford University Press. New York.

Botkin JR, Croyle RT, Smith KR et al. 1996. A model protocol for evaluating the behavioral and psychosocial effects of *BRCA1* testing. J Natl Cancer Inst 88:872–81.

Burke W, Peterson G, Lynch P et al. 1997. Recommendations for follow-up care of individuals with an inherited susceptibility to cancer. 1:HNPCC. JAMA 277: 915–9.

Burke W, Daly M, Garber J, et al. 1997. Recommendations for follow-up care of individuals with an inherited predisposition to cancer. 2:*BRCA1* and *BRCA2*. JAMA 277: 997–1003.

Ciba Foundation Symposium 149, various authors. 1990. Human genetic information: science, law and ethics. New York: John Wiley & Sons.

Clayton EW, Steinberg KK, Khoury MJ, Thomson E, Andrews L, Kahn MJE, Kopelman LM, Weiss JO. 1995. Informed consent for genetic research on stored tissue samples. JAMA 274:1786–92.

Commentary. 1994. Statement on use of DNA testing for presymptomatic identification of cancer risk. National Advisory Council for Human Genome Research JAMA 271:785.

Craufurd D, Dodge A, Kerzin–Storrar L, Harris R. 1989. Uptake of presymptomatic predictive testing for Huntington's disease. Lancet 2:603–605.

Croyle RT, Lerman C. 1993. Interest in genetic testing for colon cancer susceptibility: cognitive and emotional correlates. Prev Med 22:284–92.

Croyle RT, Smith K, Botkin JR, Baty B, Nash J. 1997. Psychological responses to *BRCA1* mutation testing. Health Psychol, in press.

Earley CL, Strong LC. 1995. Certificates of confidentiality: A valuable tool for protecting genetic data. Am J Hum Genet 57:727–31.

Gullick WJ, Handyside AH. 1994. Pre-implantation diagnosis of inherited predisposition to cancer. Eur J Cancer 30A:2030–2.

Horowitz MJ. 1976. Stress Response Syndromes. New York: Jason Aronson.

Hudson KL, Rothenberg KH, Andrews LB, Kahn MJE, Collins FS. 1995. Genetic discrimination and health insurance: an urgent need for reform. Science 270:391–3.

Institute of Medicine. 1994. Assessing genetic risks. National Academy Press, Washington, D.C.

Kash KM, Holland JC, Halper MS et al. 1992. Psychological distress and surveillance behaviors of women with a family history of breast cancer. J Natl Cancer Inst 84:24–30.

Kessler S (ed). 1979. Genetic Counseling: Psychological Dimensions. New York: Academic Press.

Kessler S. 1989. Psychological aspects of genetic counseling: VI. A critical review of the literature dealing with education and reproduction. Amer J Hum Genet 34:340–53.

Kubler-Ross E. 1969. On Death and Dying. New York: Macmillan and Company.

Lerman C, Rimer B. Trock B et al. 1990. Factors associated with repeat adherence to breast cancer screening. Prev Med 19:279–90.

Lerman C, Lustbader E, Rimer B, Daly M, Miller S, Sands C, Balshem A. 1995. Effects of individualized breast cancer risk counseling: a randomized trial. J Natl Cancer Inst 87: 286–92.

Lerman C, Narod S, Schulman K et al. 1996. *BRCA1* testing in families with hereditary breast-ovarian cancer: a prospective study of patient decision-making and outcomes. JAMA 275: 1885–92.

Lerman C, Biesecker B, Benkendorf JL, Kerner J, Gomez-Caminero A, Hughes C, Reed MM. 1997. Controlled trial of pretest education approaches to enhance informed decision-making for *BRCA1* gene testing. J Natl Cancer Inst 89:148–56.

Lynch, Watson P, Conway TA et al. 1993. DNA screening for breast/ovarian cancer susceptibility based on linked markers, a family study. Arch Intern Med 153:1979–87.

Lynch HT, Lemon SJ, Durham C et al. 1997. A descriptive study of *BRCA1* testing and reactions to disclosure of test results. Cancer 79:2219–28.

Masood E. 1996. Gene tests: who benefits from risk? Nature 379:389–92.

McEwen JE, McCarthy K, Reilly P. 1993. A survey of medical directors of life insurance companies concerning use of genetic information. Am J Hum Genet 53:33–45.

Mehler B. 1994. In genes we trust. Reform Judaism 23:10–14.

NIH Office of Protection from Research Risks. 1993. In Human Genetic Research. Protecting Human Research Subjects: Institutional Review Board Guidebook. Washington D.C.: U.S. Government Printing Office, Chapter 5H.

Pearn JH. 1973. Patients' subjective interpretation of risks offered in genetic counseling. J Med Genet 10:129–34.

Physician's Duty to Third Parties Examined. 1996. Hospital Law Newsletter. 13:6–8.

Prochaska JO. 1994. Stages of change and decisional balance for 12 problem behaviors. Health Psych 13:39–46.

Reilly PR, Boshar MF, Holtzman SH. 1997. Ethical issues in genetic research: disclosure and informed consent. Nature Genet 15:16–20.

Rogers CR. 1951. Client-Centered Therapy. Boston: Houghton-Mifflin.

Rothenberg K, Fuller B, Rothstein M et al. 1997. Genetic information and the workplace: legislative approaches and policy changes. Science 275:1755–7.

Sorenson JR. 1974. Genetic counseling: some psychological considerations. In Lipkin M Jr and Rowley PT (eds), Genetic Responsibility. New York: Plenum Press.

Struewing JP, Lerman C, Kase RG, Giambarresi TR, Tucker MA. 1995. Anticipated uptake and impact of genetic testing in hereditary breast and ovarian cancer families. Cancer Biomarkers Preven 4:169–73.

Task Force on Genetic Testing of the National Institutes of Health. 1997. Proposed Recommendations of the Task Force on Genetic Testing: Notice of Meeting and Request for Comment. Federal Register 62(20):4539–47.

Van Doren C. 1992. A History of Knowledge. New York: Ballantine Books. p. 402.

Wiggins PA, Whyte P, Huggins M et al. 1992. The psychological consequences of predictive testing for Huntington disease. New Eng J Med 327:1401–05.

Glossary

absolute risk   probability of an event over a period of time; often expressed as a cumulative incidence.

adenine   a purine base found in RNA and DNA.

alleles   different forms of the same gene found at a given locus (e.g., normal and mutant allele or two alleles, one from each parent).

allele-specific oligonucleotide   short single-stranded DNA segment that will bind (hybridize) to a normal or a mutant sequence.

amino acid   coded for by DNA triplets (codons), amino acids are the building blocks for proteins.

amplification   multiple copies of a sequence of DNA.

aneuploid   an increased number of chromosomes commonly seen in cancer cells (increase is not a multiple of the haploid number).

anticipation   the pattern of earlier age of onset, or increase in severity of the phenotype, with succeeding generations in an affected family.

apoptosis   programmed cell death.

ascertainment   collection of families with a common genetic feature.

association   the nonrandom correlation of a particular genetic marker (allele) with a phenotypic feature.

autoradiography   detection of radioactively labeled DNA fragments on radiographic film.

autosome   one of the 22 pairs of human chromosomes other than the two sex chromosomes.

base   nitrogenous base in a molecule of DNA; these include adenine, thymine, guanine, and cytosine.

base pair (bp) a pair of complementary DNA bases (e.g., adenine and thymine).

Bayes' theorem used in risk counseling where additional information is available to modify risks calculated by Mendelian probabilities; Bayesian techniques combine prior and conditional probabilities to give joint and posterior probabilities of unknown events.

case control study an epidemiologic analysis of the frequency of a risk factor (e.g., family history) in a group with the disease compared to a group free of disease.

CAT box a promotor sequence upstream of the exons of a gene.

cDNA single-stranded DNA complementary to RNA and synthesized by reverse transcription.

Centimorgan (cM) Unit of recombination used to map genetic distances; two loci are one cM apart if recombination occurs between them in 1% of meioses. One centimorgan is generally equivalent to about one megabase.

centromere the unit between the two arms of a chromosome.

chromatid during cell division, each chromosome divides into two chromatids.

chromosome bodies within the nucleus composed of protein and DNA that carry genetic information.

clone a cell or population of cells derived from a single ancestral cell.

cloning replication of a segment of DNA by propagation in a vector.

codon a triplet of nucleotides coding for an amino acid or signaling termination of a chain of amino acids (stop codon).

cohort study an epidemiologic analysis of the incidence of a disease in a group with a risk factor (e.g., family history), compared to the incidence in a group without the risk factor.

compound heterozygote an individual with two different mutant alleles at the same locus.

confounding variable is itself a risk factor for the disease as well as being associated with the risk factors under study; failure to identify potential confounders may lead to erroneous estimates of risk.

congenital an abnormality present at birth; may be genetic or induced.

consanguineous a union between blood relatives.

constitutional present in every cell in the organism.

cosmid a modified plasmid that allows large (30-46 kb) segments of DNA to be inserted into it for cloning purposes.

C-terminal the 3′ end of a gene.

cumulative incidence rate proportion of individuals developing a disease over a fixed time interval.

cytogenetics the study of chromosomes.

cytosine a pyrimidine base found in RNA and DNA.

deletion loss or absence of chromosomal material or base pairs of DNA.

DGGE (denaturing gradient gel electrophoresis) a method of mutation detection where single stranded regions of partially denatured double stranded DNA are electrophoresed in gels with increasing gradients of urea and formaldehyde.

DNA (deoxyribonucleic acid)   a nucleic acid in chromosomes composed of a sugar, nitrogenous base, and phosphate group. The order of the bases encode genetic information.

dominant   a genetic disorder in which heterozygotes express the affected phenotype.

dominant negative mutation   when a mutant gene product affects the function of the normal gene product, often by dimerizing with it.

duplication   additional chromosomal material or base pairs added to the normal sequence.

efficacy   the extent to which a medical or surgical intervention produces a beneficial result; usually determined by controlled trials.

exon   transcribed part of a gene that is not excised during transcription.

expressivity   variation in severity of a phenotype associated with a genetic mutation.

five prime (5′) end   DNA end with a 5′ phosphate group; the end of the gene where transcription starts.

founder effect   the occurrence of one or more mutations at increased frequency in a population because of the presence of the mutation—by chance—in the ancestral founders of the population.

frameshift mutation   an insertion or deletion of one or more base pairs that causes a shift in the reading frame generally resulting in a stop codon downstream.

gene   a DNA sequence of codons that encodes the amino acid composition of a protein or specifies an RNA product; the unit of heredity.

genetic heterogeneity   when multiple genetic mutations can result in the same disease phenotype.

genetic map   a map where distances between loci are measured in recombination frequency.

genotype   the genetic constitution of an individual; the specific types of alleles present at given loci.

germline mosaicism   the presence in an individual of two populations of germ cells with either normal DNA or DNA with a mutation that has occurred during the development of the germ cells.

germline mutation   mutation in DNA inherited from a parent and passed on to offspring; germline mutations may also occur as new events, which are then transmitted to progeny.

Gray (Gy)   measure of radiation dose, equivalent to 100 rads.

guanine   a purine base found in RNA and DNA.

haplotype   a configuration of alleles, closely linked, on the same chromosome.

Hardy-Weinberg law   states that gene frequency and genotype frequency remain constant in a population from one generation to the next.

hemizygous   when only one copy of a gene is present instead of two, as found in X-linked genes.

heterozygote an individual with two different alleles present at the same genetic locus on homologous chromosomes.

homologous chromosome one of two copies of the same chromosome in a cell.

homologous DNA DNA with similar sequence to another segment of DNA.

homozygote individual with identical alleles at a given genetic locus on a pair of homologous chromosomes.

hybridization complementary pairing of segments of single stranded DNA or RNA; one segment may have a radioactive "tag" for diagnostic purposes.

imprinting when the parental origin of gene influences its expression.

incidence rate the number of newly diagnosed cases of a disease over a defined time.

intron DNA that lies between exons, is excised during transcription, and is not involved in determining protein composition.

isochromosome when one chromosomal arm is duplicated, replacing the other arm.

karyotype depiction of the chromosomal complement of a cell.

kilobase (kb) 1000 base pairs.

kinase a protein that transfers phosphate groups, e.g., from ATP to side chains of serine, threonine, or tyrosine.

kindred an extended family being studied for a genetic trait.

library fragments of cDNAs or genomic DNA segments in a cloning vector.

linkage two genes located close together on a chromosome are linked if they are inherited together at a frequency that is greater than that due to chance.

linkage disequilibrium nonrandom association between two or more alleles, for example, linkage between a disease allele and a nearby locus.

locus location of a gene on a chromosome.

lod score statistical measure that two genetic loci are linked.

loss of heterozygosity loss of one or more alleles on one chromosome (often in a tumor), detected by assaying for marker alleles for which the individual is constitutionally heterozygous.

meiosis division of germ cells resulting in halving of the chromosomal complement from diploid to haploid.

messenger RNA (mRNA) RNA transcribed from DNA that is used to direct the amino acid sequence of the protein.

microsatellites repetitive elements of DNA (e.g., di-, tri-, tetranucleotides), which vary from one individual to another.

missense mutation single base pair substitution that changes a codon resulting in a different amino acid at that position.

mutagen a substance that causes a mutation in DNA.

mutation a change in the DNA sequence.

nondisjunction failure of chromatid segments to separate during meiosis or mitosis.

nonsense mutation   a single base pair substitution in DNA resulting in a premature stop codon.

Northern blot   method to measure levels of gene expression by detecting RNA fragments with complementary, radioactively labeled DNA probes.

n-terminal   the 5′ end of a gene.

nucleotide   a molecule composed of a nitrogenous base, sugar, and phosphate, it is the building block for DNA.

obligate heterozygote   an individual who may be unaffected or who may not have had DNA testing, but who is assumed to carry a mutation based on analysis of the pedigree.

odds ratio   in a case control study it approximates the relative risk (e.g., the risk of a disease, given a genetic predisposition).

oligonucleotide   a segment of DNA used as a probe or as primer for a polymerase chain reaction.

oncogene   a gene usually involved in cell growth and differentiation which, when mutated, amplified, or overexpressed, results in the neoplastic transformation of cells.

open reading frame   a sequence of codons not interrupted by a stop codon.

pedigree   a graphical depiction of the family tree utilizing standard symbols.

penetrance   the proportion with the genotype who show the expected phenotype; penetrance may vary with age.

phage (bacteriophage)   a virus that affects bacteria, used to clone segments of DNA.

phenocopy   an individual with all of the features of an hereditary syndrome but without the associated genetic alteration (e.g., affected by a sporadic breast cancer in a family with hereditary breast-ovarian cancer syndrome).

phenotype   the physical or metabolic manifestations of the genotype.

physical map   a map based on distances (e.g., in base pairs) between loci.

plasmid   circular DNA molecules in bacteria used as vectors to clone segments of DNA.

pleiotropy   multiple phenotypic features associated with the same mutation.

point mutation   single base pair change, deletion, or insertion, causing an alteration in DNA sequence.

polygenic   when a trait is determined by many genes at different loci.

polymerase chain reaction (PCR)   amplification of a short DNA sequence by use of oligonucleotide primers and DNA polymerase.

polymorphism   an allele is polymorphic in a population if it displays alternative DNA sequences at the same locus, with the least frequent allele observed at a frequency of at least 1 per hundred.

population attributable risk (per cent)   the proportion of a disease in a specified population attributable to, for example, a specific genetic risk factor.

positional cloning   isolation (cloning) of a gene based on genetic mapping, but without knowledge of the gene product.

predictive value   the probability that a person with a positive test is affected by the disease (positive predictive value) or the probability that a person with a negative test does not have the disease (negative predictive value); requires measurement of sensitivity, specificity, and disease prevalence.

prevalence   the existing cases of a disease or disorder at a point in time.

proband   the family member through which the pedigree is ascertained.

probe   a labeled DNA or RNA sequence used in hybridization reactions, e.g., for diagnostic purposes.

promotor   5′ DNA sequence that determines initiation of transcription and also the amount of mRNA formed.

propositus   the family member through which the pedigree is ascertained; same as proband.

protein truncation assay (also called *in vitro* synthesized protein assay)   a method for mutation detection by translating mRNA into a radiolabeled protein, after PCR amplification of cDNA.

purine   a nitrogenous base with connected 5- and 6-member rings (adenine, guanine).

pyrimidine   a nitrogenous base with a 6-member ring (cytosine, uracil, thymine).

rad   a measure of ionizing radiation absorbed by tissues.

recessive   a trait expressed only when both alleles are altered (homozygous) or one is absent (hemizygous).

recombination   formation of new combinations of genes by crossing over between two linked loci.

relative risk   in a cohort study it is derived as the ratio of the incidence of the disease in the group with a known risk factor divided by the incidence in the normal-risk population.

restriction fragment length polymorphism (RFLP)   polymorphisms due to presence or absence of specific sites for restriction endonucleases.

reverse genetics   positional cloning.

reverse transcriptase   an enzyme that synthesizes DNA from RNA.

ribonucleic acid (RNA)   a nucleic acid that includes the mRNA template for polypeptide synthesis, tRNA that brings amino acids to ribosomes, and ribosomal RNA that functions as the site of protein synthesis.

ribosomes   organelles where polypeptide synthesis from mRNA occurs.

ring finger   amino acid sequence surrounding a zinc atom in a protein that binds DNA (e.g., *BRCA1*).

segregation   the separation of alleles at meiosis.

segregation analysis   the fitting of observed family data to known models of inheritance.

sensitivity   proportion of truly diseased persons who are identified by a screening test; also called the true positive rate.

sequencing   direct determination of nucleotide sequence of DNA by manual or automated methods.

sibling (sib)   a brother or sister.

somatic mutation   a mutation in non-germline DNA (e.g., in a tumor).

Southern blot   technique of moving DNA fragments from an agarose gel to a nitrocellulose filter where they can be hybridized with a diagnostic probe (named after the inventor of the technique).

specificity   proportion of truly nondiseased persons who are identified by a screening test; also called the true negative test.

splice sites   locations where mRNA splices introns out and connects exons.

sporadic tumor   a cancer not due to a germline mutation.

SSCP (single strand conformational polymorphism)   a method of mutation detection based on the different mobilities of double-stranded PCR products that are denatured into single strands and electrophoresed.

stop codon   one of three codons (UAG, UAA, UGA) that terminate translation.

theta (θ)   the recombination fraction.

three prime (3′)   the end of the gene with a free 3′ hydroxyl group; the end of the gene where transcription terminates.

transcription   synthesis of RNA from DNA.

translation   synthesis of a polypeptide from mRNA.

translocation   transposition of one chromosomal segment to another.

transversion   a mutation in which a purine replaces a pyrimidine or vice versa.

tumor suppressor gene   a gene normally involved in regulation of cell growth and proliferation; loss of function of both alleles of the gene leads to malignant transformation or progression.

uracil   a pyrimidine base in RNA.

vector   a plasmid, phage, or cosmid into which a fragment of DNA can be placed as part of cloning experiments.

X-linked   genes on the X chromosome.

Western blot   a method of detection of proteins using immunologic reagents.

wild-type   normal allele or normal phenotype.

yeast artificial chromosome   cloning vector for large (200–500 kb) fragments of DNA.

Table of Inherited Disorders That May Predispose to Cancer

METHODOLOGY OF CONSTRUCTION

Sources:

Cannon-Albright LA, Bishop DT, Goldgar C, Skolnick MH. 1991. Table 3-1 in Genetic predisposition to cancer. In: Devita VT, Jr, Hellman S, Rosenberg SA (eds), Important Advances In Oncology 1991. Philadelphia: Lippincott, pp. 43–44.

Hodgson SV, Maher ER. 1993. A Practical Guide to Human Cancer Genetics. Cambridge, U.K.: Cambridge University Press.

McKusick VA, Francomano CA, Antonarakis SE. 1992. Mendelian Inheritance in Man. Baltimore: The John Hopkins University Press. (On-line Mendelian Inheritance in Man—see websites on page 384).

Mulvihill JJ. 1975. Table 3 in "Congenital and Genetic Diseases." In: Fraumeni JF Jr (ed). Persons at High Risk for Cancer: An Approach to Cancer Etiology and Control. New York: Academic Press, pp. 17–24.

Clinical descriptions of syndromes:

Emery AEH, Rimoin DL, Sofaer JA (eds). 1990. Principles and Practice of Medical Genetics. New York: Churchill Livingstone.

Isselbacher KJ, Braunwald E, Wilson J, Martin JB, Fauci AS, Kasper DL (eds). 1994. Harrison's Principles of Internal Medicine. New York: McGraw-Hill.

The four primary sources were reviewed to identify syndromes of human diseases in which one or more malignancies was a component. Syndromes were included only if the component malignancy was observed in two or more unrelated kindreds. There-fore, readers are referred to the primary sources for associations seen only in single kindreds.

HOW TO USE THIS APPENDIX

Each entry is listed alphabetically under the corresponding organ system. An index of malignancies and corresponding organ systems is listed below. Subsequently, in the table, itself, component tumors in the syndrome are listed, followed by a clinical sum-mary of salient features. At top right of each entry is the mode of inheritance, the locus of the gene, and its symbol, if known. Component tumors corresponding to the organ system under which the syndrome is listed are indicated in bold.

INDEX FOR APPENDIX A

Malignancy	Corresponding Organ System
adrenocortical adenomas	see Endocrine
adrenocortical carcinoma	see Endocrine
anal canal squamous carcinoma	see Gastrointestinal
atrial myxoma	see Cardiovascular
basal cell carcinoma	see Skin
bile duct carcinoma	see Gastrointestinal
bladder carcinoma	see Genitourinary
brain tumor	see Nervous system and eye
astrocytoma	
cerebral fibrosarcoma	
gangliocytoma	
glioblastoma multiforme	
glioma	
medulloblastoma	
meningioma	
subependymoma	
breast cancer	See Reproductive
carcinoid	
bronchial	see Respiratory
duodenal	see Gastrointestinal
carotid body tumors (chemodectoma)	see Cardiovascular
cardiac fibroma	see Cardiovascular
cervical cancer	see Reproductive
colon cancer	see Gastrointestinal
Cushing syndrome	see Endocrine
cylindroma	see Skin
desmoid	see Connective tissue

Index for Appendix A (cont.)

Index for Appendix A (cont.)

Index for Appendix A (cont.)

CANCERS OF THE CARDIOVASCULAR SYSTEM

Syndrome: BASAL CELL NEVUS (GORLIN) SYNDROME
Inheritance: AD
Locus(i): 9q31 (PTCH)

Component tumors: BASAL CELL CARCINOMA; **CARDIAC FIBROMA**; OVARIAN FIBROMATA; OVARIAN CARCINOMA; MEDULLOBLASTOMA
Clinical features: (SEE CANCERS OF THE SKIN)

Syndrome: CAROTID BODY TUMORS AND MULTIPLE EXTRA-ADRENAL PHEOCHROMOCYTOMAS
Inheritance: AD

Component tumors: **CAROTID BODY TUMORS;** MULTIPLE EXTRA-ADRENAL PHEOCHROMOCYTOMAS
Clinical features: (SEE PARAGANGLIOMATA; ALSO SEE PHEOCHROMOCY-TOMA)

Syndrome: MYXOMA, INTRACARDIAC
Inheritance: AR OR AD

Component tumors: **LEFT ATRIAL MYXOMA**; **RIGHT ATRIAL MYXOMA**; **PULMONIC VALVE MYXOMA**
Clinical features: BACTERIAL ENDOCARDITIS; MEAN AGE 20'S; MORE COMMON IN LEFT ATRIUM; SYMPTOMS DEPEND ON SITE OF TUMOR EM-BOLI, E.G. EMBOLI TO HEART (MYOCARDIAL INFARCTION), LUNGS (PUL-MONARY EMBOLISM), OR BRAIN (CEREBROVASCULAR ACCIDENT)

Syndrome: "NAME" SYNDROME (NEVI; ATRIAL MYXOMA; MUCINOSIS OF SKIN; ENDOCRINE OVERACTIVITY)

Inheritance: AD
Locus(i): LINKED TO CHROMOSOME 2p16

Component tumors: **ATRIAL MYXOID LIPOSARCOMA**; SUBCUTANEOUS MYXOID NEUROFIBROMATA; PRIMARY ADRENOCORTICAL NODULAR DYSPLASIA; VIRILIZING ADRENOCORTICAL CARCINOMA; LARGE-CELL CALCIFYING SERTOLI CELL TUMOR; PITUITARY ADENOMA; NASOPHA-RYNGEAL SCHWANNOMA; PROLACTIN-SECRETING PITUITARY ADENO-MA
Clinical features: (SEE CANCERS OF THE ENDOCRINE SYSTEM)

Syndrome: PARAGANGLIOMATA

Inheritance: AD WITH GENOMIC IMPRINTING
Locus(i): 11q22.3-q23.2; ALSO 11q13

Component tumors: **PARAGANGLIOMATA**; **CHEMODECTOMAS**; **CAROTID BODY TUMORS**; **GLOMUS JUGULAR TUMORS**
Clinical features: FAMILIAL CASES OFTEN BILATERAL; INVOLVE HEAD AND NECK, INCLUDING CAROTID BODY, UPPER MEDIASTINAL, RETROPERITONEAL OR PELVIC PARAGANGLIA; PRESENTATION DEPEN-DENT ON SITE OF TUMOR (E.G. TYMPANIC MASS, VOCAL CORD PARALY-SIS, CRANIAL NERVE ABNORMALITIES, DISPLACEMENT OF ARTERIES)

Syndrome: TELANGIECTASIA, HEREDITARY HEMORRHAGIC, OF RENDU, OSLER AND WEBER;

Inheritance: AD
Locus(i): 9q34.1; GENE ENCODES ENDOGLIN (HHT)

Component tumors: VASCULAR CANCERS
Clinical features: EPISTAXIS IN CHILDHOOD; TELANGIECTASIA OF FACE, MUCOSA, PALMS; COMPLETE PENETRANCE BY AGE 40; 62% BY AGE 16

Syndrome: TUBEROUS SCLEROSIS, TYPES I AND II

Inheritance: AD
Locus(i): 9q32-q34 (TYPE I); 16p13.3 (TYPE II)

Component tumors: **MYOCARDIAL RHABDOMYOMA**; MULTIPLE BILAT-ERAL RENAL ANGIOMYOLIPOMA; WILMS' TUMOR; **CARDIAC AND OL-FACTORY HAMARTOMAS**; EPENDYMOMA; ASTROCYTOMA; RETINAL PHAKOMAS
Clinical features: (SEE CANCERS OF CONNECTIVE TISSUES)

Syndrome: XERODERMA PIGMENTOSUM

Inheritance: AR
Locus(i): 9q34 (XPA); 3p25 (XPC); 19q13 (XPD); 15p (XPF)

Component tumors: EARLY ONSET BASAL CELL, SQUAMOUS CELL SKIN CANCER; MALIGNANT MELANOMA; KERATOACANTHOMAS; **ANGIOMAS**; INCREASED RISK OF INTERNAL MALIGNANCIES INCLUDING SARCOMAS AND ADENOCARCINOMAS
Clinical features: (SEE CANCERS OF THE SKIN)

CANCERS OF CONNECTIVE TISSUES

Syndrome: BECKWITH-WIEDEMANN SYNDROME	**Inheritance:** AD WITH INCOMPLETE PENETRANCE **Locus(i):** 11p15.5 (?IGF2/H19/p57)

Component tumors: ADRENAL CARCINOMA; NEPHROBLASTOMA (WILMS' TUMOR); HEPATOBLASTOMA; **RHABDOMYOSARCOMA**; CONGENITAL GASTRIC TERATOMA
Clinical features: (SEE CANCERS OF THE GENITOURINARY SYSTEM)

Syndrome: EXOSTOSES, MULTIPLE, TYPES 1, 2, 3	**Inheritance:** AD **Locus(i):** 8q24.1 (TYPE 1); 11p12 (TYPE 2); 19p (TYPE 3)

Component tumors: INCREASED RISK OF OSTEOSARCOMA IN EXOSTOSES; **CHONDROSARCOMA**
Clinical features: (SEE CANCERS OF THE SKELETAL SYSTEM)

Syndrome: FAMILIAL ADENOMATOUS POLYPOSIS (FAP, GARDNER SYNDROME)	**Inheritance:** AD **Locus(i):** 5q21-q22 (APC)

Component tumors: MALIGNANT TRANSFORMATION OF POLYPS; PERIAMPULLARY CARCINOMA; HEPATOBLASTOMA; BILE DUCT CARCINOMA; OSTEOSARCOMA; ADRENAL CARCINOMA WITH CUSHING SYNDROME; THYROID CARCINOMA; **DESMOIDS**
Clinical features: (SEE CANCERS OF GASTROINTESTINAL SYSTEM)

Syndrome: FAMILIAL TERATOMA	**Inheritance:** AD **Locus(i):** LINKED TO 7q36; MAY BE HETEROGENEOUS WITH SECOND LOCUS AT 13q OR 20p

Component tumors: SACROCOCCYGEAL TERATOMA
Clinical features: RARE SYNDROME OF SACROCOCCYGEAL TERATOMAS WITH CONGENITAL MALFORMATIONS OF SACRUM, VERTBRAE, SOMETIMES WITH ANORECTAL MALFORMATION AND OTHER URINARY OR NEUROLOGIC MALFORMATIONS

Syndrome: FIBROMATOSIS, CONGENITAL GENERALIZED	**Inheritance:** AR

Component tumors: FIBROBLASTIC TUMORS AT SEVERAL SITES
Clinical features: FIBROBLASTIC TUMORS OF SKIN, STRIATED MUSCLES, BONES, AND VISCERA

Syndrome: FIBROMATOSIS, GINGIVAL	**Inheritance:** AD, AR

Component tumors: GINGIVAL FIBROMATOSIS
Clinical features: FIBROMAS OF GINGIVA, WITH OR WITHOUT HYPERTRI-CHOSIS; VARIANT WITH SPLENOMEGALY AND FINGER ABNORMALITIES

Syndrome: KAPOSI SARCOMA	**Inheritance:** AD

Component tumors: KAPOSI SARCOMA
Clinical features: RED-PURPLE NODULES, PLAQUES, AND MACULES ON EXTREMITIES; EDEMA DUE TO LYMPHATIC INVASION; RARE FAMILIES REPORTED

Syndrome: LI-FRAUMENI SYNDROME	**Inheritance:** AD **Locus(i):** 17p13.1 (p53)

Component tumors: RHABDOMYOSARCOMA; SOFT TISSUE SARCOMA; BREAST CANCER; BRAIN TUMORS; OSTEOSARCOMA; LEUKEMIA; AD-RENOCORTICAL CARCINOMA; LYMPHOCYTIC LYMPHOMA; LUNG ADE-NOCARCINOMA; MELANOMA; GONADAL GERM CELL TUMORS; PROS-TATE CARCINOMA; PANCREATIC CARCINOMA; LARYNGEAL CARCINOMA
Clinical features: EARLY AGE OF ONSET OF COMPONENT TUMORS AND MULTIPLE PRIMARIES (SEE TEXT)

Syndrome: LIPOMATOSIS, FAMILIAL	**Inheritance:** AD **Locus(i):** MAPPED TO 12q

Component tumors: MULTIPLE LIPOMAS
Clinical features: LIPOMAS OF EXTREMITIES AND TRUNK; RARE MALIG-NANT DEGENERATION

Syndrome: MULTIPLE ENCHONDRO-MATOSIS (OLLIER'S DISEASE)	**Inheritance:** ?AD FORM

Component tumors: CHONDROSARCOMA; RARELY ASSOCIATED WITH OVARIAN JUVENILE GRANULOSA CELL TUMOR
Clinical features: CALLED MAFUCCI'S SYNDROME WHEN ASSOCIATED WITH HEMANGIOMATA; PRESENTS AS DEFORMITY OF LONG BONES DUE TO ENCHONDROMAS WHICH MAY DEGENERATE INTO CHONDRO-SARCOMA

Syndrome: MULTIPLE ENDOCRINE NEOPLASIA, TYPE I	**Inheritance:** AD **Locus(i):** 11q13 (MEN1)

Component tumors: ISLET CELL TUMORS OF PANCREAS; PARATHYROID ADENOMAS; PITUITARY ADENOMAS; ADRENOCORTICAL ADENOMAS; **LIPOMAS**

Clinical features: (SEE CANCERS OF THE ENDOCRINE SYSTEM)

Syndrome: "NAME" SYNDROME (NEVI; ATRIAL MYXOMA; MUCINOSIS OF SKIN; ENDOCRINE OVERACTIVITY)	**Inheritance:** AD **Locus(i):** LINKED TO CHROMOSOME 2p16

Component tumors: MYXOID LIPOSARCOMA; SUBCUTANEOUS MYXOID NEUROFIBROMATA; PRIMARY ADRENOCORTICAL NODULAR DYSPLASIA; VIRILIZING ADRENOCORTICAL CARCINOMA; LARGE-CELL CALCIFYING SERTOLI CELL TUMOR; PITUITARY ADENOMA; NASOPHARYNGEAL SCHWANNOMA; PROLACTIN-SECRETING PITUITARY ADENOMA
Clinical features: (SEE CANCERS OF THE ENDOCRINE SYSTEM)

Syndrome: NEUROFIBROMATOSIS TYPE I	**Inheritance:** AD **Locus(i):** 17q11.2 (NF1)

Component tumors: PHEOCHROMOCYTOMA; OPTIC GLIOMA; HYPOTHAL-AMIC TUMOR; NEUROFIBROSARCOMA; **RHABDOMYOSARCOMA**; DUO-DENAL CARCINOID; SOMATOSTATINOMA; PARATHYROID ADENOMA; LISCH NODULES (IRIS HAMARTOMAS); NEUROFIBROMAS; PLEXIFORM NEUROMA
Clinical features: (SEE CANCERS OF THE NERVOUS SYSTEM AND EYE)

Syndrome: NOONAN-LIKE/MULTI-PLE GIANT CELL LESION SYNDROME	**Inheritance:** AD

Component tumors: GIANT CELL GRANULOMAS OF BONE AND SOFT TISSUES
Clinical features: (SEE CANCERS OF THE SKELETAL SYSTEM)

Syndrome: RHABDOMYOSARCOMA	**Inheritance:** AD

Component tumors: RHABDOMYOSARCOMA
Clinical features: (SEE LI-FRAUMENI SYNDROME; SEE BECKWITH-WIEDE-MANN SYNDROME)

Syndrome: TUBEROUS SCLEROSIS, TYPES I AND II	**Inheritance:** AD **Locus(i):** 9q32-q34 (TSI);16p13.3 (TSII)

Component tumors: MYOCARDIAL RHABDOMYOMA; MULTIPLE BILAT-ERAL RENAL ANGIOMYOLIPOMAS; WILMS' TUMOR; CARDIAC AND OL-FACTORY HAMARTOMAS; EPENDYMOMA; ASTROCYTOMA; RETINAL PHAKOMAS
Clinical features: MENTAL RETARDATION; SEIZURES; BRAIN AND RETINAL HAMARTOMAS; ADENOMA SEBACEUM; SHAGREEN PATCH; UNGUAL FI-BROMAS; HYPOMELANOTIC SKIN MACULES (ASH LEAF SHAPED); RENAL ANGIOMYOLIPOMA; SUBEPENDYMAL GLIAL NODULE (ON CT OR MRI SCAN)

Syndrome: WERNER SYNDROME   **Inheritance:** AR

Component tumors: OSTEOSARCOMA; **SARCOMAS AND OTHER CONNEC-TIVE TISSUES TUMORS**; OTHER RARE TUMORS
Clinical features: (SEE CANCERS OF THE SKELETAL SYSTEM)

CANCERS OF THE ENDOCRINE SYSTEM

Syndrome: ACROMEGALY   **Inheritance:** AD

Component tumors: SOMATOSTATINOMA (PITUITARY TUMOR)
Clinical features: ACANTHOSIS NIGRICANS, GALACTORRHEA; DISTINCT FROM MEN1

Syndrome: ADRENOCORTICAL   **Inheritance:** AR
CARCINOMA, HEREDITARY

Component tumors: ADRENOCORTICAL CARCINOMA
Clinical features: VIRILISM; HEREDITARY SYNDROME DISTINCT FROM LI-FRAUMENI SYNDROME; DESCRIBED IN SIB PAIRS

Syndrome: BECKWITH-WIEDEMANN   **Inheritance:** AD WITH INCOMPLETE
SYNDROME   PENETRANCE
                                  Locus(i): 11p15.5/(?IGF2/H19/p57)

Component tumors: ADRENAL CARCINOMA; NEPHROBLASTOMA
(WILMS' TUMOR); HEPATOBLASTOMA; RHABDOMYOSARCOMA; CON-GENITAL GASTRIC TERATOMA
Clinical features: (SEE CANCERS OF THE GENITOURINARY SYSTEM)

Syndrome: CAROTID BODY TUMORS **Inheritance:** AD
AND MULTIPLE EXTRA-ADRENAL
PHEOCHROMOCYTOMAS

Component tumors: CAROTID BODY TUMORS; **MULTIPLE EXTRA-ADRENAL PHEOCHROMOCYTOMAS**
Clinical features: (SEE CANCERS OF THE CARDIOVASCULAR SYSTEM)

Syndrome: CHOLESTASIS WITH   **Inheritance:** AD
PERIPHERAL PULMONARY   **Locus(i):** ?CONTIGUOUS GENE SYN-
STENOSIS   DROME IN 20p11.23-p12.1

Component tumors: HEPATOCELLULAR CARCINOMA; **PAPILLARY THY-ROID CARCINOMA**
Clinical features: (SEE CANCERS OF THE GASTROINTESTINAL SYSTEM)

Syndrome: DEXAMETHASONE-SENSITIVE ALDOSTERONISM
Inheritance: AD
Locus(i): 8q21 (CYP11B1) AND 8q21 (CYP11B2) GENES

Component tumors: MULTIPLE ADRENOCORTICAL ADENOMAS
Clinical features: HYPERTENSION, LOW PLASMA RENIN ACTVITY, INCREASED ALDOSTERONE SECRETION RESPONSIVE TO DEXAMETHASONE

Syndrome: FAMILIAL ADENOMATOUS POLYPOSIS (FAP, GARDNER SYNDROME)
Inheritance: AD
Locus(i): 5q21-q22 (APC)

Component tumors: MALIGNANT TRANSFORMATION OF POLYPS; PERIAMPULLARY CARCINOMA; HEPATOBLASTOMA; BILE DUCT CARCINOMA; OSTEOSARCOMA; **ADRENAL CARCINOMA** WITH CUSHING SYNDROME; **THYROID CARCINOMA**; DESMOIDS
Clinical features: (SEE CANCERS OF GASTROINTESTINAL SYSTEM)

Syndrome: FAMILIAL CUSHING DISEASE
Inheritance: AR IN SOME FAMILIES

Component tumors: VIRILIZING ADRENOCORTICAL CARCINOMA, HYPERPLASIA, OR MICRONODULAR DYSPLASIA
Clinical features: SYMPTOMS OF CUSHING SYNDROME INCLUDING; INCREASED WEIGHT, WEAKNESS, HYPERTENSION, HIRSUTISM, AMENORRHEA, STRIAE, PERSONALITY CHANGES, EDEMA, ETC.

Syndrome: FAMILIAL EXTRA-ADRENAL PHEOCHROMOCYTOMA
Inheritance: AD

Component tumors: PRIMARY EXTRA-ADRENAL PHEOCHROMOCYTOMA; **PHEOCHROMOCYTOMA** OF ORGAN OF ZUCKERKANDL; **PHEOCHROMOCYTOMA** AT THE AORTIC BIFURCATION; **PHEOCHROMOCYTOMA** OF LOWER URINARY TRACT; **PHEOCHROMOCYTOMA** OF RENAL HILUM
Clinical features: SWEATING; HYPERTENSIVE RETINOPATHY; EPISODIC HYPERTENSION, TACHYCARDIA, CHF; CEREBRAL HEMORRHAGE; PROTEINURIA; HYPERCALCEMIA

Syndrome: FAMILIAL HYPERPARATHYROIDISM
Inheritance: AD
Locus(i): ONE FORM LINKED TO 1q21-q31 WITH LOD=6.1

Component tumors: CYSTIC PARATHYROID ADENOMAS
Clinical features: HYPERCALCEMIA; CAN HAVE MAXILLARY OR MANDIBULAR OSSIFYING FIBROMAS

Syndrome: FAMILIAL MEDULLARY THYROID CARCINOMA
Inheritance: AD
Locus(i): 10q11.2 (RET)

Component tumors: MEDULLARY THYROID CARCINOMA
Clinical features: NO EXTRATHYROID MANIFESTATIONS OF MEN2a

Syndrome: FAMILIAL PHEO-
CHROMOCYTOMA

Inheritance: AD

Component tumors: PHEOCHROMOCYTOMA
Clinical features: SWEATING; HYPERTENSIVE RETINOPATHY; TACHYCAR-
DIA; CONGESTIVE HEART FAILURE; HYPERTENSION; HYPERCALCEMIA;
RARELY WITH CAFÉ AU LAIT SPOTS AND OTHER STIGMATA OF NF1

Syndrome: FAMILIAL PROLACTIN-
OMA

Inheritance: FAMILIAL TENDENCY
INDEPENDENT OF ASSOCIATION
WITH MEN1

Component tumors: PROLACTIN-SECRETING PITUITARY ADENOMA;
PROLACTINOMA
Clinical features: 4 FAMILIES DESCRIBED; DISTINCT FROM MEN; IRREGU-
LAR MENSES; AMENORRHEA; GALACTORRHEA; SEXUAL DYSFUNCTION

Syndrome: FAMILIAL THYROID
GOITER, NONTOXIC, WITH INTRA-
THYROIDAL CALCIFICATION

Inheritance: AD (DIMINISHED
PENETRANCE IN MALES)

Component tumors: MULTIPLE THYROID ADENOMATA
Clinical features: NONTOXIC GOITER

Syndrome: LI-FRAUMENI
SYNDROME

Inheritance: AD
Locus(i): 17p13.1 (p53)

Component tumors: RHABDOMYOSARCOMA; SOFT TISSUE SARCOMA;
BREAST CANCER; BRAIN TUMORS; OSTEOSARCOMA; LEUKEMIA;
ADRENOCORTICAL CARCINOMA; LYMPHOCYTIC LYMPHOMA; LUNG
ADENOCARCINOMA, MELANOMA, GONADAL GERM CELL TUMORS;
PROSTATE CARCINOMA; PANCREATIC CARCINOMA; LARYNGEAL CARCI-
NOMA
Clinical features: (SEE CANCERS OF CONNECTIVE TISSUES)

Syndrome: McCUNE-ALBRIGHT
SYNDROME

Inheritance: AD
Locus(i): 20q13.2 (GNAS1), SPORADIC
CASES DUE TO SOMATIC MUTATION

Component tumors: PITUITARY ADENOMA
Clinical features: VERY RARELY FAMILIAL; PROLIFERATION OF FIBROUS
TISSUES; BONE DESTRUCTION; CAFÉ AU LAIT SPOTS; ENDOCRINE AB-
NORMALITIES; DEAFNESS OR BLINDNESS DUE TO CRANIAL NERVE IM-
PINGEMENT

Syndrome: MULTIPLE ENDOCRINE
NEOPLASIA, TYPE I

Inheritance: AD
Locus(i): 11q13 (MEN1)

Component tumors: ISLET CELL TUMORS OF PANCREAS; **PARATHYROID ADENOMAS**; **PITUITARY ADENOMAS**; **ADRENOCORTICAL ADENOMAS**; LIPOMAS; BRONCHIAL CARCINOMA, THYMIC CARCINOMA, DUODENAL CARCINOID, BRONCHIAL CARCINOID, MALIGNANT SCHWANNOMA
Clinical features: SKIN RASH; PEPTIC ULCER; ULCERATIVE GASTRITIS; DIARRHEA; STEATORRHEA; HYPOGLYCEMIA; HYPERCALCEMIA; GLUCOSE INTOLERANCE; CUSHING SYNDROME; BONE PAIN

Syndrome: MULTIPLE ENDOCRINE NEOPLASIA, TYPE 2A	**Inheritance:** AD **Locus(i):** 10q11.2 (RET)

Component tumors: **PHEOCHROMOCYTOMA**; **MEDULLARY THYROID CARCINOMA**; **PARATHYROID ADENOMA OR HYPERPLASIA**
Clinical features: HYPERCALCEMIA; HYPERTENSION; PALPITATIONS; HEADACHES; SWEATING; HYPOPHOSPHATEMIA; HYPERCALCURIA

Syndrome: MULTIPLE ENDOCRINE NEOPLASIA, TYPE 2B	**Inheritance:** AD **Locus(i):** 10q11.2 (RET)

Component tumors: MULTIPLE TRUE NEUROMAS; **PHEOCHROMOCYTOMA**; **MEDULLARY THYROID CARCINOMA**
Clinical features: MARFANOID HABITUS; ENLARGED NODULAR LIPS; MUCOSAL NEUROMAS; INTESTINAL GANGLIONEUROMATOSIS CAUSING BOWEL DYSFUNCTION; NEUROLOGICAL ABNORMALITIES; CAFÉ AU LAIT SPOTS; SKIN FEATURES MAY RESEMBLE NFI

Syndrome: MULTIPLE HAMARTOMA (COWDEN) SYNDROME	**Inheritance:** AD **Locus(i):** 10q22-q23 (PTEN)

Component tumors: DYSPLASTIC CEREBELLAR GANGLIOCYTOMA; BREAST CANCERS; PRIMARY NEUROENDOCRINE (MERKEL CELL) TUMORS; SKIN CARCINOMA; RENAL CELL CARCINOMA; **THYROID CANCER**
Clinical features: (SEE CANCERS OF THE REPRODUCTIVE SYSTEM)

Syndrome: "NAME" SYNDROME (NEVI; ATRIAL MYXOMA; MUCINOSIS OF SKIN; ENDOCRINE OVERACTIVITY)	**Inheritance:** AD **Locus(i):** LINKED TO CHROMOSOME 2p16

Component tumors: MYXOMAS OF THE HEART (ATRIUM); MYXOID LIPOSARCOMA; SUBCUTANEOUS MYXOID NEUROFIBROMATA; **PRIMARY ADRENOCORTICAL NODULAR DYSPLASIA**; **VIRILIZING ADRENOCORTICAL CARCINOMA**; LARGE-CELL CALCIFYING SERTOLI CELL TUMOR; **PITUITARY ADENOMA**; NASOPHARYNGEAL SCHWANNOMA
Clinical features: CARDIAC, BREAST, AND CUTANEOUS MYXOMAS; PIGMENTED SKIN LESIONS USUALLY ON FACE LOOK LIKE PEUTZ-JEGHERS SYNDROME; CARDIAC TUMORS MAY BE LIFE THREATENING

Syndrome: NEUROFIBROMATOSIS TYPE I	**Inheritance:** AD **Locus(i):** 17q11.2 (NF1)

Component tumors: PHEOCHROMOCYTOMA; OPTIC GLIOMA; HYPOTHAL-AMIC TUMOR; NEUROFIBROSARCOMA; RHABDOMYOSARCOMA; DUO-DENAL CARCINOID; **SOMATOSTATINOMA**; **PARATHYROID ADENOMA**; LISCH NODULES (IRIS HAMARTOMAS); NEUROFIBROMAS; PLEXIFORM NEUROMA
Clinical features: (SEE CANCERS OF THE NERVOUS SYSTEM AND EYE)

Syndrome: NEUROFIBROMATOSIS-PHEOCHROMOCYTOMA-DUODENAL CARCINOID SYNDROME | **Inheritance:** AD

Component tumors: DUODENAL CARCINOID TUMOR; NEUROFIBROMA-TOSIS; **PHEOCHROMOCYTOMA**
Clinical features: (SEE CANCERS OF THE NERVOUS SYSTEM AND EYE)

Syndrome: PAPILLARY CARCINOMA OF THE THYROID | **Inheritance:** AD

Component tumors: **PAPILLARY CARCINOMA OF THYROID**; REPORTED COLON CANCERS IN RELATIVES
Clinical features: ONSET EARLIER THAN IN SPORADIC CASES

Syndrome: PENDRED SYNDROME | **Inheritance:** AR
Locus(i): 7q21-34

Component tumors: **THYROID CARCINOMA**
Clinical features: GOITER AND CONGENITAL NEUROSENSORY DEAFNESS

Syndrome: PHEOCHROMOCYTOMA-ISLET CELL TUMOR SYNDROME | **Inheritance:** AD

Component tumors: **PHEOCHROMOCYTOMA**; PANCREATIC ISLET CELL TUMOR
Clinical features: SWEATING; HYPERTENSIVE RETINOPATHY; TACHYCAR-DIA; CHF; FAMILIAL PHEOCHROMOCYTOMA, USUALLY BILATERAL; EPISODIC HYPERTENSION; PROTEINURIA; HYPERCALCEMIA; (THIS SYN-DROME APPEARS TO BE DISTINCT FROM MEN AND VHL)

Syndrome: RETINOBLASTOMA | **Inheritance:** AD
Locus(i): 13q14 (RB1)

Component tumors: RETINOBLASTOMA; OSTEOSARCOMA; **PINEALOMA**
Clinical features: (see NERVOUS SYSTEM AND EYE)

Syndrome: VON HIPPEL-LINDAU SYNDROME | **Inheritance:** AD
Locus(i): 3p26-p25 (VHL)

Component tumors: **PHEOCHROMOCYTOMA**; CEREBELLAR HEMAN-GIOBLASTOMA; HYPERNEPHROMA; **ADRENAL HEMANGIOMAS**; PUL-MONARY HEMANGIOMAS; LIVER HEMANGIOMAS; PANCREATIC CARCI-NOMA; PANCREATIC ISLET CELL TUMOR; INTRACRANIAL HEMANGIO-BLASTOMA; SPINAL CORD HEMANGIOMA
Clinical features: (SEE CANCERS OF THE NERVOUS SYSTEM AND EYE)

CANCERS OF THE GASTROINTESTINAL SYSTEM

Syndrome: AGAMMAGLOBULINEMIA **Inheritance:** XL; ALSO OTHER TYPES
(BRUTON DISEASE)

Component tumors: INCREASED RISK OF COLORECTAL CANCER
Clinical features: ONSET IN INFANTS; RECURRENT PYOGENIC INFEC-
TIONS; RHEUMATOID-LIKE ARTHRITIS; HEMOLYTIC ANEMIA; HYPOGAM-
MAGLOBULINEMIA

Syndrome: ALPHA1-ANTITRYPSIN **Inheritance:** AD
DEFICIENCY **Locus(i):** 14q32.1

Component tumors: HEPATOCELLULAR CARCINOMA
Clinical features: PANACINAR EMPHYSEMA; SCLEROSING ALVEOLITIS; JU-
VENILE CIRRHOSIS; JUVENILE LIVER DISEASE (INCLUDING PORTAL HY-
PERTENSION AND VARICES); BLEEDING DISORDER (PITTSBURGH AL-
LELE)

Syndrome: ANAL CANAL **Inheritance:** AD
CARCINOMA

Component tumors: ANAL CANAL SQUAMOUS CARCINOMA
Clinical features: CANCER PREDISPOSITION TO ANAL CARCINOMA

Syndrome: BARRET ESOPHAGUS **Inheritance:** AD

Component tumors: ADENOCARCINOMA OF ESOPHAGUS (RISK 10%)
Clinical features: ULCERATING ESOPHAGUS; GASTROESOPHAGEAL RE-
FLUX; COLUMNAR EPITHELIAL-LINED DISTAL ESOPHAGUS

Syndrome: BECKWITH-WIEDEMANN **Inheritance:** AD WITH INCOMPLETE
SYNDROME PENETRANCE
Locus(i): 11p15.5

Component tumors: ADRENAL CARCINOMA; NEPHROBLASTOMA (WILMS'
TUMOR); **HEPATOBLASTOMA**; RHABDOMYOSARCOMA; **CONGENITAL
GASTRIC TERATOMA**
Clinical features: (SEE CANCERS OF THE GENITOURINARY SYSTEM)

Syndrome: BLOOM SYNDROME **Inheritance:** AR
Locus(i): 15q26.1 (BLM)

Component tumors: LEUKEMIAS; LYMPHOMAS; **GASTROINTESTINAL TU-
MORS**; LARYNGEAL AND CERVICAL CANCERS
Clinical features: (SEE CANCERS OF THE HEMATOLOGIC AND LYMPHATIC
SYSTEM)

Syndrome: CELIAC SPRUE

Inheritance: AR VS. MULTI-FACTORIAL

Component tumors: SMALL BOWEL CANCER AND OTHER GI CANCERS;
LYMPHOMA
Clinical features: GLUTEN SENSITIVITY; DIARRHEA; ANEMIA;
ANTIGLANDIN ANTIBODY

Syndrome: CHOLESTASIS WITH
PERIPHERAL PULMONARY
STENOSIS

Inheritance: AD
Locus(i): CONTIGUOUS GENE
SYNDROME IN 20p11.23-p12.1

Component tumors: HEPATOCELLULAR CARCINOMA; PAPILLARY THY-
ROID CARCINOMA
Clinical features: FAILURE TO THRIVE; CHARACTERISTIC FACIES; OCULAR
ABNORMALITIES; CARDIAC ANOMALIES; RENAL DYSPLASIA; RENAL
ARTERY STENOSIS; CIRRHOSIS AND PORTAL HYPERTENSION; INTRAHEP-
ATIC CHOLESTASIS; PERIPHERAL PULMONARY STENOSIS; ABSENT RE-
FLEXES; MILD MENTAL RETARDATION; VERTEBRAL AND SKELETAL AB-
NORMALITIES; HYPERCHOLESTEROLEMIA; HYPERLIPIDEMIA

Syndrome: CYSTIC FIBROSIS

Inheritance: AR
Locus(i): 7q31.2 (CFTR)

Component tumors: ADENOCARCINOMA OF THE ILEUM
Clinical features: CHRONIC LUNG INFECTIONS; COR PULMONALE; INFER-
TILITY; PANCREATIC INSUFFICIENCY; MECONIUM ILEUS IN NEONATES;
BILIARY CIRRHOSIS; DISTAL INTESTINAL OBSTRUCTION SYNDROME;
RECURRENT EPISODES OF ABDOMINAL PAIN; PALPABLE MASS IN RIGHT
ILIAC FOSSA; BILIARY TRACT OBSTRUCTION; DISTAL COMMON BILE
DUCT STRICTURE; EMPHYSEMA; MICROSCOPIC NEPHROCALCINOSIS;
HYPERCALCINURIA; DECREASE IN PANCREATIC FLUID AND SALT SE-
CRETION; DIAGNOSED BY MEASUREMENT OF SWEAT ELECTROLYTES

Syndrome: DYSKERATOSIS
CONGENITA

Inheritance: XLR
Locus(i): Xq28 (DKC)

Component tumors: SQUAMOUS CELL CANCER OF MUCOSA OR SKIN;
PANCREATIC ADENOCARCINOMA; OTHER INTERNAL MALIGNANCIES;
ESOPHAGEAL CANCER
Clinical features: (SEE CANCERS OF THE SKIN)

Syndrome: FAMILIAL ADENOMA-
TOUS POLYPOSIS (FAP, GARDNER
SYNDROME)

Inheritance: AD
Locus(i): 5q21-q22 (APC)

**Component tumors: COLORECTAL CANCER; PERIAMPULLARY CARCI-
NOMA; HEPATOBLASTOMA; BILE DUCT CARCINOMA**; OSTEOSARCO-
MA; ADRENAL CARCINOMA; THYROID CARCINOMA; MANDIBULAR OS-
TEOMA

Clinical features: DESMOIDS; EPIDERMOID CYSTS; SEBACEOUS CYSTS; CONGENITAL HYPERTROPHY OF RETINAL PIGMENT EPITHELIUM (CHRPE); MULTIPLE COLON POLYPS; MULTIPLE DUODENAL POLYPS; MESENTERIC FIBROMATOSIS

Syndrome: FAMILIAL GASTRIC CANCER	**Inheritance:** AD

Component tumors: GASTRIC CANCER
Clinical features: GASTRIC DYSPLASIA; CHRONIC ATROPHIC GASTRITIS; INTESTINAL METAPLASIA

Syndrome: GLYCOGEN STORAGE DISEASE I	**Inheritance:** AR

Component tumors: HEPATOCELLULAR CARCINOMA; HEPATOBLAS-TOMA
Clinical features: OBESITY; ABNORMAL DISTENSION DUE TO HE-PATOSPLENOMEGALY; HEPATIC ADENOMAS; RENAL FAILURE; HYPO-GLYCEMIA; PANCREATITIS; PULMONARY HYPERTENSION; GOUT; HYPER-LIPIDEMIA

Syndrome: GLYCOGEN STORAGE DISEASE IV	**Inheritance:** AR

Component tumors: POSTCIRRHOTIC HEPATOCELLULAR CARCINOMA; HEPATOCELLULAR CARCINOMA
Clinical features: HEPATIC FAILURE; CARDIOMYOPATHY; DEATH BY AGE 4

Syndrome: HEMOCHROMATOSIS	**Inheritance:** AR **Locus(i):** 6p21.3 (HLA-H)

Component tumors: PRIMARY HEPATOCELLULAR CARCINOMA
Clinical features: HEPATOSPLENOMEGALY; HYPERMELANOTIC PIGMENTA-TION; CARDIOMYOPATHY; CIRRHOSIS; DIABETES; HYPOGONADISM; ARTHROPATHY; DIAGNOSED BY INCREASED FERRITIN, SERUM IRON, AND TIBC; INCREASED URINARY IRON EXCRETION AFTER DEFEROXAM-INE

Syndrome: HEREDITARY BREAST-OVARIAN CANCER SYNDROME	**Inheritance:** AD **Locus(i):** 17q21 (BRCA1) AND 13q12-13 (BRCA2)

Component tumors: BREAST CANCER; OVARIAN CANCER; INCREASED RISK FOR PROSTATE CANCER AND **COLORECTAL CANCER**
Clinical features: (SEE CANCERS OF THE REPRODUCTIVE SYSTEM)

Syndrome: HEREDITARY HEPATO-CELLULAR CARCINOMA	**Inheritance:** AD (SEGREGATION ANALYSIS OF 490 FAMILIES)

Component tumors: HEPATOCELLULAR CARCINOMA
Clinical features: MICRONODULAR CIRRHOSIS; SUBACUTE VIRAL HEPATITIS; HBV ASSOCIATED

Syndrome: HEREDITARY NONPOLY-POSIS COLORECTAL CANCER	**Inheritance:** AD **Locus(i):** MULTIPLE LOCI ON CHROM 2, 3 AND 7 (MLH1, MSH2, PMS1, PMS2)

Component tumors: CARCINOMAS OF THE COLON, ENDOMETRIUM, **STOMACH**, OVARY, **HEPATOBILIARY SYSTEM**, KIDNEY, AND BREAST (SEE CHAPTER 4)
Clinical features: EARLY AGE OF ONSET; BILATERAL AND MULTIFOCAL

Syndrome: HEREDITARY PANCREATITIS	**Inheritance:** AD

Component tumors: PANCREATIC CARCINOMA
Clinical features: ABDOMINAL PAIN DUE TO PANCREATITIS AND ITS COMPLICATIONS; INCREASED AMYLASE; PORTAL AND SPLENIC THROMBOSIS

Syndrome: KERATOSIS PALMARIS ET PLANTARIS WITH ESOPHAGEAL CANCER	**Inheritance:** AD

Component tumors: ESOPHAGEAL CANCER
Clinical features: KERATOSIS PALMARIS; KERATOSIS PLANTARIS; ORAL LEUKOPLAKIA

Syndrome: LI-FRAUMENI SYNDROME	**Inheritance:** AD **Locus(i):** 17p13.1 (p53)

Component tumors: RHABDOMYOSARCOMA; SOFT TISSUE SARCOMA; BREAST CANCER; BRAIN TUMORS; OSTEOSARCOMA; LEUKEMIA; ADRENOCORTICAL CARCINOMA; LYMPHOCYTIC LYMPHOMA; LUNG ADENOCARCINOMA, MELANOMA, GONADAL GERM CELL TUMORS; PROSTATE CARCINOMA; **PANCREATIC CARCINOMA**; LARYNGEAL CARCINOMA
Clinical features: (SEE CANCERS OF CONNECTIVE TISSUES)

Syndrome: MACROCEPHALY, MULTIPLE LIPOMAS AND HEMANGIOMATA (RUVALCABA-MYHRE-SMITH SYNDROME)	**Inheritance:** AD **Locus(i):** 10q22 (PTEN)

Oncology: INTESTINAL HAMARTOMATOUS POLYPS
Clinical features: MACROCEPHALY; HAMARTOMATOUS INTESTINAL POLYPS; CAFÉ AU LAIT SPOTS ON THE PENIS; LIPOMAS

Syndrome: MELANOMA, HEREDITARY	**Inheritance:** AD **Locus(i):** 1p36, 9p21 (CDKN2), 6q (CDK4)

Component tumors: MELANOMA, PANCREATIC CANCER
Clinical features: (SEE CANCERS OF THE SKIN)

Syndrome: MUIR-TORRE SYNDROME	**Inheritance:** AD **Locus(i):** MULTIPLE LOCI ON CHROM 2, 3 AND 7 (MLH1, MSH2, PMS1, PMS2)

Component tumors: SEBACEOUS SKIN TUMORS; **SMALL BOWEL CARCI-NOMA; CANCER OF THE COLON, STOMACH,** ENDOMETRIUM, KIDNEY, OVARIES, BLADDER, BREAST, LARYNX; KERATOACANTHOMATA

Syndrome: MULTIPLE ENDOCRINE NEOPLASIA, TYPE I	**Inheritance:** AD **Locus(i):** 11q13 (MEN1)

Component tumors: ISLET CELL TUMORS OF PANCREAS; PARATHYROID ADENOMAS; PITUITARY ADENOMAS; ADRENOCORTICAL ADENOMAS; LIPOMAS
Clinical features: (SEE CANCERS OF THE ENDOCRINE SYSTEM)

Syndrome: NEUROFIBROMATOSIS TYPE I	**Inheritance:** AD **Locus(i):** 17q11.2 (NF1)

Component tumors: PHEOCHROMOCYTOMA; MENINGIOMA; OPTIC GLIOMA; VESTIBULAR SCHWANNOMA (ACOUSTIC NEUROMA); HYPO-THALAMIC TUMOR; NEUROFIBROSARCOMA; RHABDOMYOSARCOMA; **DUODENAL CARCINOID**; SOMATOSTATINOMA; PARATHYROID ADENO-MA; LISCH NODULES (IRIS HAMARTOMAS); NEUROFIBROMAS; PLEXI-FORM NEUROMA
Clinical features: (SEE CANCERS OF THE NERVOUS SYSTEM AND EYE)

Syndrome: NEUROFIBROMATOSIS-PHEOCHROMOCYTOMA-DUODENAL CARCINOID SYNDROME	**Inheritance:** AD

Component tumors: DUODENAL CARCINOID TUMOR; NEUROFIBRO-MATOSIS; PHEOCHROMOCYTOMA
Clinical features: (SEE CANCERS OF THE NERVOUS SYSTEM AND EYE)

Syndrome: PANCREATIC CARCINOMA	**Inheritance:** AD

Component tumors: PANCREATIC CARCINOMA
Clinical features: FAMILIAL CLUSTERS OBSERVED (SEE TEXT)

Syndrome: PAPILLARY CARCINOMA OF THE THYROID	**Inheritance:** AD

Component tumors: PAPILLARY CARCINOMA OF THYROID; **COLORECTAL CANCERS** (REPORTED IN RELATIVES)
Clinical features: (SEE CANCERS OF THE ENDOCRINE SYSTEM)

Syndrome: PHEOCHROMOCYTOMA-ISLET CELL TUMOR SYNDROME   **Inheritance:** AD

Component tumors: PHEOCHROMOCYTOMA; **PANCREATIC ISLET CELL TUMOR**
Clinical features: SWEATING; HYPERTENSIVE RETINOPATHY; TACHYCARDIA; CHF; FAMILIAL PHEOCHROMOCYTOMA, USUALLY BILATERAL; EPISODIC HYPERTENSION; PROTEINURIA; HYPERCALCEMIA; (THIS SYNDROME APPEARS TO BE DISTINCT FROM MEN AND VHL)

Syndrome: POLYPOSIS, GASTRIC   **Inheritance:** AD

Component tumors: **GASTRIC ADENOCARCINOMA**; PROPENSITY TOWARD ADENOCARCINOMA
Clinical features: MULTIPLE GASTRIC POLYPS

Syndrome: POLYPOSIS, HAMARTO-MATOUS INTESTINAL (PEUTZ-JEGHERS SYNDROME, POLYPS AND SPOTS SYNDROME)   **Inheritance:** AD
Locus(i): 1p34-p36

Component tumors: **RARE MALIGNANT TRANSFORMATION OF SMALL INTESTINAL POLYPS;** INCREASED RISK FOR BREAST AND **PANCREATIC CARCINOMA**, BENIGN OVARIAN TUMORS, TESTICULAR TUMORS, AND PANCREATIC CANCER
Clinical features: MELANIN SPOTS: LIPS, BUCCAL MUCOSA, AND DIGITS; PIGMENTED MACULES WITHIN PREEXISTING PSORIATIC PLAQUES; NASAL POLYPS; GYNECOMASTIA WITH TESTIS TUMORS; URETERAL POLYPS; BLADDER POLYPS; RENAL PELVIS POLYPS; MULTIPLE INTESTINAL POLYPS; JEJUNAL POLYPS; INTUSSUSCEPTION; GI BLEEDING; BRONCHIAL POLYPS

Syndrome: POLYPOSIS COLI, JUVENILE TYPE   **Inheritance:** AD

Component tumors: **COLORECTAL CANCER** (NOT ARISING FROM POLYPS)
Clinical features: HAMARTOMATOUS POLYPS; MELENOTIC STOOLS; CONGENITAL CARDIAC ABNORMALITIES; MALROTATION OF THE GUT

Syndrome: SCLEROATROPHIC AND KERATOTIC DERMATOSIS OF LIMBS (SCLEROTYLOSIS)   **Inheritance:** AD
Locus(i): 4q28-q31

Component tumors: SQUAMOUS CELL CANCER AND **BOWEL CANCER**
Clinical features: (SEE CANCERS OF THE SKIN)

Syndrome: TURCOT SYNDROME   **Inheritance:** AD AND AR
Locus(i): MULTIPLE LOCI (MLH1, MSH2, APC)

Component tumors: COLORECTAL CANCER; GLIOBLASTOMA; ASTROCY-TOMA; MEDULLOBLASTOMA; **GASTRIC CANCER**; SCALP BASAL CELL CARCINOMAS
Clinical features: AVERAGE AGE 18; COLON POLYPS; CAFÉ AU LAIT SPOTS; HEPATIC NODULAR HYPERPLASIA

Syndrome: TYROSINEMIA, TYPE I   **Inheritance:** AR

Component tumors: HEPATOCELLULAR CARCINOMA
Clinical features: GROWTH FAILURE; NODULAR CIRRHOSIS; RENAL TUBU-LAR NEPHROPATHY; HYPOGLYCEMIA; HYPOPHOSPHATEMIC RICKETS; INCREASED EXCRETION OF TYROSINE METABOLITES; INCREASED SERUM ALPHA-FETOPROTEIN POSTNATALLY

Syndrome: VON HIPPEL-LINDAU   **Inheritance:** AD
SYNDROME   **Locus(i):** 3p25-p26 (VHL)

Component tumors: PHEOCHROMOCYTOMA; CEREBELLAR HEMAN-GIOBLASTOMA; HYPERNEPHROMA; ADRENAL HEMANGIOMAS; PUL-MONARY HEMANGIOMAS; LIVER HEMANGIOMAS; **PANCREATIC CARCI-NOMA**; **PANCREATIC ISLET CELL TUMOR**; INTRACRANIAL HEMANGIOBLASTOMA; SPINAL CORD HEMANGIOMA
Clinical features: (SEE CANCERS OF THE NERVOUS SYSTEM AND EYE)

CANCERS OF THE GENITOURINARY SYSTEM

Syndrome: BECKWITH-WIEDEMANN   **Inheritance:** AD WITH
SYNDROME   INCOMPLETE PENETRANCE
     Locus(i): 11p15.5 (?IGF2, H19, p57)

Component tumors: ADRENOCORTICAL CARCINOMA; **NEPHROBLAS-TOMA (WILMS' TUMOR)**; HEPATOBLASTOMA; RHABDOMYOSARCOMA; CONGENITAL GASTRIC TERATOMA
Clinical features: UMBILICAL HERNIA (EXOMPHALOS); MACROGLOSSIA; GIGANTISM; HEMIHYPERTROPHY; ABNORMAL FACIAL FEATURES; OVER-GROWTH OF EXTERNAL GENITALIA; VISCEROMEGALY; HEPATOMEGALY; ADVANCED BONE AGE; NEONATAL HYPOGLYCEMIA; ADRENOCORTICAL CYTOMEGALY; CARDIAC DEFECTS AND OTHER ABNORMALITIES

Syndrome: FAMILIAL HEMIHY-   **Inheritance:** AD VS. MULTI-
PERTROPHY   FACTORIAL

Component tumors: WILMS' TUMOR
Clinical features: HEMIHYPERTROPHY; IPSILATERAL RENAL ENLARGE-MENT; CYSTS; HYDRONEPHROSIS; SCOLIOSIS; MYELOMENINGOCELE

Syndrome: FAMILIAL
HYDRONEPHROSIS

Inheritance: AD
Locus(i): LINKED TO 6p

Component tumors: CONGENITAL RENAL SARCOMA
Clinical features: HYDRONEPHROSIS; CONGENITAL MEGALOURETERS
DUE TO PELVIURETERIC JUNCTION OBSTRUCTION

Syndrome: FAMILIAL RENAL CELL
CARCINOMA

Inheritance: AD
Locus(i): 3p14 translocations

Component tumors: RENAL CELL CARCINOMA
Clinical features: BILATERAL OR MULTIPLE PRIMARY TUMORS; PAPIL-
LARY TYPE ASSOCIATED WITH GERMLINE MET MUTATIONS

Syndrome: HEREDITARY BLADDER
CANCERS

Inheritance: AD
Locus(i): 11p

Component tumors: TRANSITIONAL CELL BLADDER CARCINOMA
Clinical features: DESCRIBED IN FOUR FAMILIES

Syndrome: HEREDITARY BREAST-
OVARIAN CANCER SYNDROME

Inheritance: AD
Locus(i): 17q21 (BRCA1) AND
13q12-13 (BRCA2)

Component tumors: BREAST CANCER; OVARIAN CANCER; INCREASED
RISK FOR **PROSTATE CANCER** AND COLON CANCER
Clinical features: (SEE CANCERS OF THE REPRODUCTIVE SYSTEM)

Syndrome: HEREDITARY NONPOLY-
POSIS COLON CANCER

Inheritance: AD
Locus(i): MULTIPLE LOCI ON
CHROM 2,3 AND 7 (MLH1, MSH2,
PMS1, PMS2)

Component tumors: CARCINOMAS OF THE COLON, ENDOMETRIUM, STOM-
ACH, OVARIES, HEPATOBILIARY SYSTEM, **KIDNEY (RENAL CELL CARCI-
NOMA AND TRANSITIONAL CELL RENAL PELVIC TUMORS)** AND
BREAST
Clinical features: (SEE CANCERS OF THE GASTROINTESTINAL SYSTEM)

Syndrome: LI-FRAUMENI
SYNDROME

Inheritance: AD
Locus(i): 17p13.1 (p53)

Component tumors: RHABDOMYOSARCOMA; SOFT TISSUE SARCOMA;
BREAST CANCER; BRAIN TUMORS; OSTEOSARCOMA; LEUKEMIA;
ADRENOCORTICAL CARCINOMA; LYMPHOCYTIC LYMPHOMA; LUNG
ADENOCARCINOMA; MELANOMA; GONADAL GERM CELL TUMORS;
PROSTATE CARCINOMA; PANCREATIC CARCINOMA; LARYNGEAL CAR-
CINOMA
Clinical features: (SEE CANCERS OF CONNECTIVE TISSUES)

Syndrome: MUIR-TORRE SYNDROME **Inheritance:** AD
Locus(i): MULTIPLE LOCI ON
CHROM 2, 3 AND 7 (MLH1, MSH2,
PMS1, PMS2)

Component tumors: SEBACEOUS SKIN TUMORS; SMALL BOWEL CARCINO-
MA; CARCINOMA OF THE COLON, STOMACH, ENDOMETRIUM, **KIDNEY
(RENAL CELL CARCINOMA AND TRANSITIONAL CELL RENAL PELVIC
TUMORS)**, OVARIES, BLADDER, BREAST, LARYNX; KERATOACAN-
THOMATA
Clinical features: (SEE CANCERS OF THE GASTROINTESTINAL SYSTEM)

Syndrome: MULTIPLE HAMARTOMA **Inheritance:** AD
(COWDEN) SYNDROME **Locus(i):** 10q22-q23 (PTEN)

Component tumors: DYSPLASTIC CEREBELLAR GANGLIOCYTOMA;
BREAST CANCER; PRIMARY NEUROENDOCRINE (MERKEL CELL) TUMOR;
SKIN CARCINOMA; **RENAL CELL CARCINOMA**; THYROID CANCER
Clinical features: (SEE CANCERS OF THE REPRODUCTIVE SYSTEM)

Syndrome: RENAL HAMARTOMAS, **Inheritance:** AR
NEPHROBLATOMATOSIS, AND
FETAL GIGANTISM

Component tumors: WILMS' TUMOR; BILATERAL RENAL HAMARTOMAS
Clinical features: DYSMORPHIC FEATURES; MACROSOMIA; BACKWARD
DISPLACEMENT OF EYEBALL (ENOPTHALMOS); BROAD DEPRESSED
NASAL BRIDGE; ANTEVERTED UPPER LIP; VISCEROMEGALY; CRYP-
TORCHIDISM IN MALES

Syndrome: TUBEROUS SCLEROSIS, **Inheritance:** AD
TYPES I AND II **Locus(i):** 9q32-q34 (TSC1); 16p13.3
(TSC2)

Component tumors: MYOCARDIAL RHABDOMYOMA; MULTIPLE BILATER-
AL RENAL ANGIOMYOLIPOMA; **WILMS' TUMOR**; CARDIAC AND OLFAC-
TORY HAMARTOMAS; EPENDYMOMA; ASTROCYTOMA; RETINAL PHAKO-
MAS
Clinical features: (SEE CANCERS OF CONNECTIVE TISSUES)

Syndrome: VON HIPPEL-LINDAU **Inheritance:** AD
SYNDROME **Locus(i):** 3p25-p26 (VHL)

Component tumors: PHEOCHROMOCYTOMA; SPORADIC CEREBELLAR
HEMANGIOBLASTOMA; **RENAL CELL CARCINOMAS**; ADRENAL HE-
MANGIOMAS; PULMONARY HEMANGIOMAS; LIVER HEMANGIOMAS;
PANCREATIC CARCINOMA; PANCREATIC ISLET CELL TUMOR; INTRACRA-
NIAL HEMANGIOBLASTOMA; SPINAL CORD HEMANGIOMA
Clinical features: (SEE CANCERS OF THE NERVOUS SYSTEM AND EYE)

Syndrome: WAGR SYNDROME   **Inheritance:** AD
Locus(i): 11p13

Component tumors: WILMS' TUMOR
Clinical features: ANIRIDIA; GENITOURINARY ABNORMALITIES; MENTAL RETARDATION; (CONTIGUOUS GENE SYNDROME WITH SYMPTOMS DEPENDENT ON SIZE OF DELETION)

Syndrome: WILMS' TUMOR AND   **Inheritance:** AD
PSEUDOHEMAPHRODITISM

Component tumors: WILMS' TUMOR; GONADOBLASTOMA
Clinical features: MALE PSEUDOHEMAPHRODITISM

Syndrome: WILMS' TUMOR, OTHER   **Inheritance:** AD
HEREDITARY TYPES   **Locus(i):** 11p15.5; 17q12-21

Component tumors: WILMS' TUMOR

CANCERS OF THE HEMATOLOGIC AND LYMPHATIC SYSTEMS

Syndrome: ATAXIA-PANCYTOPENIA   **Inheritance:** AD
SYNDROME

Component tumors: ACUTE MYELOMONOCYTIC LEUKEMIA
Clinical features: CEREBELLAR ATAXIA;HYPOPLASTIC ANEMIA AND OTHER NEUROLOGIC ABNORMALITIES; LEUKEMIA DESCRIBED IN TWO FAMILIES

Syndrome: ATAXIA TELANGIEC-   **Inheritance:** AR
TASIA; AT   **Locus(i):** 11q22.3 (ATM)

Component tumors: LEUKEMIA; EPITHELIAL CANCERS; MEDULLOBLASTOMAS; GLIOMAS; INCREASED BREAST CANCER RISK IN HETEROZYGOTES
Clinical features: CEREBELLAR ATAXIA; OCULOMOTOR APRAXIA; DYSTONIA; PROGRESSIVE NEUROLOGIC IMPAIRMENT; OCULOCUTANEOUS TELANGIECTASIA; PULMONARY AND SINUS INFECTIONS

Syndrome: BERLIN BREAKAGE   **Inheritance:** AR
SYNDROME

Component tumors: STRONG PREDISPOSITION TO MALIGNANCY; **LEUKEMIA**; INCREASED CANCER RISK IN HETEROZYGOTES
Clinical features: SEE NIJMEGAN SYNDROME (SEMANOVA SYNDROME) PAGE 351; PROBABLY DISTINCT FROM ATAXIA-TELANGIECTASIA

Syndrome: BLOOM SYNDROME

Inheritance: AR
Locus(i): 15q26.1 (BLM)

Component tumors: LEUKEMIAS; LYMPHOMAS; GASTROINTESTINAL, LARYNGEAL, AND CERVICAL CANCERS
Clinical features: GROWTH DEFICIENCY; TELANGIECTASIA; ERYTHEMA; LONG THIN FACE; MEDIAL DEVIATION OF FINGERS (CLINODACTYLY); IMMUNE DEFICIENCY CAUSING MULTIPLE INFECTIONS; OTHER ABNORMALITIES

Syndrome: CARTILAGE-HAIR-HYPOPLASIA SYNDROME

Inheritance: AR WITH INCOMPLETE PENETRANCE

Component tumors: INCREASED RISK OF MALIGNANCY; **LYMPHOMA**
Clinical features: SHORT LIMBED DWARFISM; HYPOPLASIA OF CARTILAGE AND HAIR; CHARACTERISTIC IMMUNODEFICIENCY AND OTHER FEATURES; ORGINALLY DESCRIBED BY McKUSICK

Syndrome: CELIAC SPRUE

Inheritance: AR VS. MULTI-FACTORIAL

Component tumors: SMALL BOWEL AND OTHER GI CANCERS; **LYMPHOMA**
Clinical features: (SEE CANCERS OF THE GASTROINTESTINAL SYSTEM)

Syndrome: CHEDIAK-HIGASHI SYNDROME

Inheritance: AR

Component tumors: MALIGNANT LYMPHOMA; LEUKEMIA
Clinical features: ALBINISM; NYSTAGMUS; UVEAL HYPOPIGMENTATION; PERIPHERAL NEUROPATHY; DEFECTIVE NEUTROPHILS CAUSING INFECTION; BLEEDING DIATHESIS; PATIENTS RARELY SURVIVE PAST AGE 20

Syndrome: CHRONIC MYELOCYTIC LEUKEMIA-LIKE SYNDROME, FAMILIAL

Inheritance: ?AD

Component tumors: FAMILIAL CHRONIC MYELOCYTIC LEUKEMIA-LIKE SYNDROME
Clinical features: FAMILIAL SYNDROME WITH LEUKOCYTOSIS, LEADING TO DEATH IN SEVERAL FAMILIES DESCRIBED; NO PHILADELPHIA CHROMOSOME

Syndrome: DIAMOND-BLACKFAN SYNDROME

Inheritance: AR, ALSO DOMINANT FORMS

Component tumors: INCREASED RISK FOR LEUKEMIA
Clinical features: SHORT STATURE; THICK UPPER LIP; HYPERTELORISM; "SNUB" NOSE; CONGENITAL HYPOPLASTIC ANEMIA WITH NORMAL WHITE BLOOD CELL AND PLATELET COUNTS

Syndrome: DOWN SYNDROME   **Inheritance:** AUTOSOMAL

Component tumors: ACUTE LEUKEMIA
Clinical features: CHARACTERISTIC FACIAL FEATURES; SINGLE PALMAR CREASE; CARDIAC ANOMALIES; SHORT STATURE

Syndrome: DUNCAN SYNDROME   **Inheritance:** XLR
(X-LINKED LYMPHOPROLIFERATIVE
DISEASE)

Component tumors: LYMPHOMA
Clinical features: PHARYNGITIS; HEPATOSPLENOMEGALY; FEVER; LYMPHADENOPATHY; FATAL INFECTIOUS MONONUCLEOSIS; COMBINED VARIABLE IMMUNODEFICIENCY; NATURAL KILLER CELL DEFICIENCY; HYPOGAMMAGLOBULINEMIA

Syndrome: ERYTHROLEUKEMIA,   **Inheritance:** AD
FAMILIAL

Component tumors: ERYTHROID LEUKEMIA
Clinical features: INEFFECTIVE HYPERPLASTIC ERYTHROPOIESIS; MEGALOBLASTOSIS; MYELODYSPLASIA WITH SIDEROBLASTOSIS

Syndrome: FAMILIAL HISTIO-   **Inheritance:** AR OR XL
CYTOSIS (LETTERER-SIWE DISEASE)

Component tumors: LEUKEMIA OR LYMPHOMA
Clinical features: FAILURE TO THRIVE; ANEMIA; NEUTROPENIA; DIARRHEA; HEPATOSPLENOMEGALY; OCCASIONAL RASH; HYPERLIPIDEMIA; HISTIOCYTIC INFILTRATION INVOLVING NERVOUS SYSTEM

Syndrome: FAMILIAL HODGKIN'S   **Inheritance:** ?AR
DISEASE

Component tumors: HODGKIN'S DISEASE
Clinical features: MULTIPLE FAMILIES DESCRIBED

Syndrome: FANCONI ANEMIA   **Inheritance:** AR
    Locus(i): 16q24 (FACA); 9q22 (FACC);
    3p22-26 (FACD)

Component tumors: LEUKEMIA
Clinical features: PANCYTOPENIA; SMALL STATURE; BRUISABILITY; HYPERPIGMENTATION; CAFÉ AU LAIT SPOTS; MICROCEPHALY; STRABISMUS; MICROPHTHALMIA; EAR ANOMALY; DEAFNESS; CONGENITAL HEART DEFECT; KIDNEY MALFORMATION; HYPERGONADOTROPIC HYPOGONADISM; CRYTORCHIDISM; MENTAL RETARDATION; RADIAL APLASIA; THUMB APLASIA; OTHER PHENOTYPIC ABNORMALITIES; CHROMOSOMAL BREAKAGE SYNDROME

Syndrome: KOSTMANN SYNDROME   **Inheritance:** AR

Component tumors: ACUTE MONOCYTIC LEUKEMIA
Clinical features: LETHAL BEFORE AGE 3 YEARS; AGRANULOCYTOSIS; IN-
FECTIONS; HYPERGAMMAGLOBULINEMIA; TREATED WITH G-CSF

Syndrome: LEUKEMIA, ACUTE   **Inheritance:** AD
MYELOCYTIC   **Locus(i):** 21q, 16q

Component tumors: ACUTE LEUKEMIA
Clinical features: MULTIPLE FAMILIES DESCRIBED

Syndrome: LI-FRAUMENI   **Inheritance:** AD
SYNDROME   **Locus(i):** 17p13.1 (p53)

Component tumors: RHABDOMYOSARCOMA; SOFT TISSUE SARCOMA;
BREAST CANCER; BRAIN TUMORS; OSTEOSARCOMA; LEUKEMIA;
ADRENOCORTICAL CARCINOMA; **LYMPHOCYTIC LYMPHOMA**; LUNG
ADENOCARCINOMA, MELANOMA, GONADAL GERM CELL TUMORS;
PROSTATE CARCINOMA; PANCREATIC CARCINOMA; LARYNGEAL CARCI-
NOMA
Clinical features: (SEE CANCERS OF CONNECTIVE TISSUES)

Syndrome: MACROGLOBULINEMIA,   **Inheritance:** AD
WALDENSTRÖM'S

Component tumors: LUNG ADENOCARCINOMA; **OTHER LYMPHOPROLIF-
ERATIVE DISEASES**
Clinical features: POLYNEUROPATHY; WALDENSTRÖM'S MACROGLOBU-
LINEMIA; HYPERCOAGUABLE STATE; FAMILIES WITH WALDENSTRÖM'S
MACROGLOBULINEMIA AND LUNG CANCER HAVE BEEN DESCRIBED;
LUNG CANCERS MAY BE ON THE BASIS OF IMMUNE DEFICIT

Syndrome: MAST CELL DISEASE   **Inheritance:** AD

Component tumors: MAST CELL LEUKEMIA
Clinical features: PRURITIS; FLUSHING; TACHYCARDIA; UTICARIA PIG-
MENTOSA; CUTANEOUS MASTOCYTOSIS; BULLOUS MASTOCYTOSIS;
SYSTEMIC MASTOCYTOSIS MAY AFFECT BONE, GI, LYMPHATICS,
SPLEEN, AND LIVER

Syndrome: MICROCEPHALY WITH   **Inheritance:** AR
NORMAL INTELLIGENCE, IMMUNO-
DEFICIENCY, AND LYMPHORETICU-
LAR MALIGNANCIES (SEMANOVA
SYNDROME / NIJMEGAN BREAKAGE
SYNDROME)

Component tumors: INCREASED RISK FOR **ACUTE LYMPHOBLASTIC
LEUKEMIA; MALIGNANT LYMPHOMA**

Clinical features: MICROCEPHALY; GROWTH RETARDATION; "BIRD-LIKE" FACE; HUMORAL AND CELLULAR IMMUNODEFICIENCY; MAY HAVE FEATURES OF ATAXIA-TELANGIECTASIA

Syndrome: MYELOMA, MULTIPLE   **Inheritance:** AR OR AD

Component tumors: MULTIPLE MYELOMA
Clinical features: FAMILIAL CLUSTERS AND SIB PAIRS IN MULTIPLE CASE REPORTS; SOMETIMES INCLUDES INCREASED M COMPONENT AS ONLY FEATURE

Syndrome: N SYNDROME   **Inheritance:** XL
                                  Locus(i): Xp21.1-22.3

Component tumors: LYMPHOBLASTIC LEUKEMIA WITH MEDIASTINAL MASS
Clinical features: VERY RARE SYNDROME; VISUAL IMPAIRMENT; LATERALLY OVERLAPPING UPPER EYELIDS; DEAFNESS; ABNORMAL AURICLES; OTHER ABNORMALITIES; INCREASED CHROMOSOME BREAKAGE

Syndrome: NUCLEOSIDE PHOS-   **Inheritance:** AD
PHORYLASE DEFICIENCY   **Locus(i):** 14q13.1 (NP)

Component tumors: B-IMMUNOBLASTIC TYPE MALIGNANT LYMPHOMA
Clinical features: IMMUNE DEFICIENCY WITH NEUROLOGICAL ABNORMALITIES (SPASTIC TETRAPARESIS); HYPOURICEMIA

Syndrome: PANCREATIC INSUFFI-   **Inheritance:** AR
CIENCY AND BONE MARROW
DYSFUNCTION (SCHWACHMAN
SYNDROME)

Component tumors: PREDISPOSITION TO LEUKEMIAS
Clinical features: PANCYTOPENIA; PANCREATIC INSUFFICIENCY AND DWARFISM; SKELETAL ABNORMALITIES; RECURRENT INFECTIONS

Syndrome: POLYCYTHEMIA RUBRA   **Inheritance:** ?AR
VERA; PRV

Component tumors: HEMATOLOGIC CANCERS
Clinical features: RARE FAMILIES WITH POLYCYTHEMIA VERA, ERYTHROCYTOSIS AND OTHER SYMPTOMS

Syndrome: SEVERE COMBINED   **Inheritance:** XLR AND AR
IMMUNODEFICIENCY DISEASE,
X-LINKED (INCLUDING ADENOSINE
DEAMINASE DEFICIENCY)

Component tumors: INCREASED RISK FOR LYMPHOMA
Clinical features: COMBINED IMMUNODEFICIENCY; PAUCITY OF LYMPHOID TISSUE; RECURRENT SINUSITIS, OTITIS MEDIA, BRONCHITIS,

PNEUMONIA; SEVERE VARICELLA; CHRONIC PAPILLOMAVIRUS INFEC-
TIONS; NORMAL CONCENTRATIONS OF SERUM Ig's; DECREASED NUM-
BERS OF CD4(+) AND CD8(+) T-LYMPHOCYTES

Syndrome: WISKOTT-ALDRICH SYNDROME	**Inheritance:** AR; MOST CASES X-LINKED

Component tumors: LYMPHOMA AND OTHER LYMPHOID CANCERS
Clinical features: ECZEMA; THROMBOCYTOPENIA; BLOODY DIARRHEA;
DEATH IN FIRST DECADE DUE TO INFECTIONS; LOW IgM AND DEFEC-
TIVE ANTIBODY PRODUCTION

Syndrome: WT LIMB-BLOOD SYNDROME	**Inheritance:** AD

Component tumors: LEUKEMIA
Clinical features: IRREGULAR HYPERPIGMENTATION; SENSORINEURAL
HEARING LOSS; RADIOULNAR SYNOSTOSIS; FIFTH FINGER CLIN-
ODACTYLY; RADIAL DEFECTS; HYPOPLASTIC/ABSENT THUMBS; FINGER
FLEXION CONTRACTURES; HYPOPLASTIC ANEMIA; PANCYTOPENIA; NO
CHROMOSOME BREAKAGE; SIMILAR PHENOTYPE TO FANCONI'S ANE-
MIA BUT DOMINANT TRANSMISSION

CANCERS OF THE NERVOUS SYSTEM AND EYE

Syndrome: ATAXIA TELANGIEC-TASIA; AT	**Inheritance:** AR **Locus(i):** 11q22.3 (ATM)

Component tumors: LEUKEMIA; EPITHELIAL CANCERS; **MEDULLOBLAS-
TOMAS; GLIOMAS;** INCREASED BREAST CANCER RISK IN HETEROZY-
GOTES
Clinical features: (SEE CANCERS OF THE HEMATOLOGIC AND LYMPHATIC
SYSTEMS)

Syndrome: BASAL CELL NEVUS (GORLIN) SYNDROME	**Inheritance:** AD **Locus(i):** 9q31 (PTCH)

Component tumors: BASAL CELL CARCINOMA; CARDIAC FIBROMA; OVAR-
IAN FIBROMATA; OVARIAN CARCINOMA; **MEDULLOBLASTOMA**
Clinical features: (SEE CANCERS OF THE SKIN)

Syndrome: BLUE RUBBER BLEB NEVUS	**Inheritance:** AD

Component tumors: CEREBELLAR MEDULLOBLASTOMA
Clinical features: PAINFUL BLEEDING SKIN HEMANGIOMAS, MAY ALSO BE
VISCERAL

Syndrome: CEREBRAL SARCOMA   **Inheritance:** AD

Component tumors: CEREBRAL FIBROSARCOMA
Clinical features: FOUR CASES IN TWO FAMILIES DESCRIBED

Syndrome: FAMILIAL GLIOMAS   **Inheritance:** AD VS. AR

**Component tumors: GLIOBLASTOMA MULTIFORME (OR OTHER ASTRO-
CYTOMA) OF BRAIN**
Clinical features: FAMILIAL GLIOMAS DESCRIBED IN MULTIPLE SIB PAIRS
AND IN MULTIPLEX FAMILIES (SEE TEXT)

Syndrome: FAMILIAL MENINGIOMA   **Inheritance:** AD
                                                       Locus(i): 22q12.3-qter

Component tumors: MENINGIOMA
Clinical features: CAN OCCUR WITHOUT CLINICAL FEATURES OF NEU-
ROFIBROMATOSIS

Syndrome: LI-FRAUMENI   **Inheritance:** AD
SYNDROME   **Locus(i):** 17p13.1 (p53)

Component tumors: RHABDOMYOSARCOMA; SOFT TISSUE SARCOMA;
BREAST CANCER; **BRAIN TUMORS**; OSTEOSARCOMA; LEUKEMIA; AD-
RENOCORTICAL CARCINOMA; LYMPHOCYTIC LYMPHOMA; LUNG ADE-
NOCARCINOMA, MELANOMA, GONADAL GERM CELL TUMORS; PROS-
TATE CARCINOMA; PANCREATIC CARCINOMA; LARYNGEAL CARCINOMA
Clinical features: (SEE CANCERS OF CONNECTIVE TISSUES)

Syndrome: MELANOMA-ASTRO-   **Inheritance:** AD
CYTOMA SYNDROME

Component tumors: CUTANEOUS MALIGNANT MELANOMA; **CEREBRAL
ASTROCYTOMA; OTHER CNS TUMORS**
Clinical features: (SEE CANCERS OF THE SKIN)

Syndrome: MULTIPLE ENDOCRINE   **Inheritance:** AD
NEOPLASIA, TYPE 2B   **Locus(i):** 10q11.2 (RET)

Component tumors: MULTIPLE NEUROMAS; PHEOCHROMOCYTOMA;
MEDULLARY THYROID CARCINOMA; (NO PARATHYROID DISEASE)
Clinical features: (SEE CANCERS OF THE ENDOCRINE SYSTEM)

Syndrome: MULTIPLE HAMARTOMA   **Inheritance:** AD
(COWDEN) SYNDROME   **Locus(i):** 10q22-q23 (PTEN)

Component tumors: DYSPLASTIC CEREBELLAR GANGLIOCYTOMA;
BREAST CANCERS; PRIMARY NEUROENDOCRINE (MERKEL CELL) TU-
MORS; SKIN CARCINOMA; RENAL CELL ADENOCARCINOMA; THYROID
CANCER
Clinical features: (SEE CANCERS OF THE REPRODUCTIVE SYSTEM)

Syndrome: NAME SYNDROME (NEVI; **Inheritance:** AD
ATRIAL MYXOMA; MUCINOSIS OF **Locus(i):** LINKED TO CHROMOSOME
SKIN; ENDOCRINE OVERACTIVITY) 2p16

Component tumors: MYXOID LIPOSARCOMA; SUBCUTANEOUS MYXOID
NEUROFIBROMATA; PRIMARY ADRENOCORTICAL NODULAR DYSPLASIA;
VIRILIZING ADRENOCORTICAL CARCINOMA; LARGE-CELL CALCIFYING
SERTOLI CELL TUMOR; PITUITARY ADENOMA; **NASOPHARYNGEAL
SCHWANNOMA**; PROLACTIN-SECRETING PITUITARY ADENOMA
Clinical features: (SEE CANCERS OF THE ENDOCRINE SYSTEM)

Syndrome: NEUROBLASTOMA   **Inheritance:** AR

Component tumors: NEUROBLASTOMA
Clinical features: ABDOMINAL, PELVIC, HEAD AND NECK OR MEDIASTI-
NAL MASS; SUBCUTANEOUS BLUE TINGED NODULES; OPSOCLONUS-
POLYMYOCLONUS SYNDROME

Syndrome: NEUROFIBROMATOSIS   **Inheritance:** AD
TYPE I   **Locus(i):** 17q11.2 (NF1)

Component tumors: PHEOCHROMOCYTOMA; **OPTIC GLIOMA**; HYPO-
THALAMIC TUMOR; **NEUROFIBROSARCOMA**; RHABDOMYOSARCOMA;
DUODENAL CARCINOID; SOMATOSTATINOMA; PARATHYROID ADENO-
MA; LISCH NODULES (IRIS HAMARTOMAS); **NEUROFIBROMAS**; **PLEXI-
FORM NEUROMA**
Clinical features: NEUROFIBROMAS, CAFÉ AU LAIT SPOTS; AXILLARY
FRECKLING; LISCH NODULES; MACROCEPHALY; KYPHOSCOLIOSIS;
PSEUDOARTHROSES; RENAL ARTERY STENOSIS; MENTAL RETARDATION
(MILD IN 30%, MODERATE IN 3%)

Syndrome: NEUROFIBROMATOSIS   **Inheritance:** AD
TYPE II   **Locus(i):** 22q12.2 (NF2)

**Component tumors: BILATERAL VESTIBULAR SCHWANNOMAS
(ACOUSTIC NEUROMA); MENINGIOMA; GLIOMA; SCHWANNOMA**;
MACULAR HAMARTOMA
Clinical features: RARE CAFÉ AU LAIT SPOTS; "NF2" PLAQUES (i.e., RAISED
PIGMENTED SKIN LESIONS WITH EXCESS HAIR); SUBCUTANEOUS TU-
MORS ON PERIPHERAL NERVES; PAPILLARY SKIN NEUROFIBROMA; POS-
TERIOR SUBCAPSULAR OR NUCLEAR CATARACT; MACULAR HAMAR-
TOMA; HEARING LOSS; TINNITUS

Syndrome: NEUROFIBROMATOSIS   **Inheritance:** AD
TYPE III

**Component tumors: BILATERAL VESTIBULAR SCHWANNOMAS; POSTE-
RIOR FOSSA AND UPPER CERVICAL MENINGIOMAS; SPINAL/
PARASPINAL NEUROFIBROMAS**

Clinical features: PALMAR NEUROFIBROMAS, FEW PALE RELATIVELY LARGE CAFÉ AU LAIT SPOTS; RAPID AND FATAL CLINICAL COURSE

Syndrome: NEUROFIBROMATOSIS-PHEOCHROMOCYTOMA-DUODENAL CARCINOID SYNDROME	**Inheritance:** AD

Component tumors: DUODENAL CARCINOID TUMOR; **NEUROFIBRO-MATOSIS**; PHEOCHROMOCYTOMA
Clinical features: CAN PRESENT WITH OBSTRUCTIVE JAUNDICE SECONDARY TO DUODENAL CARCINOID; ?VARIANT OF NFI

Syndrome: PARAGANGLIOMATA	**Inheritance:** AD WITH GENOMIC IMPRINTING **Locus(i):** 11q22.3-q23.2

Component tumors: **PARAGANGLIOMATA**; CHEMODECTOMAS, CAROTID BODY TUMORS, GLOMUS JUGULAR TUMORS
Clinical features: (SEE CANCERS OF THE CARDIOVASCULAR SYSTEM)

Syndrome: RETINOBLASTOMA	**Inheritance:** AD **Locus(i):** 13q14

Component tumors: **RETINOBLASTOMA**; OSTEOSARCOMA; PINEALOMA
Clinical features: TUMORS MORE FREQUENTLY BILATERAL

Syndrome: MICROCEPHALY WITH NORMAL INTELLIGENCE, IMMUNO-DEFICIENCY, AND LYMPHORETIC-ULAR MALIGNANCIES (SEMANOVA SYNDROME / NIJMEGAN BREAKAGE SYNDROME)	**Inheritance:** AR

Component tumors: INCREASED RISK FOR ACUTE LYMPHOBLASTIC LEUKEMIA, MALIGNANT LYMPHOMA, ACUTE UNDIFFERENTIATED HE-MOBLASTOMA AND **NEUROBLASTOMA**
Clinical features: (SEE CANCERS OF THE HEMATOLOGIC AND LYMPHATIC SYSTEMS)

Syndrome: SUBEPENDYMOMA	**Inheritance:** ?AD

Component tumors: **SUBEPENDYMOMA**
Clinical features: RARE, SLOW-GROWING TUMOR DESCRIBED IN SEVERAL FAMILIAL CLUSTERS

Syndrome: TUBEROUS SCLEROSIS, TYPES I AND II	**Inheritance:** AD **Locus(i):** 9q32-q34 (TSC1);16p13.3 (TSC2)

Component tumors: MYOCARDIAL RHABDOMYOMA; MULTIPLE BILATER-AL RENAL ANGIOMYOLIPOMA; WILMS' TUMOR; CARDIAC AND OLFAC-TORY HAMARTOMAS; **EPENDYMOMA; ASTROCYTOMA; RETINAL PHAKOMAS**
Clinical features: (SEE CANCERS OF CONNECTIVE TISSUES)

Syndrome: TURCOT SYNDROME	**Inheritance:** AD AND AR **Locus(i):** MULTIPLE LOCI (MLH1, PMS2, APC)

Component tumors: COLON CANCER; **GLIOBLASTOMA; MEDULLOBLAS-TOMA; ASTROCYTOMA;** GASTRIC CANCER; SCALP BASAL CELL CARCI-NOMAS
Clinical features: (SEE CANCERS OF THE GASTROINTESTINAL SYSTEM)

Syndrome: VON HIPPEL-LINDAU SYNDROME	**Inheritance:** AD **Locus(i):** 3p25-p26 (VHL)

Component tumors: PHEOCHROMOCYTOMA; **CEREBELLAR HEMAN-GIOBLASTOMA**; RENAL CELL CARCINOMA; ADRENAL HEMANGIOMAS; PULMONARY HEMANGIOMAS; LIVER HEMANGIOMAS; PANCREATIC CARCINOMA; PANCREATIC ISLET CELL TUMOR; **INTRACRANIAL HE-MANGIOBLASTOMA; SPINAL CORD HEMANGIOMA**
Clinical features: MANIFESTATIONS INCLUDE: HEADACHES, VOMITING, AND NEUROLOGIC SYMPTOMS DUE TO CEREBELLAR LESIONS; NEURO-LOGIC SYMPTOMS DUE TO SPINAL CORD HEMANGIOBLASTOMAS; VIS-UAL IMPAIRMENT DUE TO RETINAL ANGIOMA; HEMATURIA DUE TO RE-NAL CARCINOMA; HYPERTENSION DUE TO PHEOCHROMOCYTOMA; TESTICULAR MASS DUE TO EPIDIDYMAL CYSTADENOMA

CANCERS OF THE REPRODUCTIVE SYSTEM

Syndrome: ATAXIA-TELANGIEC-TASIA; AT	**Inheritance:** AR **Locus(i):** 11q22.3 (ATM)

Component tumors: LEUKEMIA; EPITHELIAL CANCERS; MEDULLOBLAS-TOMAS; GLIOMAS; **INCREASED BREAST CANCER RISK IN HETEROZY-GOTES**
Clinical features: (SEE CANCERS OF THE HEMATOLOGIC AND LYMPHATIC SYSTEMS)

Syndrome: BASAL CELL NEVUS (GORLIN) SYNDROME	**Inheritance:** AD **Locus(i):** 9q31 (PTCH)

Component tumors: BASAL CELL CARCINOMA; CARDIAC FIBROMA; **OVARIAN FIBROMATA; OVARIAN CARCINOMA**; MEDULLOBLASTOMA
Clinical features: (SEE CANCERS OF THE SKIN)

Syndrome: BLOOM SYNDROME   **Inheritance:** AR
Locus(i): 15q26.1 (BLM)

Component tumors: LEUKEMIAS; LYMPHOMAS; GASTROINTESTINAL, LA-RYNGEAL, AND **CERVICAL CANCERS**
Clinical features: (SEE CANCERS OF THE HEMATOLOGIC AND LYMPHATIC SYSTEM)

Syndrome: BREAST CANCER, 11;22   **Inheritance:** AD
TRANSLOCATION ASSOCIATED

Component tumors: **BREAST CANCER**
Clinical features: BREAST CANCER DESCRIBED IN 5 OF 8 FAMILIES WITH CONSTITUTIONAL TRANSLOCATION t(11;22)(q23;q11)

Syndrome: COWDEN SYNDROME   **Inheritance:** AD
Locus(i): 10q22-q23 (PTEN)

Component tumors: DYSPLASTIC CEREBELLAR GANGLIOCYTOMA; **BREAST CANCER**; PRIMARY NEUROENDOCRINE (MERKEL CELL) TU-MORS; SKIN CARCINOMA; RENAL CELL CARCINOMA; THYROID CANCER
Clinical features: CUTANEOUS FACIAL PAPULES; MULTIPLE PAPILLOMAS APPEARING AS COBBLESTONE PAPULES; KERATOSES; NUMEROUS OTH-ER FEATURES; 50% RISK FOR BREAST CANCER AND POSSIBLY IN-CREASED RISK FOR OTHER CANCERS

Syndrome: GONADAL DYSGENESIS   **Inheritance:** AR, XL, YL, AD
SYNDROMES

Component tumors: **GONADOBLASTOMA; DYSGERMINOMA**
Clinical features: PHENOTYPIC FEMALES OR PHENOTYPIC MALES WITH ABNORMALITIES OF GENITALIA OR UNDESCENDED TESTES; TUMORS MAY FORM FROM DYSGENETIC GONADS; NUMEROUS SYNDROMES

Syndrome: HEREDITARY BREAST-   **Inheritance:** AD
OVARIAN CANCER SYNDROME   **Locus(i):** 17q21 (BRCA1) AND
13q12-13 (BRCA2)

Component tumors: **BREAST CANCER; OVARIAN CANCER;** INCREASED RISK FOR PROSTATE CANCER AND COLON CANCER
Clinical features: FREQUENT BILATERAL DISEASE; EARLY AGE OF ONSET

Syndrome: HEREDITARY NONPOLY-   **Inheritance:** AD
POSIS COLORECTAL CANCERS   **Locus(i):** MULTIPLE LOCI ON
CHROM 2, 3 AND 7 (MLH1, MSH2,
PMS1, PMS2)

Component tumors: CARCINOMAS OF THE COLON, ENDOMETRIUM, STOM-ACH, **OVARY**, HEPATOBILIARY SYSTEM, KIDNEY (RENAL CELL AND TRANSITIONAL CELL RENAL PELVIC TUMORS), AND **BREAST**
Clinical features: (SEE CANCERS OF THE GASTROINTESTINAL SYSTEM)

Syndrome: LEIOMYOMATA, HEREDI-TARY MULTIPLE, OF SKIN **Inheritance:** AD

Component tumors: MULTIPLE CUTANEOUS LEIOMYOMATA; **UTERINE LEIOMYOMATA**
Clinical features: MALIGNANT TRANSFORMATION RARE

Syndrome: LI-FRAUMENI SYNDROME **Inheritance:** AD
Locus(i): 17p13.1 (p53)

Component tumors: RHABDOMYOSARCOMA; SOFT TISSUE SARCOMA; **BREAST CANCER**; BRAIN TUMORS; OSTEOSARCOMA; LEUKEMIA; ADRENOCORTICAL CARCINOMA; LYMPHOCYTIC LYMPHOMA; LUNG ADENOCARCINOMA, MELANOMA, **GONADAL GERM CELL TUMORS**; PROSTATE CARCINOMA; PANCREATIC CARCINOMA; LARYNGEAL CARCINOMA
Clinical features: (SEE CANCERS OF CONNECTIVE TISSUES)

Syndrome: LICHEN SCLEROSIS ET ATROPHICUS (LSA) **Inheritance:** AD

Component tumors: **VULVAR** LSA MAY PREDISPOSE TO **SQUAMOUS CELL CARCINOMA;**
Clinical features: LICHEN SCLEROSIS ET ATROPHICUS, IVORY-COLORED POLYGONAL FLAT-TOPPED LICHENOID PLAQUES, PAPULES MAY COALESCE INTO ATROPHIC PLAQUES;

Syndrome: MUIR-TORRE SYNDROME **Inheritance:** AD
Locus(i): MULTIPLE LOCI ON CHROM 2, 3 AND 7 (MLH1, MSH2, PMS1, PMS2)

Component tumors: SEBACEOUS SKIN TUMORS; SMALL BOWEL CARCINOMA; CARCINOMA OF THE COLON, STOMACH, ENDOMETRIUM, KIDNEY, **OVARIES**, BLADDER, **BREAST**, LARYNX; KERATOACANTHOMATA
Clinical features: (SEE CANCERS OF THE GASTROINTESTINAL SYSTEM)

Syndrome: MULTIPLE ENCHONDRO-MATOSIS (OLLIER'S DISEASE) **Inheritance:** ?AD FORM

Component tumors: CHONDROSARCOMA; **RARELY ASSOCIATED WITH OVARIAN JUVENILE GRANULOSA CELL TUMOR**
Clinical features: (SEE CANCERS OF CONNECTIVE TISSUES)

Syndrome: MULTIPLE ENDOCRINE NEOPLASIA, TYPE I **Inheritance:** AD
Locus(i): 11q13 (MEN1)

Component tumors: BRONCHIAL CARCINOMA; THYMIC CARCINOMA; DUODENAL CARCINOID; BRONCHIAL CARCINOID; MALIGNANT SCHWANNOMA; **OVARIAN TUMOR;** LIPOMAS; GLUCAGANOMA; INSULINOMA; VASOINTESTINAL PEPTIDE TUMOR
Clinical features: (SEE CANCERS OF THE ENDOCRINE SYSTEM)

Syndrome: NAME SYNDROME (NEVI; **Inheritance:** AD
ATRIAL MYXOMA; MUCINOSIS OF **Locus(i):** LINKED TO CHROMOSOME
SKIN; ENDOCRINE OVERACTIVITY) 2p16

Component tumors: MYXOID LIPOSARCOMA; SUBCUTANEOUS MYXOID
NEUROFIBROMATA; PRIMARY ADRENOCORTICAL NODULAR DYSPLASIA;
VIRILIZING ADRENOCORTICAL CARCINOMA; **LARGE-CELL CALCIFY-
ING SERTOLI CELL TUMOR**; PITUITARY ADENOMA; NASOPHARYNGEAL
SCHWANNOMA; PROLACTIN-SECRETING PITUITARY ADENOMA
Clinical features: (SEE CANCERS OF THE ENDOCRINE SYSTEM)

Syndrome: OVARIAN TERATOMA   **Inheritance:** AD

Component tumors: OVARIAN TERATOMA
Clinical features: DERMOID CYSTS, USUALLY BILATERAL IN YOUNG
WOMEN

Syndrome: OVARIAN CANCER   **Inheritance:** AD
SYNDROME (SITE SPECIFIC)

Component tumors: OVARIAN EPITHELIAL CARCINOMA
Clinical features: MAY BE DISTINCT FROM HEREDITARY BREAST-OVARIAN
CANCER SYNDROME

Syndrome: POLYPOSIS, HAMARTO-   **Inheritance:** AD
MATOUS INTESTINAL (PEUTZ-   **Locus(i):** 1p34-36
JEGHERS SYNDROME, POLYPS AND
SPOTS SYNDROME)

Component tumors: RARE MALIGNANT TRANSFORMATION OF SMALL IN-
TESTINAL POLYPS; INCREASE IN **BREAST CARCINOMA, BENIGN OVARI-
AN TUMORS, TESTICULAR TUMORS**, AND PANCREATIC CANCERS
Clinical features: (SEE CANCERS OF THE GASTROINTESTINAL SYSTEM)

Syndrome: REIFENSTEIN   **Inheritance:** XLR
SYNDROME   **Locus(i):** (AR)

Component tumors: MALE BREAST CANCER
Clinical features: NORMAL XY KARYOTYPE; HYPOGONADISM; GYNECO-
MASTIA; HYPOSPADIAS

Syndrome: TESTICULAR TUMORS   **Inheritance:** ?AR

**Component tumors: MALE GERM CELL TUMORS; SEMINOMA; TESTICU-
LAR TERATOMA**
Clinical features: FAMILIAL CLUSTERS DESCRIBED; USUALLY SIB PAIRS
AFFECTED (SEE TEXT)

Syndrome: WILMS' TUMOR AND   **Inheritance:** AD
PSEUDOHEMAPHRODITISM

Component tumors: WILMS' TUMOR; **GONADOBLASTOMA**
Clinical features: (SEE CANCERS OF THE GENITOURINARY SYSTEM)

CANCERS OF THE RESPIRATORY SYSTEM

| **Syndrome:** BLOOM SYNDROME | **Inheritance:** AR |
| | **Locus(i):** 15q26.1 (BLM) |

Component tumors: LEUKEMIAS; LYMPHOMAS; GASTROINTESTINAL, **LA-RYNGEAL**, AND CERVICAL CANCERS
Clinical features: (SEE CANCERS OF THE HEMATOLOGIC AND LYMPHATIC SYSTEMS)

| **Syndrome:** ENDOCRINE ADENO-MATOSIS, MULTIPLE (WERMER SYNDROME, MEN1) | **Inheritance:** AD |
| | **Locus(i):** 11q13 (MEN1) |

Component tumors: ISLET CELL TUMORS; PARATHYROID ADENOMAS; PI-TUITARY ADENOMAS; **BRONCHIAL CARCINOID**; SCHWANNOMA; LIPO-MAS; ADRENOCORTICAL CARCINOMA
Clinical features: (SEE CANCERS OF THE ENDOCRINE SYSTEM)

| **Syndrome:** FAMILIAL ALVEOLAR CELL CARCINOMA | **Inheritance:** ? |

Component tumors: ALVEOLAR CELL LUNG CANCERS
Clinical features: POSSIBLE SENSITIVITY TO ENVIRONMENTAL CARCINO-GENS (SEE TEXT); CASE REPORTS OF TWO FAMILIES WITH ALVEOLAR CELL SUBTYPE OF LUNG CANCERS

| **Syndrome:** LI-FRAUMENI SYNDROME | **Inheritance:** AD |
| | **Locus(i):** 17p13.1 (p53) |

Component tumors: RHABDOMYOSARCOMA; SOFT TISSUE SARCOMA; BREAST CANCER; BRAIN TUMORS; OSTEOSARCOMA; LEUKEMIA; ADRENOCORTICAL CARCINOMA; LYMPHOCYTIC LYMPHOMA; **LUNG ADENOCARCINOMA**; MELANOMA , GONADAL GERM CELL TUMORS; PROSTATE CARCINOMA; PANCREATIC CARCINOMA; LARYNGEAL CARCI-NOMA
Clinical features: (SEE CANCERS OF CONNECTIVE TISSUES)

| **Syndrome:** MACROGLOBULINEMIA, WALDENSTRÖM'S | **Inheritance:** AD |

Component tumors: LUNG ADENOCARCINOMA; OTHER LYMPHOPROLIF-ERATIVE DISEASES
Clinical features: (SEE CANCERS OF THE HEMATOLOGIC AND LYMPHATIC SYSTEMS)

Syndrome: MESOTHELIOMA, MALIGNANT   **Inheritance:** ?AD

Component tumors: MALIGNANT MESOTHELIOMA
Clinical features: SEVERAL SIBSHIPS AND FAMILIES REPORTED; MAY BE THE RESULT OF ASBESTOS EXPOSURE THROUGH CLOTHING BROUGHT HOME; SEEN IN ONE INFANT WITHOUT ASBESTOS EXPOSURE

Syndrome: MUIR-TORRE SYNDROME   **Inheritance:** AD
Locus(i): MULTIPLE LOCI ON CHROM 2, 3 AND 7 (MLH1, MSH2, PMS1, PMS2)

Component tumors: SEBACEOUS SKIN TUMORS; SMALL BOWEL CARCINOMA; CANCER OF THE COLON, STOMACH, ENDOMETRIUM, KIDNEY, OVARIES, BLADDER, BREAST, **LARYNX**; KERATOACANTHOMATA
Clinical features: (SEE CANCERS OF THE GASTROINTESTINAL SYSTEM)

Syndrome: PULMONARY FIBROSIS, FAMILIAL (FIBROCYSTIC PULMONARY DYSPLASIA)   **Inheritance:** AD

Component tumors: ALVEOLAR CELL LUNG CARCINOMA
Clinical features: IDIOPATHIC PULMONARY FIBROSIS; DIGITAL CLUBBING; SEVERAL FAMILIES WITH PULMONARY FIBROSIS AND ALVEOLAR CELL CARCINOMA HAVE BEEN DESCRIBED; FIBROSIS MAY PRESENT IN CHILDHOOD

Syndrome: VON HIPPEL-LINDAU SYNDROME   **Inheritance:** AD
Locus(i): 3p25-p26 (VHL)

Component tumors: PHEOCHROMOCYTOMA; CEREBELLAR HEMANGIOBLASTOMA; RENAL CELL CARCINOMA; ADRENAL HEMANGIOMAS; **PULMONARY HEMANGIOMAS**; LIVER HEMANGIOMAS; PANCREATIC CARCINOMA; PANCREATIC ISLET CELL TUMOR; INTRACRANIAL HEMANGIOBLASTOMA; SPINAL CORD HEMANGIOMA
Clinical features: (SEE CANCERS OF THE NERVOUS SYSTEM AND EYE)

CANCERS OF THE SKELETAL SYSTEM

Syndrome: BONE DYSPLASIA WITH MEDULLARY FIBROSARCOMA   **Inheritance:** AD

Component tumors: MALIGNANT FIBROUS HISTIOCYTOMA
Clinical features: DIAPHYSEAL MEDULLARY STENOSIS WITH OVERLYING CORTICAL BONE THICKENING; SKELETAL DYSPLASIA FOLLOWING MINIMAL TRAUMA;

Syndrome: EXOSTOSES, MULTIPLE, TYPES 1,2,3

Inheritance: AD
Locus(i): 8q24.1 (TYPE 1); 11p12 (TYPE 2); 19p (TYPE 3)

Component tumors: INCREASED **OSTEOSARCOMA** IN EXOSTOSES; CHONDROSARCOMA
Clinical features: EXOSTOSES OF RIBS, SCAPULA, LONG BONES, PELVIS, WITH SPARING OF SKULL AND VERTEBRAE; EXOSTOSES MAY UNDERGO MALIGNANT DEGENERATION IN <10% OF CASES.

Syndrome: FAMILIAL ADENOMATOUS POLYPOSIS (FAP, GARDNER SYNDROME)

Inheritance: AD
Locus(i): 5q21-q22 (APC)

Component tumors: COLON CANCER; PERIAMPULLARY CARCINOMA; HEPATOBLASTOMA; BILE DUCT CARCINOMA; **OSTEOSARCOMA**; ADRENAL CARCINOMA; THYROID CARCINOMA; MANDIBULAR OSTEOMA
Clinical features: (SEE CANCERS OF THE GASTROINTESTINAL SYSTEM)

Syndrome: LI-FRAUMENI SYNDROME

Inheritance: AD
Locus(i): 17p13.1 (p53)

Component tumors: RHABDOMYOSARCOMA; SOFT TISSUE SARCOMA; BREAST CANCER; BRAIN TUMORS; **OSTEOSARCOMA**; LEUKEMIA; ADRENOCORTICAL CARCINOMA; LYMPHOCYTIC LYMPHOMA; LUNG ADENOCARCINOMA, MELANOMA, GONADAL GERM CELL TUMORS; PROSTATE CARCINOMA; PANCREATIC CARCINOMA; LARYNGEAL CARCINOMA
Clinical features: (SEE CANCERS OF CONNECTIVE TISSUES)

Syndrome: NOONAN-LIKE/ MULTIPLE GIANT CELL LESION SYNDROME

Inheritance: AD

Component tumors: **GIANT CELL GRANULOMAS OF BONE AND SOFT TISSUES**
Clinical features: SYMPTOMS OF NOONAN SYNDROME (SHORT STATURE, OCULAR HYPERTELORISM, SHORT WEBBED NECK, ETC.) WITH GIANT CELL GRANULOMAS IN RARE FAMILIES

Syndrome: OSLAM SYNDROME

Inheritance: AD

Component tumors: **OSTEOSARCOMA**
Clinical features: CLINODACTYLY; ABSENT DIGITAL RAY IN FOOT; RADIOULNAR FUSION OF BONES (SYNOSTOSIS); MACROCYTOSIS WITHOUT ANEMIA; LIMB ANOMALIES

Syndrome: PAGET'S DISEASE OF BONE

Inheritance: AD
Locus(i): LINKED TO 6p21.3

Component tumors: **GIANT CELL TUMOR; OSTEOSARCOMA**

Clinical features: SWELLING OR DEFORMITY OF LONG BONE; BONE PAIN; LYTIC AND SCLEROTIC LESIONS BY RADIOGRAPHIC EXAM; NEUROLOGIC COMPLICATIONS

| **Syndrome:** RETINOBLASTOMA | **Inheritance:** AD |
| | **Locus(i):** 13q14 (RB1) |

Component tumors: RETINOBLASTOMA; **OSTEOSARCOMA**; PINEALOMA
Clinical features: (SEE CANCERS OF THE NERVOUS SYSTEM AND EYE)

| **Syndrome:** ROTHMUND-THOMSON SYNDROME | **Inheritance:** AR |

Component tumors: **OSTEOSARCOMA**
Clinical features: SKIN ABNORMALITIES INCLUDING ATROPHY, HYPERPIGMENTATION AND TELANGIECTASIA WITH SHORT STATURE AND CATARACTS; **OSTEOSARCOMAS** (RARE COMPLICATION)

| **Syndrome:** WERNER SYNDROME | **Inheritance:** AR |

Component tumors: **OSTEOSARCOMA**; SARCOMAS AND OTHER CONNECTIVE TISSUES TUMORS; OTHER RARE TUMORS
Clinical features: SHORT STATURE; DECREASED FAT AND MUSCLE; PREMATURE "AGING": LOSS OF HAIR, ARTERIOSCLEROSIS, OSTEOPOROSIS

CANCERS OF THE SKIN

| **Syndrome:** ALBINISM I (TYROSINE NEGATIVE OCULOCUTANEOUS) | **Inheritance:** AR |
| | **Locus(i):** 11q14-21 |

Component tumors: **BASAL CELL CARCINOMA; MELANOMA** (RARE)
Clinical features: ALBINISM; NYSTAGMUS; VISUAL LOSS; PHOTOPHOBIA; TYROSINASE DEFICIENCY

| **Syndrome:** ALBINISM II (TYROSINE POSITIVE) | **Inheritance:** AR |
| | **Locus(i):** 15q11.2-12 |

Component tumors: **BASAL CELL CARCINOMA; MELANOMA** (RARE)
Clinical features: ALBINISM; NYSTAGMUS; VISUAL LOSS; PHOTOPHOBIA; NORMAL TYROSINASE

| **Syndrome:** ALBINISM WITH HEMORRHAGIC DIATHESIS AND PIGMENTED RETICULOENDOTHELIAL CELLS (HERMANSKY-PUDLAKS SYNDROME) | **Inheritance:** AR |
| | **Locus(i):** 10q23.1-23.3 |

Component tumors: **BASAL CELL CARCINOMA; MELANOMA** (RARE)

Clinical features: ALBINISM; NYSTAGMUS; VISUAL LOSS; LIFELONG BLEEDING TENDENCY; DEPOSITION OF CEROID-LIKE MATERIAL IN TISSUES; OTHER CARDIAC AND PULMONARY FEATURES; FREQUENT IN PUERTO RICANS

Syndrome: BASAL CELL CARCI-NOMAS WITH MILIA AND COARSE SPARSE HAIR | **Inheritance:** AD VS. XLD

Component tumors: BASAL CELL CARCINOMAS
Clinical features: COARSE AND SPARSE HAIR; MILIA ON FACE AND LIMBS IN CHILDHOOD; LIKE BAZEX SYNDROME

Syndrome: BASAL CELL NEVUS (GORLIN) SYNDROME | **Inheritance:** AD
Locus(i): 9q31 (PTCH)

Component tumors: BASAL CELL CARCINOMA; CARDIAC FIBROMA; OVARIAN FIBROMATA; OVARIAN CARCINOMA; MEDULLOBLASTOMA
Clinical features: PITS ON ARMS AND SOLES; ODONTOGENIC KERATO-CYSTS OF JAWS; HYPERTELORISM; LAMELLAR CALCIFICATION OF FALX CEREBRI; BRIDGING OF SELLA TURCICA; ABNORMAL CERVICAL VERTE-BRAE; RIB ANOMALIES; EPIDERMAL CYSTS OF SKIN

Syndrome: BAZEX SYNDROME | **Inheritance:** XLD

Component tumors: BASAL CELL CARCINOMAS
Clinical features: MULTIPLE 'ICE-PICK' MARKS ON DORSUM OR HANDS AND ELBOWS AT INFANCY; BASAL CELL CARCINOMAS OF FACE AGES 15 TO 26 YEARS

Syndrome: CHEILITIS GLANDULARIS | **Inheritance:** AD

Component tumors: INCREASED **LOWER LIP SQUAMOUS CELL CARCI-NOMA**
Clinical features: ENLARGED EVERTED LOWER LIP; LABIAL MUCOUS GLAND HYPERTROPHY; DILATATION OF EXCRETORY DUCTS; RARE SYN-DROME

Syndrome: DYSKERATOSIS CONGENITA | **Inheritance:** XLR
Locus(i): Xq28 (DKC)

Component tumors: SQUAMOUS CELL CANCERS OF MUCOSA OR SKIN; PANCREATIC ADENOCARCINOMA; OTHER INTERNAL MALIGNANCIES; ESOPHAGEAL CANCER
Clinical features: CUTANEOUS PIGMENTATION; DYSTROPHY OF NAILS; ORAL LEUKOPLAKIA; ATRESIA OF LACRIMAL DUCTS; TESTICULAR AT-ROPHY; ANEMIA; OTHER SIGNS

Syndrome: EPIDERMODYSPLASIA VERRUCIFORMIS | **Inheritance:** XL OR AR

Component tumors: SQUAMOUS OR BASAL CELL CARCINOMA

Clinical features: OFTEN ASSOCIATED WITH HUMAN PAPILLOMA VIRUS INFECTION; WARTS ON FACE, HANDS, NECK, BACK; CAN HAVE MALIGNANT DEGENERATION OF WARTS

Syndrome: EPIDERMOLYSIS BULLOSA DYSTROPHICA, HALLOPEAU-SIEMENS TYPE

Inheritance: AR
Locus(i): 3p21.3

Component tumors: SQUAMOUS CELL CARCINOMA
Clinical features: BULLAE; SEVERE SCARRING; ESOPHAGEAL STRICTURE; MALNUTRITION; ALSO DOMINANT FORM OF EPIDERMOLYSIS BULLOSA, BUT CANCERS LESS FREQUENT

Syndrome: EPITHELIOMA, MULTIPLE BENIGN CYSTIC OF BROOKE (MULTIPLE CYLINDRO-MATOSIS)

Inheritance: AD ?ALSO XL
Locus(i): 16q12-13

Component tumors: MULTIPLE EPITHELIOMAS; SALIVARY GLAND TUMORS
Clinical features: CUTANEOUS TUMORS ON FACE WITH CYLINDROMAS OF SALIVARY GLANDS

Syndrome: EPITHELIOMA, SELF-HEALING SQUAMOUS (FURGESON-SMITH TYPE)

Inheritance: AD
Locus(i): 9q31

Component tumors: EPITHELIOMAS, SIMILAR TO SQUAMOUS CELL CARCINOMAS
Clinical features: STARTS WITH CUTANEOUS TUMORS RESEMBLING SQUAMOUS CARCINOMAS, WHICH ULCERATE AND LEAVE SCARS; MOST OFTEN IN INDIVIDUALS OF SCOTTISH DESCENT

Syndrome: FIBROMATOSIS, JUVENILE HYALINE

Inheritance: AR

Component tumors: MULTIPLE SUBCUTANEOUS TUMORS
Clinical features: MULTIPLE RECURRING SUBCUTANEOUS SCALP TUMORS; GINGIVAL HYPERPLASIA; SKELETAL LESIONS

Syndrome: GIANT PIGMENTED HAIRY NEVUS

Inheritance: AD

Component tumors: MALIGNANT MELANOMA
Clinical features: LARGE PIGMENTED NEVI IN NEWBORNS; RARELY FAMILIAL

Syndrome: HYPERKERATOSIS LENTICULARIS PERSTANS (HLP); (FLEGEL DISEASE)

Inheritance: AD

Component tumors: SQUAMOUS AND BASAL CELL CARCINOMA

Clinical features: HYPERKERATOTIC PINK OR REDDISH-BROWN SCALY 1–5 mm PAPULES OF LOWER LEG AND DORSUM OF FOOT

Syndrome: KERATITIS-ICHTHYOSIS-DEAFNESS   **Inheritance:** AD FORM HETEROGENEOUS

Component tumors: SQUAMOUS CELL CARCINOMAS
Clinical features: HYPERKERATOTIC PLAQUES; ICTHYOSIS; NEUROSENSORY HEARING LOSS; FUNGAL INFECTIONS; CORNEAL OPACIFICATION

Syndrome: LEIOMYOMATA, HEREDITARY MULTIPLE, OF SKIN   **Inheritance:** AD

Component tumors: MULTIPLE CUTANEOUS LEIOMYOMATA; UTERINE LEIOMYOMATA
Clinical features: (SEE CANCERS OF THE REPRODUCTIVE SYSTEM)

Syndrome: LI-FRAUMENI SYNDROME   **Inheritance:** AD
Locus(i): 17p13.1 (p53)

Component tumors: RHABDOMYOSARCOMA; SOFT TISSUE SARCOMA; BREAST CANCER; BRAIN TUMORS; OSTEOSARCOMA; LEUKEMIA; ADRENOCORTICAL CARCINOMA; LYMPHOCYTIC LYMPHOMA; LUNG ADENOCARCINOMA, **MELANOMA,** GONADAL GERM CELL TUMORS; PROSTATE CARCINOMA; PANCREATIC CARCINOMA; LARYNGEAL CARCINOMA
Clinical features: (SEE CANCERS OF CONNECTIVE TISSUES)

Syndrome: LIPOMATOSIS, FAMILIAL BENIGN CERVICAL   **Inheritance:** AD

Component tumors: MULTIPLE LIPOMATA
Clinical features: MALIGNANT DEGENERATION IS RARE; NECK COLLAR OF FAT

Syndrome: LIPOMATOSIS, MULTIPLE   **Inheritance:** AD

Component tumors: LIPOMATOSIS
Clinical features: MULTIPLE SOFT FLESHY LESIONS

Syndrome: MALIGNANT MELANOMA (BK MOLE; FAMM SYNDROME)   **Inheritance:** AD
Locus(i): 1p36,9p21 (CDKN2^{p16}), 6q (CDK4)

Component tumors: MALIGNANT MELANOMA; DYSPLASTIC NEVI (VARIABLE IN SIZE, OUTLINE AND COLOR)
Clinical features: IN ADDITION TO MELANOMAS, PANCREATIC CANCER HAS BEEN OBSERVED IN RARE FAMILIES

Syndrome: MELANOMA-ASTROCYTOMA SYNDROME   **Inheritance:** AD

Component tumors: CUTANEOUS MALIGNANT MELANOMA; CEREBRAL ASTROCYTOMA; OTHER CNS TUMORS
Clinical features: ASTROCYTOMA AND OTHER CNS TUMORS IN EPIDEMIO-LOGIC SERIES AND CASE REPORTS

Syndrome: MUIR-TORRE SYNDROME	**Inheritance:** AD **Locus(i):** MULTIPLE LOCI ON CHROM 2, 3 AND 7 (MLH1, MSH2, PMS1, PMS2)

Component tumors: SEBACEOUS SKIN TUMORS; SMALL BOWEL CARCI-NOMA; CARCINOMA OF THE COLON, STOMACH, ENDOMETRIUM, KID-NEY, OVARIES, BLADDER, BREAST, LARYNX; KERATOACANTHOMATA
Clinical features: (SEE CANCERS OF THE GASTROINTESTINAL SYSTEM)

Syndrome: MULTIPLE HAMARTOMA (COWDEN) SYNDROME	**Inheritance:** AD **Locus(i):** 10q22-q23 (PTEN)

Component tumors: DYSPLASTIC CEREBELLAR GANGLIOCYTOMA; BREAST CANCER; PRIMARY NEUROENDOCRINE (MERKEL CELL) TU-MORS; **SKIN CARCINOMA**; RENAL CELL CARCINOMA; THYROID CANCER
Clinical features: (SEE CANCERS OF THE REPRODUCTIVE SYSTEM)

Syndrome: PACHYONYCHIA CONGENITA	**Inheritance:** AD **Locus(i):** ?17q12-q21

Component tumors: CYLINDROMA
Clinical features: HYPERKERATOSIS (PALMS, SOLES, KNEES, ELBOWS); THICKENED NAILS AT BIRTH; HAIR AND DENTAL ABNORMALITIES

Syndrome: PIEBALD TRAIT	**Inheritance:** AD **Locus(i):** 4q11-q12

Component tumors: FREQUENT **EPITHELIOMAS**
Clinical features: WHITE SCALP HAIR; ABSENT PIGMENTATION (MEDIAL FOREHEAD, EYEBROWS, CHIN, VENTRAL CHEST, ABDOMEN, LIMBS)

Syndrome: POROKERATOSIS OF MIBELLI	**Inheritance:** AD FORM

Component tumors: FREQUENT **SKIN CANCERS**
Clinical features: 7% DEVELOP SKIN CANCERS; CHILDHOOD ONSET OF CENTRIFUGALLY SPREADING PATCHES SURROUNDED BY NARROW HORNY RIDGES WITH CENTRAL ATROPHY; OTHER MALIGNANCIES MAY ALSO BE MORE COMMON

Syndrome: SCLEROATROPHIC AND KERATOTIC DERMATOSIS OF LIMBS (SCLEROTYLOSIS)	**Inheritance:** AD **Locus(i):** 4q28-q31

Component tumors: SQUAMOUS CELL CANCERS AND BOWEL CANCERS

Clinical features: ATROPHY OF SKIN ON HANDS AND FEET; HYPOPLASTIC NAILS; SQUAMOUS CELL CANCERS METASTATIC IN ONE CASE; DESCRIBED IN FRENCH FAMILIES

Syndrome: TURCOT SYNDROME	**Inheritance:** AR AND AR
	Locus(i): MULTIPLE LOCI (MLH1, MSH2, APC)

Component tumors: COLON CANCER; GLIOBLASTOMA; ASTROCYTOMA; MEDULLOBLASTOMA; GASTRIC CANCER; **SCALP BASAL CELL CARCINOMAS**
Clinical features: (SEE CANCERS OF THE GASTROINTESTINAL SYSTEM)

Syndrome: XERODERMA PIGMENTOSUM	**Inheritance:** AR
	Locus(i): 9q34 (XPA); 3p25 (XPC); 19q13 (XPD); 15p (XPF)

Component tumors: EARLY ONSET BASAL CELL, SQUAMOUS CELL SKIN CANCERS; MALIGNANT MELANOMA; KERATOACANTHOMAS; ANGIOMAS; INCREASED RISK OF INTERNAL MALIGNANCIES INCLUDING SARCOMAS AND ADENOCARCINOMAS
Clinical features: PHOTOPHOBIA AND CONJUNCTIVITIS IN CHILDHOOD; SKIN PHOTOSENSITIVITY; SKIN ERYTHEMA AND BLISTERING PROGRESSING TO POIKILODERMA (ATOPIC SKIN CHANGES); ACTINIC KERATOSIS; EARLY ONSET SKIN NEOPLASMS; ECTROPION; LOW IQ; MENTAL DETERIORATION; DEAFNESS; NEUROLOGIC ABNORMALITIES

Practical Materials for Clinical Cancer Genetics Consultations: Clinical Laboratories and Internet Resources

METHOD OF CONSTRUCTION

The first part of the appendix (B-1) consists of a list of clinical laboratories offering cancer genetic testing. The list of academic laboratories was compiled by inquiring directly, browsing available internet resources, and utilizing the Test Directory of the Association for Molecular Pathology (AMP), 1996 edition. The address for the Association for Molecular Pathology is: 9650 Rockville Pike, Bethesda, Maryland, 20814-3993. The second part of this appendix (B-2) consists of a list of software available for pedigree drawing and data storage. Appendix B-3 lists the National Cancer Institute Website and the phone number for the NCI Cancer Information Service. Both sources can provide lists of names of individuals offering cancer genetic counseling services in your region. In addition the National Society of Genetic Counselors maintains a Cancer Risk Counseling Special Interest Group. Further information is available from Ms. Bea Leopold, NSGC, 233 Canterbury Drive, Wallingford PA, 19086-6617. Since not every individual on these lists will be experienced in all aspects of clinical cancer genetics, specialized resources are available through the NCI designated Comprehensive Cancer Centers. The locations of these Centers can be provided by the NCI Cancer Information Service. The final part of the appendix (B-4) consists of internet resources relevant to clinical cancer genetics. It was compiled by searching various sites.

B-1 LABORATORIES PROVIDING CLINICAL CANCER GENETIC TESTING

a. Testing for Cancer Predisposition Genes

An internet reference to laboratories offering testing for patients with heritable disorders is provided by HELIX, a computer-based directory funded by the National Center for Biotechnology Information and the National Library of Medicine. The database is restricted to health care professionals by password-protection. Individuals may register on-line. The internet address is:

(hhtp://www.hslib.washington.edu/helix)

As surveyed in 1996, HELIX had successfully identified laboratory information for 81% of more than 19,000 inquiries. [Pagon RA, Covington ML, Fuller S, Tarczy-Hornoch P. 1996. Helix: a directory of medical genetics laboratories. Amer J Hum Genet 59: 1970 (abstr)].

Listed below are selected clinical laboratories that offer genetic testing for cancer predisposition. Inclusion in this list does not signify that the laboratory has passed CLIA inspection or ACP certification (see Chapter 7). That information should be obtained directly from the laboratory or by consulting the Test Directory of the Association for Molecular Pathology. In some cases, the laboratories offer testing primarily, or exclusively, as part of research protocols. In addition to the laboratories listed, University-affiliated laboratories offer a number of these tests as part of investigational studies. Regardless of laboratory requirements, testing should only be offered in the context of counseling and after informed consent based on an understanding of risks, benefits, and alternatives to testing (see Chapter 10). The fees for tests are approximated as of mid-1997, and will vary as technologies continue to change.

Methods of mutation identification are summarized in Chapter 7. "ASO" refers to allele specific oligonucleotide, "CDGE" refers to constant denaturant gel electrophoresis, "PCR" refers to polymerase chain reaction. "Jewish Panel" refers to screening for the following mutations: 185delAG, 5382insC *BRCA1*, and 6174delT *BRCA2* mutations. Some labs also include the rarer 188del11 *BRCA1* mutation.

Breast Cancer

LAB	LOCATION	CONTACT	TEST	METHOD	FEE
Boston University School of Medicine Center for Human Genetics	Boston, MA 02118-2394	Alexis Poss, MS (617) 638-7083	*BRCA1* 185delAG *BRCA2* 6174delT	ASO restriction enzyme	$150 prices not yet established

LAB	LOCATION	CONTACT	TEST	METHOD	FEE
Genetics; IVF Institute Molecular Genetics Lab	Fairfax, VA 22031	Client Response Center (800) 654-4363	"Jewish Panel"	allele-specific assay	$295
Myriad Genetic Laboratories, Inc.	Salt Lake City, UT 84108	Client Services (800) 469-7423	"Jewish Panel"	sequencing	$450
			BRCA1 + *BRCA2* unknown mutation	sequencing	$2400
			known mutation	sequencing	$395
Oncor Med	Gaithersburg, MD 20877	Joan Scott, MS (800) 662-6763 (301) 208-1888	"Jewish Panel"	ASO	$350
			BRCA1	ASO/sequencing	$420-1995
			BRCA2	ASO/sequencing	$420-1195
University of Pennsylvania School of Medicine The Genetic Diagnostic Lab	Philadelphia, PA 19104-6145	Lynn Godmilow, MSW (800) 669-2172	*BRCA 1* unknown mutation	CDGE + sequencing	$680
			known mutation	CDGE + sequencing	$260
			BRCA 2 unknown mutation	CDGE + sequencing	$920**
			"Jewish Panel"	CDGE + sequencing	$440
University of Utah School of Medicine DNA Diagnostic Lab	Salt Lake City, UT 84112	Stephanie Hallam, PhD (801) 581-8334	"Jewish Panel"	ASO	$250
Yale University School of Medicine DNA Diagnostics Lab	New Haven, CT 06520-8005	Dr. Michael Glynn (203) 785-5745	"Jewish Panel"	PCR- restriction enzyme	$200

**$860 if sample also analyzed for BRCA1

Hereditary non-Polyposis Colorectal Cancer

LAB	LOCATION	CONTACT	TEST	METHOD	FEE
Lab Corporation of America Center of Molecular Biology and Pathology	Research Triangle Park, NC 27709	Genetic Services (800) 345-4363	*MSH2* *MLH1*	truncated protein (known mutation)	$550
				truncated protein (unknown mutation)	$750
Oncor Med	Gaithersburg, MD 20877	Client Services (800) 662-6763	*MSH2* *MLH1* RER	sequencing	$2350
				microsatellite instability	$570 (frozen tumor)
					$720 (paraffin tumor)

Familial Adenomatous Polyposis

LAB	LOCATION	CONTACT	TEST	METHOD	FEE
Boston University School of Medicine Center for Human Genetics	Boston, MA 02118-2394	Alexis Poss, MS (617) 638-7083	*APC*	linkage	$1500 per family
Lab Corporation of America Center of Molecular Biology and Pathology	Research Triangle Park, NC 27709	Genetic Services (800) 345-4363	*APC*	truncated protein	$500 unknown mutation
					$350 known mutation
Mayo Clinic Molecular Genetics Lab	Rochester, MN 55905	Stephen Thibodeau, PhD (507) 284-9185	*APC*	linkage	$248 per individual

LAB	LOCATION	CONTACT	TEST	METHOD	FEE
University of Utah School of Medicine DNA Diagnostic Lab	Salt Lake City, UT 84112	Stephanie Hallam, PhD (801) 581-8334	*APC*	linkage	$235 per individual $600 per family
Washington School of Medicine Molecular Diagnostic Lab	St. Louis, MO 63110	Barbara Zehnbauer, PhD (314) 362-1700	*APC*	truncated protein	[under development]

Multiple Endocrine Endoplasia 2A/2B

LAB	LOCATION	CONTACT	TEST	METHOD	FEE
Children's Hospital of LA Molecular Diagnostic Lab	Los Angeles, CA 90027	Lee-Jun Wong, PhD (213) 669-5619	*RET* exon 10, 11, 16	sequencing	$250
Dartmouth-Hichcock Medical Center Molecular Diagnostics	Lebanon, NH 03756	Walter Noll, MD (603) 650-8257	*RET* exons 10, 11, 16	sequencing	$250
Henry Ford Hospital DNA Diagnostic Lab	Detroit, MI 48202	Gerald Feldman, MD, PhD (313) 876-7681	*RET* exons 10, 11, 13 exon 14, 16	sequencing	$305 $145
Mayo Clinic Molecular Genetics Lab	Rochester, MN 55905	Stephen Thibodeau, PhD (507) 284-9185	*RET* exons 10, 11, exon 16	sequencing	$300 $246
Oncor Med	Gaithersburg, MD 20877	Client Services (800) 662-6763/ (301) 208-1888	*RET* exons 10, 11, 16 exon 13	sequencing	$450 $150

Multiple Endocrine Endoplasia 2A/2B *(continued)*

LAB	LOCATION	CONTACT	TEST	METHOD	FEE
UCLA Diagnostic Molecular Pathology Lab	Los Angeles, CA 90024-1110	Wayne Grody MD, PhD (310) 206-5294	*RET* exons 10, 11, 13, 16	sequencing	$275
University of Pennsylvania School of Medicine Genetic Diagnostic Lab	Philadelphia, PA 19104-6145	Lynn God-milow, MSW (800) 669-2172	*RET* exons 10, 11, 13, 14 exon 16	sequencing	$320 $260
University of Pittsburgh School of Medicine Molecular Diagnostic Lab	Pittsburgh, PA 15261	Jeffrey Kant, MD, PhD (412) 648-8519	*RET* exons 10, 11, 16	sequencing	prices not yet established
Washington University School of Medicine Molecular Diagnostic Lab	St. Louis, MO 63110	Barbara Zehn-bauer, PhD (314) 362-1700	*RET* exons 10, 11, 13, 16	sequencing	$360 unknown mutations $260 known mutation
Yale School of Medicine DNA Diagnostics Lab	New Haven, CT 06520-8005	Dr. Michael Glynn (203) 785-5745	*RET* exons 10, 11, 13, 14 16	sequencing	$330 $330

Multiple Endocrine Neoplasia 1

LAB	LOCATION	CONTACT	TEST	METHOD	FEE
Yale University School of Medicine	New Haven, CT 06520-8005	Dr. Michael Glynn (203) 785-5745	*MEN1*	linkage sequencing	$330 per sample

von Hippel-Lindau

LAB	LOCATION	CONTACT	TEST	METHOD	FEE
Johns Hopkins Hospital DNA Diagnostic Lab	Baltimore, MD 21287	Corinne Boehm, MS (410) 955-0483	*VHL* mutation	Southern blot, ASO	$270 per sample
University of Pennsylvania School of Medicine The Genetic Diagnostic Lab	Philadelphia, PA 19104-6145	Lynn Godmilow, MSW (800) 669-2172	*VHL*	Southern blot sequencing	$220 $540
Boston University School of Medicine Center for Human Genetics	Boston, MA 02118-2394	Alexis Poss, MS (617) 638-7083	*VHL*	Southern blot & sequencing	$500 1st person $150 additional person

Retinoblastoma

LAB	LOCATION	CONTACT	TEST	METHOD	FEE
University of Vermont Molecular Diagnostic Lab	Burlington, VT 05405	Sandy Thompson May (802) 656-4553	*RBI*	haplotype (if known mutation) sequencing (unknown mutation)	approx. $200 approx. $4000

Melanoma

LAB	LOCATION	CONTACT	TEST	METHOD	FEE
Oncor Med	Gaithersburg, MD 20877	Client Services (800) 662-6763 (301) 208-1888	*p16*	sequencing	$550

Li-Fraumeni Syndrome

LAB	LOCATION	CONTACT	TEST	METHOD	FEE
Oncor Med	Gaithersburg, MD 20877	Client Services (800) 662-6763 (301) 208-1888	*p53*	functional assay sequencing	$650 $650-1300

b. Molecular Diagnostic Testing for Cancer

Note: Only those Association for Molecular Pathology member laboratories that are CLIA approved and/or certified by the College of American Pathology are listed. Where available, telephone number is a general access number. In some cases, telephone number is for the laboratory director. The menu of tests varies by laboratory. "GR" signifies gene rearrangement analysis, generally by Southern blot or PCR, for immunoglobulin, T cell receptor, *BCL2*/IG, and/or *BCR/ABL* gene rearrangement. "MC" signifies molecular cytogenetic analysis for diagnostic rearrangements in leukemia, sarcomas, and/or selected solid tumors. "NM" signifies *NMYC* gene amplification for staging of neuroblastoma.

University-affiliated laboratories

Armed Forces Institute of Pathology Washington, D.C.	202 782 2877	GR, MC
Beth Israel Hospital New York, NY	212 420 3831	GR
Cedars-Sinai Medical Center Los Angeles, CA	310 855 2369	GR
The Children's Hospital Denver, CO	303 837 2725	GR, MC
Children's Hospital Columbus, OH	614 722 5350	GR, NM
Children's Hospital of Los Angeles Los Angeles, CA	213 669 5611	GR, MC, NM
Columbia Michael Reese Hospital Chicago, IL	312 791 2928	GR
Cook County Hospital Chicago, IL	312 633 7151	GR
Dartmouth Hitchcock Medical Center Hanover, NH	603 650 7171	GR
Emory University School of Medicine Atlanta, GA	404 712 7297	GR

Evanston Hospital		
Evanston IL	847 570 2857	GR
Hartford Hospital		
Hartford, CT	860 545 3409	GR
Henry Ford Hospital		
Detroit, MI	313 876 2840	GR, MC
H. Lee Moffitt Cancer Center		
Tampa, FL	813 979 3001	GR
Hospital of the University of Pennsylvania		
Philadelphia, PA	215 898 0884	MC
Illinois Masonic Medical Center		
Chicago, IL	773 296 7900	GR
Indiana University Medical Center		
Indianapolis, IN	317 274 4606	GR, NM
J.L. McClellan Memorial Veterans Hospital		
Little Rock, AR	501 660 2045	GR
John Hopkins Medical Institutions		
Baltimore, MD	410 955 8363	GR
Lutheran General Hospital		
Park Ridge, IL	847 723 7536	GR
Maine Medical Center		
South Portland, ME	207 761 9090	GR
Mayo Clinic		
Rochester MN	507 284 4169	GR, NM
Medical College of Virginia Hospital		
Richmond, VA	804 828 9564	GR
Medical College of Wisconsin		
Milwaukee, WI	414 456 7605	GR
Medical University of South Carolina		
Charlston, SC	803 792 5356	GR
Memorial Sloan-Kettering Cancer Center		
New York, NY	212 639 8895	GR, MC
	212 639 8280	
The Methodist Hospital		
Houston TX	713 790 3520	GR
Miami Children's Hospital		
Miami, FL	305 666 3556	GR
Oregon Health Sciences University DNA Diagnostic Lab		
Portland, OR	503 494 7821	GR
Rush Presbyterian		
Chicago, IL	312 942 3724	GR
Saint Barnabas Medical Center		
Livingston, NJ	201 533 8248	GR

St. John Hospital and Medical Center		
Detroit, MI	313 343 3520	GR
SUNY Health Science Center at Syracuse		
Syracuse, NY	315 464 6808	GR
UCLA Medical Center		
Los Angeles, CA	310 825 5648	GR
UMC Health Sciences Center		
Columbia, MO	573 882 1305	GR, MC
University Hospital SUNY at Stony Brook		
Stony Brook, NY	516 444 3747	GR
University of California, San Diego		
San Diego, CA	619 534 8955	GR
University of Chicago Hospitals		
Chicago, IL	773 702 4542	GR, MC
University of Illinois at Chicago		
Chicago, IL	312 996 1737	GR
University of Iowa Hospital and Clinics		
Iowa City, IO	319 356 2591	GR
University of Maryland		
Baltimore, MD	410 706 0513	GR
University of Minnesota		
Minneapolis, MN	612 624 8445	GR, MC, NM
University of Nebraska Medical Center		
Omaha, NE	402 559 4186	GR, MC
University of New Mexico		
Albuquerque, NM	505 272 4783	GR, MC
University of Pittsburgh Medical Center		
Pittsburgh, PA	412 648 2186	GR, MC, NM
University of Rochester		
Rochester, NY	716 275 7574	GR
University of Texas Health Science Center at San Antonio		
San Antonio, TX	210 567 3100	GR, MC
University of Texas M.D. Anderson Cancer Center		
Houston, TX	713 794 1292	GR, MC
University of Texas Southwestern Medical Center		
Dallas, TX	214 648 4075	GR
University of Utah Health Sciences Center		
Salt Lake City, UT	801 581 8334	GR, MC
University of Virginia		
Charlottesville, VA	804 982 0973	GR
Vanderbilt University Medical Center		
Nashville, TN	615 343 8121	GR, NM

Washington University School of Medicine
St. Louis, MO 314 362 1700 GR

William Beaumont Hospital
Royal Oak, MI 810 551 0073 GR

Yale University School of Medicine
New Haven, CT 203 785 4492 GR

Note: Listed below are commercial laboratories that provide molecular testing services for cancer diagnosis. "(*)" indicates those labs that were 1996 members of the Association for Molecular Pathology.

Commercial Laboratories Providing Molecular Diagnostic Testing for Cancer

Cancer Genetics
Providence, RI 888 978 9945

Cytometry Associates
Nashville, TN 615 370 8393

(*) Diagnostic and Biologic Technologies, Inc.
San Antonio, TX 800 336 3060

Dianon Systems
Stratford, CT 203 381 4000

Genzyme Genetics
Santa Fe, NM 505 438 1111

IMPATH
New York, NY 800 447 5816

Lab Corporation of America
Research Triangle Park, NC 800 345 4363

(*) Laboratory for Molecular Diagnostic Testing in
Microbiology and Oncology
Philadelphia, PA 215 503 1036

Quest Diagnostics
Teterboro, NJ 201 393 5000

Smith Kline Beecham
Van Nuys, CA 610 631 4300

B-2 PEDIGREE DRAWING SOFTWARE

A number of software systems for generating pedigrees are available. Some of these applications also allow information storage in a relational database. Examples of software programs currently available are included below.

	Telephone number
Cyrillic/Cherwell Scientific Oxford, U.K.	44(0) 1865 784800
Megadats/Helios Software Works Hilo, HI	317 253 6965
Molecular Machines Sebastapol, CA	800 294 1024
Pedigree Draw/SW Foundation for Biomedical Research San Antonio, TX	210 674 1410
Progeny/Genetic Data Systems Notre Dame, IN	219 257 4000

B-3 PROVIDERS OF CANCER RISK COUNSELING SERVICES

Resources for referral to individuals providing cancer risk counseling include:

- Website of the National Cancer Institute:
  http://cancernet.nci.nih.goc/wwwprot/genetic/genesrch.html
- The National Cancer Institute Cancer Information Service:
  phone: (800) 4-CANCER (9 A.M. until 4:30 P.M. Monday to Friday)
- The National Society of Genetic Counselors
  FAX: 610-872-1192

B-4 INTERNET RESOURCES FOR CLINICAL CANCER GENETICS CONSULTATIONS

There are an increasing number of internet resources in human genetics. The following Websites are useful for the clinical cancer geneticist. Most sites are readily accessed; however, some require passwords or subscription.

- Mutation Databases

Note: There are some databases that catalog reported mutations in cancer predisposition genes. Reporting is generally voluntary, so information is not complete.

ATM Mutational Database (Virginia Mason Research Center)	http://www.vmmc.org/vmrc/atm.htm
ATM Mutational Database (Johns Hopkins)	http://www.med.jhu.edu/ataxia/mutate.htm

APC Mutation Database
(current to 1993)   http://www.mayo.edu/research/papers/
                                           P53%20Mutations/

Breast Cancer Information Core
(*BRCA1, BRCA2* mutational   http://www.nhgri.nih.gov/Intramural_
database)   research/Lab_transfer/Bic/index.html

Fanconi Anemia Mutation Database http://www.rockefeller.edu/fanconi/mutate/

Human Genome Mutation Database
(Cardiff)   http://www.cf.ac.uk/uwcm/mg/hgmd0.html

p53 Mutational Database
(current to 1993)   http://www.mayo.edu/research/papers/
                                           P53%20Mutations/

- Support Groups

Note: The Alliance of Genetic Support Groups maintains an up-to-date Directory of National Genetic Voluntary Organizations. For some syndromes (e.g. neurofibromatosis, breast cancer) there are several well-organized support groups, and groups also exist for some of the less common syndromes (e.g. von Hippel-Lindau syndrome, Nevoid Basal Cell Carcinoma Syndrome). These organizations can be invaluable resources for affected families. Information, including addresses of these organizations, is available in the Website.

http://medhelp.org/www/agsg.htm

- Web Index Sites

Note: These are primarily links to other Websites; they are useful for browsing

Genetics professional societies: FASEB
(professional organization updates)   http://www.faseb.org/genetics/mainmenu.html

Human Genome Project Resources
(Johns Hopkins)   http://gdbwww.gdb.org/gdb/hgbResources.html

Human Genome Project Resources
(U.S. Dept of Energy)   http://www.ornl.gov/TechResources/Human_
                                           Genome/links.html

Yahoo Human Genetics Links
(commercial Web search engine)   http://www.yahoo.com/Science/Biology/
                                           Molecular_Biology/Genetics/Human_Genetics/

- Bibliography/Information

Note: In addition to MEDLINE, and CANCERLIT, these sources focus on references in genetics. OMIM is an encyclopedic source of data on clinical genetic syndromes.

OMIM: On-line Mendelian Inheritance in Man
(on-line classic textbook, updated)   http://www3.ncbi.nlm.nih.gov/Omim/

Journal Links: Rockefeller University
(current contents and abstracts)   http://linkage.rockefeller.edu/outside/journals.html

Classic papers in Genetics
(texts in Adobe Acrobat format)   http://www.gdb.org/rjr/history.html

Healthfinder: Government guide
to health-related sites   http://www.healthfinder.gov

- Databases

Note: These are technical databases for use primarily by researchers; however, they can be used to check gene sequences and other data

ENTREZ: National Center for
Biotechnology Information   http://www3.ncbi.nlm.gov/Entrez/

GenBank:National Center for
Biotechnology Information   http://www.ncbi.nlm.nih.gov/Web/
                               Genbank/index.html

Genethon   http://www.genethon.fr/genethon_en.html

Genome Database:Johns Hopkins
University   http://gdbwww.gdb.org/gdb/

- Genealogy Sites

These databases are useful for locating specific individuals needed for clinical or research genetic studies, confirming date of death, or browsing federal, state, and other genealogy resources (see Cunningham J, Pillow P, Claffey J, Cunningham S. Overcoming faulty memory: using genealogic sources in epidemiologic research. Am J Epidemiol 145: S43.)

Genealogical Database Index of
all searchable Web databases   http:///www.genealogy.org

US Census Bureau general
information   http:///www.census.gov

US Gen Web project listing state,
national and international   http:///www.//www.usgenweb.com
resources

Ancestry genealogy search site for
US Social Security Death Data   http:///www.ancestry.com
Index, etc.

Cyndi's list of genealogy sites on
the internet (highly recommended   http:///www.oz.net/~cydihow/sites.htm
by experts)

Four 11 to search white pages
telephone directories and   http:///www.four11.com
government directories

Tables of Familial Risk Due to Breast, Ovarian, and Colon Cancer

Tables C-1 through C-9:

Claus EB, Risch N, Thompson WD. 1994. Autosomal dominant inheritance of early onset breast cancer: Implications for risk prediction. Cancer 73: 643–51.

Claus EB, Risch NR, Thompson WD. 1993. The calculation of breast cancer risk for women with a first degree family history of ovarian cancer. Breast Cancer Res and Treatment 28: 115–20.

Tables C-10 and Figures C-1, C-2, C-3 from:

Benichou J, Gail M, Mulvihill J. 1996. Graphs to estimate an individualized risk of breast cancer. Jour Clin Oncol 14: 103–10.

Figure C-4 from:

St. John DJB, McDermott FT, Hopper JL, et al. 1993. Cancer risk in relatives of patients with colorectal cancer. Ann Intern Med 118: 785–790.

Figure C-5 from:

Winawer SJ, Zauber AG, Gerdes H et al. 1996. Risk of colorectal cancer in families of people with adenomatous polyps. New Engl J Med 334: 82–7.

METHODOLOGY OF CONSTRUCTION

The empiric risk tables are taken from analyses of the Cancer and Steroid Hormone Study (The "Claus model") and from the Breast Cancer Detection and Demonstration Project (the "Gail model"), both described in Chapter 6. The colon cancer risk data are derived from the National Polyp Study. Additional empiric data for first degree relatives of those affected by colon cancer at various ages is presented in Table 6-3.

HOW TO USE THE "CLAUS" MODEL

Use the table appropriate for the family history and read the appropriate risks.

Example: A 39-year-old woman has a mother who developed breast cancer at age 46. Her mother's sister had breast cancer diagnosed at age 44. Looking at Table C-4, we find the column corresponding to maternal aunt's age of 40–49, under the section "age of mother 40–49." For the proband, her risk to age 79 is 33.8%. 4.6% of this risk occurs by age 39. [Note: Values in tables are multiplied by 100 to give the woman's % cumulative risk by ages shown in left-hand column.]

TABLE C-1   Predicted Cumulative Probability of Breast Cancer for a Woman Who Has One First-Degree Relative Affected with Breast Cancer, by Age of Onset of the Affected Relative

Age of Woman (yr)	First-Degree Relative with Age of Onset (yr)					
	20–29	*30–39*	*40–49*	*50–59*	*60–69*	*70–79*
29	.007	.005	.003	.002	.002	.001
39	.025	.017	.012	.008	.006	.005
49	.062	.044	.032	.023	.018	.015
59	.116	.086	.064	.049	.040	.035
69	.171	.130	.101	.082	.070	.062
79	.211	.165	.132	.110	.096	.088

TABLE C-2   Predicted Cumulative Probability of Breast Cancer for a Woman Who Has One Second-Degree Relative Affected with Breast Cancer, by Age of Onset of the Affected Relative

Age of Woman (yr)	Second-Degree Relative with Age of Onset (yr)					
	20–29	*30–39*	*40–49*	*50–59*	*60–69*	*70–79*
29	.004	.003	.002	.001	.001	.001
39	.014	.010	.007	.006	.005	.004
49	.035	.027	.021	.017	.017	.013
59	.070	.056	.045	.038	.038	.032
69	.110	.090	.076	.067	.067	.058
79	.142	.120	.104	.094	.094	.083

TABLE C-3 Predicted Cumulative Probability of Breast Cancer for a Woman Who Has Two First-Degree Relatives Affected with Breast Cancer, by Age of Onset of the Affected Relatives

	Age of Onset of First Relative (yr)										
	20–29						30–39				
	Age of Onset of Second Relative (yr)										
Age of Woman (yr)	20–29	30–39	40–49	50–59	60–69	70–79	30–39	40–49	50–59	60–69	70–79
29	.021	.020	.018	.016	.014	.012	.018	.016	.014	.012	.009
39	.069	.066	.061	.055	.048	.041	.062	.056	.048	.040	.032
49	.166	.157	.146	.133	.117	.099	.148	.134	.116	.096	.077
59	.295	.279	.261	.238	.210	.179	.265	.239	.209	.175	.143
69	.412	.391	.366	.335	.297	.256	.371	.337	.296	.251	.207
79	.484	.460	.434	.397	.354	.308	.437	.399	.353	.302	.252

	Age of Onset of First Relative (yr)								
	40–49				50–59			60–69		70–79
	Age of Onset of Second Relative (yr)								
Age of Woman (yr)	40–49	50–59	60–69	70–79	50–59	60–69	70–79	60–69	70–79	70–79
29	.014	.012	.009	.007	.009	.006	.005	.004	.003	.002
39	.048	.039	.030	.023	.030	.022	.016	.016	.012	.008
49	.117	.096	.075	.058	.075	.056	.042	.041	.030	.023
59	.210	.174	.139	.108	.138	.105	.081	.080	.061	.049
69	.298	.249	.202	.161	.200	.157	.124	.122	.098	.081
79	.354	.300	.246	.200	.245	.195	.158	.156	.128	.109

TABLE C-4 Predicted Cumulative Probability of Breast Cancer for a Woman Who Has Mother and Maternal Aunt Affected With Breast Cancer, by Age of Onset of the Affected Relatives

Age of Woman (yr)	Age of Onset of Mother (yr)											
	20–29						30–39					
	Age of Onset of Maternal Aunt (yr)											
	20–29	30–39	40–49	50–59	60–69	70–79	20–29	30–39	40–49	50–59	60–69	70–79
29	.019	.018	.017	0.16	.014	.012	.018	.017	.016	.014	.011	.009
39	.064	.062	.058	.054	.047	.040	.061	.058	.053	.046	.039	.031
49	.153	.148	.141	.129	.115	.098	.147	.139	.128	.112	.094	.076
59	.273	.265	.251	.232	.206	.178	.262	.249	.229	.203	.172	.140
69	.382	.371	.353	.327	.293	.254	.367	.350	.323	.287	.246	.204
79	.450	.437	.417	.388	.349	.305	.433	.414	.383	.343	.296	.248

Age of Onset of Mother (yr)

| | 40–49 | | | | | | | 50–59 | | | | | |
| Age of Woman (yr) | Age of Onset of Maternal Aunt (yr) | | | | | | | | | | | | |
	20–29	30–39	40–49	50–59	60–69	70–79	20–29	30–39	40–49	50–59	60–69	70–79
29	.017	.015	.013	.011	.009	.006	.015	.013	.011	.008	.006	.004
39	.057	.052	.046	.038	.030	.022	.051	.044	.036	.028	.021	.016
49	.137	.125	.110	.092	.073	.056	.122	.107	.089	.070	.053	.040
59	.245	.225	.199	.167	.134	.106	.220	.194	.162	.130	.101	.078
69	.344	.317	.282	.240	.196	.158	.311	.275	.233	.190	.151	.121
79	.407	.377	.338	.289	.239	.196	.369	.329	.281	.233	.188	.154

Age of Onset of Mother (yr)

| | 60–69 | | | | | | | 70–79 | | | | | |
| Age of Woman (yr) | Age of Onset of Maternal Aunt (yr) | | | | | | | | | | | | |
	20–29	30–39	40–49	50–59	60–69	70–79	20–29	30–39	40–49	50–59	60–69	70–79
29	.013	.010	.008	.006	.004	.003	.010	.008	.006	.004	.003	.002
39	.043	.035	.027	.020	.015	.011	.034	.026	.019	.014	.010	.008
49	.104	.086	.067	.051	.038	.029	.082	.065	.049	.036	.027	0.21
59	.187	.157	.125	.096	.075	.059	.151	.121	.093	.071	.056	.046
69	.267	.226	.183	.145	.116	.094	.218	.178	.141	.111	.090	.077
79	.320	.274	.225	.182	.148	.124	.264	.219	.177	.143	.120	.105

TABLE C-5 Predicted Cumulative Probability of Breast Cancer for a Woman Who Has Mother and Paternal Aunt Affected with Breast Cancer, by Age of Onset of the Affected Relatives

Age of Woman (yr)	Age of Onset of Mother (yr)											
	20–29						30–39					
	Age of Onset of Paternal Aunt (yr)											
	20–29	30–39	40–49	50–59	60–69	70–79	20–29	30–39	40–49	50–59	60–69	70–79
29	.010	.009	.008	.008	.007	.007	.008	.007	.006	.005	.005	.005
39	.033	.030	.028	.026	.025	.025	.026	.023	.021	.019	.018	.018
49	.080	.073	.068	.065	.063	.062	.064	.057	.052	.048	.046	.045
59	.148	.136	.127	.121	.117	.115	.119	.108	.097	.092	.089	.086
69	.214	.198	.186	.178	.173	.170	.176	.160	.148	.140	.134	.131
79	.260	.241	.228	.219	.214	.210	.257	.185	.180	.176	.170	.166

Age of Onset of Mother (yr)

Age of Woman (yr)	40–49						50–59					
	20–29	30–39	40–49	50–59	60–69	70–79	20–29	30–39	40–49	50–59	60–69	70–79
29	.006	.005	.004	.004	.004	.003	.005	.004	.003	.003	.002	.002
39	.021	.018	.016	.014	.013	.012	.018	.014	.012	.010	.009	.009
49	.053	.045	.040	.036	.034	.032	.045	.037	.032	.028	.026	.024
59	.100	.087	.078	.071	.068	.065	.087	.074	.064	.058	.054	.051
69	.150	.132	.120	.111	.106	.102	.132	.114	.101	.093	.087	.084
79	.216	.197	.154	.144	.138	.134	.187	.167	.152	.123	.116	.113

Age of Onset of Paternal Aunt (yr)

Age of Onset of Mother (yr)

Age of Woman (yr)	60–69						70–79					
	20–29	30–39	40–49	50–59	60–69	70–79	20–29	30–39	40–49	50–59	60–69	70–79
29	.004	.003	.003	.002	.002	.002	.004	.003	.002	.002	.001	.001
39	.016	.012	.010	.008	.007	.007	.015	.011	.009	.007	.006	.005
49	.041	.033	.027	.023	.021	.019	.038	.030	.024	.020	.018	.016
59	.079	.065	.055	.049	.042	.042	.074	.060	.050	.044	.039	.037
69	.121	.103	.090	.081	.076	.072	.116	.097	.083	.074	.068	.065
79	.168	.147	.132	.122	.103	.100	.148	.127	.112	.101	.095	.092

Age of Onset of Paternal Aunt (yr)

TABLE C-6 Predicted Cumulative Probability of Breast Cancer for a Woman Who Has One Maternal and One Paternal Second-Degree Relative Affected with Breast Cancer, by Age of Onset of the Affected Relatives

Age of Onset of First Relative (yr)

Age of Woman (yr)	20–29						30–39				
	Age of Onset of Second Relative (yr)										
	20–29	30–39	40–49	50–59	60–69	70–79	30–39	40–49	50–59	60–69	70–79
29	.007	.006	.005	.004	.004	.004	.005	.004	.003	.003	.003
39	.023	.020	.017	.016	.015	.014	.016	.014	.012	.011	.010
49	.057	.050	.044	.040	.038	.037	.042	.036	.032	.030	.029
59	.108	.095	.085	.079	.075	.073	.081	.071	.065	.061	.058
69	.160	.143	.130	.121	.116	.113	.124	.111	.102	.097	.094
79	.199	.179	.164	.155	.149	.145	.179	.144	.134	.128	.124

Age of Onset of First Relative (yr)

Age of Woman (yr)	40–49				50–59			60–69		70–79
	Age of Onset of Second Relative (yr)									
	40–49	50–59	60–69	70–79	50–59	60–69	70–79	60–69	70–79	70–79
29	.003	.003	.002	.002	.002	.002	.002	.002	.001	.001
39	.011	.010	.009	.008	.008	.007	.006	.006	.005	.005
49	.030	.026	.024	.023	.022	.020	.019	.018	.016	.015
59	.061	.055	.050	.048	.048	.044	.041	.039	.037	.034
69	.098	.089	.083	.080	.080	.074	.071	.068	.065	.062
79	.128	.118	.112	.108	.108	.102	.098	.095	.091	.087

TABLE C-7 Predicted Cumulative Probability of Breast Cancer for a Woman Who Has Two Second-Degree Relatives (Both Maternal or Both Paternal) Affected with Breast Cancer, by Age of Onset of the Affected Relatives

	Age of Onset of First Relative (yr)										
	20–29						30–39				
Age of Woman (yr)	Age of Onset of Second Relative (yr)										
	20–29	30–39	40–49	50–59	60–69	70–79	30–39	40–49	50–59	60–69	70–79
29	.010	.009	.009	.008	.007	.006	.009	.008	.007	.006	.005
39	.033	.032	.030	.028	.025	.021	.030	.028	.025	.021	.017
49	.081	.079	.075	.069	.062	.054	.075	.069	.061	.052	.043
59	.149	.145	.138	.129	.116	.102	.138	.128	.115	.099	.084
69	.216	.210	.201	.188	.171	.152	.201	.188	.170	.149	.128
79	.262	.256	.245	.231	.211	.189	.245	.230	.200	.186	.162

	Age of Onset of First Relative (yr)									
	40–49				50–59			60–69		70–79
Age of Woman (yr)	Age of Onset of Second Relative (yr)									
	40–49	50–59	60–69	70–79	50–59	60–69	70–79	60–69	70–79	70–79
29	.007	.006	.005	.004	.005	.003	.003	.002	.002	.001
39	.024	.020	.016	.013	.016	.012	.010	.009	.007	.006
49	.061	.052	.042	.034	.052	.042	.033	.026	.020	.017
59	.114	.098	.082	.067	.081	.066	.054	.053	.044	.038
69	.169	.147	.124	.105	.124	.104	.088	.087	.075	.067
79	.209	.184	.159	.137	.158	.135	.117	.116	.103	.094

TABLE C-8   Predicted Cumulative Probability of Breast Cancer for a Woman Who Has One or Two First-Degree Relatives Affected with Ovarian Cancer

Age in Years of Woman	Number of First-Degree Relatives Affected with Ovarian Cancer	
	One	Two
29	.002	.011
39	.010	.037
49	.026	.090
59	.054	.164
69	.088	.236
79	.117	.285
89	.135	.308

TABLE C-9   Predicted Cumulative Probability of Breast Cancer for a Woman Who Has One First-Degree Relative Affected with Ovarian Cancer and One First-Degree Relative Affected with Breast Cancer, by Age at Onset of the Relative Affected with Breast Cancer

Age in Years of Woman	First-Degree Relative with Age at Onset of Breast Cancer between:						
	20–29	30–39	40–49	50–59	60–69	70–79	80–89
29	.017	.015	.013	.010	.007	.005	.004
39	.057	.050	.042	.034	.025	.019	.014
49	.136	.122	.103	.082	.063	.048	.036
59	.244	.219	.186	.151	.118	.091	.072
69	.343	.309	.266	.218	.174	.138	.112
79	.406	.367	.319	.265	.214	.174	.144
89	.434	.394	.344	.288	.236	.193	.163

HOW TO USE THE GAIL MODEL

First use Table C-10 to fill in relative risks for your patient. Multiply these together. Multiply by 1.82 if atypical hyperplasia is present. Go to appropriate graph for 30-year risk (Figure C-1) or 10-year risk (Figure C-2), and interpolate, if necessary, for the age of the patient. Check confidence intervals from Figure C-3.

Example: A 35-year-old woman whose mother was just diagnosed with breast cancer. Her first menstruation was age 12. She has had one biopsy, which showed atypical hyperplasia. She had her first birth (live-born) at age 31.

From Table C-10, the relative risks are:

age of menarche 12	1.10
one biopsy < age 50	1.70
> 30 at first live birth with one first-degree relative with breast cancer	2.83

The product of above = (1.1)(1.7)(2.83) = 5.29. Multiply this by 1.82 because of presence of atypical hyperplasia, getting (5.29)(1.82) = 9.6.

Next consult Figure C-1, panel E because of biopsy showing atypical hyperplasia. Read 9.6 from X-axis, and go up to midpoint between lines for ages 30 and 40. This corresponds to 27%, which is risk of developing breast cancer over next 30 years. Confidence intervals can be read from Figure C-3, looking at the brackets between the dashed lines at 27% (17%–41% confidence interval).

TABLE C-10 Relative Risks for Selected Risk Factors

Risk Factor		Relative Risk
A. Age at menarche, years		
≥ 14		1.00
12–13		1.10
< 12		1.21
B. No. of breast biopsies		
Age at counseling < 50 years		
0		1.00
1		1.70
≥ 2		2.88
Age at counseling ≥ 50 years		
0		1.00
1		1.27
≥ 2		1.62

	No. of first-degree relatives with breast cancer	
C. Age at first term live birth, years		
< 20	0	1.00
	1	2.61
	≥ 2	6.80
20–24	0	1.24
	1	2.68
	≥ 2	5.78
25–29 or nulliparous	0	1.55
	1	2.76
	≥ 2	4.91
≥ 30	0	1.93
	1	2.83
	≥ 2	4.17

Recommendations for use: Be sure the counselee does not have a single gene trait that predisposes to breast cancer. Select one number each from risk factor groups A, B, and C. Multiply the three numbers together to get the summary relative risk. If atypical hyperplasia is absent on all biopsies, multiply the summary relative risk by 0.93, then go to Fig C-1A, B, or C; if atypical hyperplasia is present, multiply by 1.82 and then go to Fig C-1E or F.

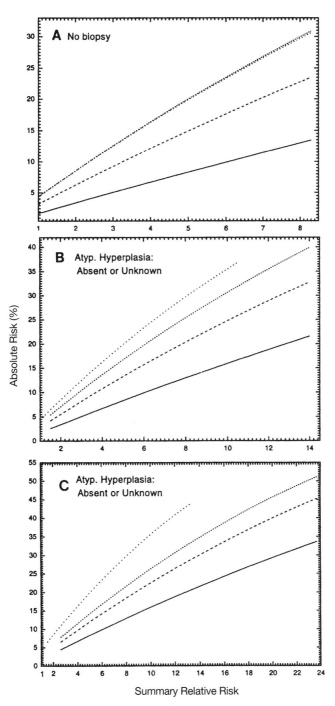

FIGURE C-1 Curves show absolute risk of developing breast cancer in 30 years for a white woman whose summary relative risk is estimated from Table C-10 and who intends to follow an annual screening program. Each panel has curves for four different ages at evaluation (50, · · ·; 40, - - -; 30, – – –; 20, ———). Different panels represent curves for no history of a breast biopsy (A and D) or a history of one biopsy (B and E), or of more than one (C and F); separate curves are used if (at least) one biopsy shows atypical hyperplasia (E and F), or *(continued on next page)*

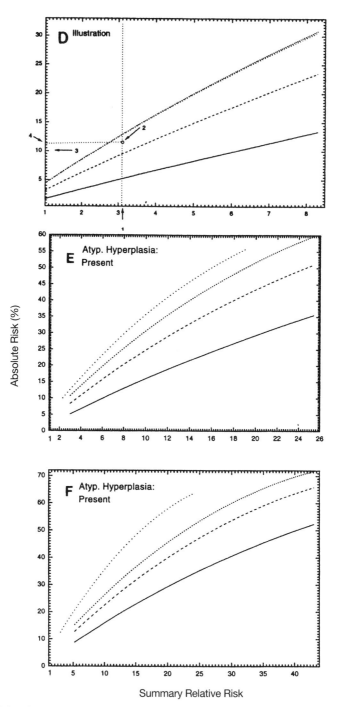

FIGURE C-1 *(continued)* all biopsies either show no atypical hyperplasia or have an unknown result (B and C). (D) The four steps in reading any panel. For a hypothetical woman (not the example in text): (1) the summary relative risk is first calculated from Table C-10 and located on the X-axis (e.g., 3.1), then (2) that number is projected to the specific age at evaluation curve, with linear interpolation between the flanking curves, if needed (e.g., age 35 years), then (3) that point is projected onto the Y-axis, where (4) the absolute risk can be read (e.g., 11).

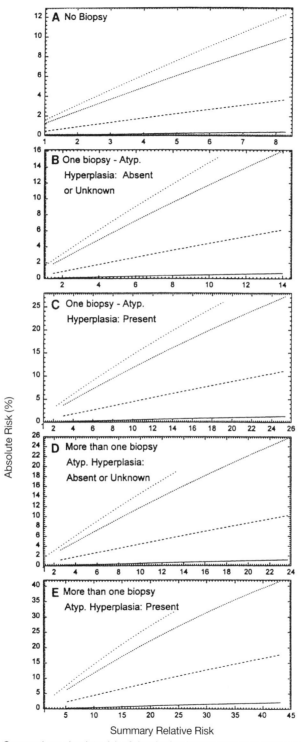

FIGURE C-2 Curves show absolute risk of developing breast cancer in 10 years (A to E) and 20 years (F to J) for a white woman whose summary relative risk is estimated from Table C-10 and who intends to follow an annual screening program. Each panel has curves for four different ages at evaluation (50, · · ·; 40 - - -; 30 – – –; 20, ———). Different panels *(continued on next page)*

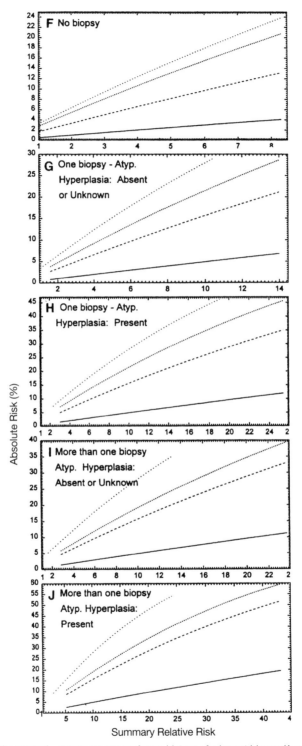

FIGURE C-2 *(continued)*   represent curves for no history of a breast biopsy (A and F) or a history of one biopsy (B, C, G, and H) or of more than one (D, E, I, and J); separate curves are used if (at least) one biopsy shows atypical hyperplasia (C, E, H, and J), or all biopsies either show no atypical hyperplasia or have an unknown result (B, D, G, and I).

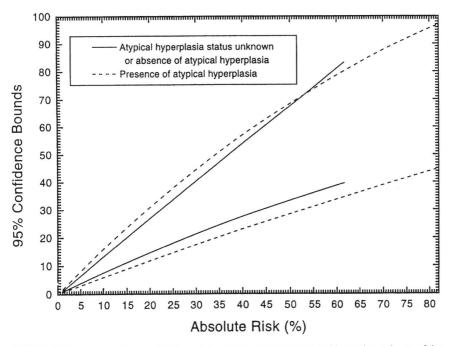

FIGURE C-3 Lower and upper 95% confidence bounds associated with a point estimate of the absolute risk (the Y-axes from Figs. C-1 and C-2) for two different conditions: when (at least) one biopsy shows atypical hyperplasia (- - -) and for all other biopsy results (no biopsy, all biopsies either without atypical hyperplasia or with an unknown result) (——).

HOW TO USE THE CUMULATIVE INCIDENCE FIGURES OF ST. JOHN ET AL., AND WINAWER ET AL.

Figure C-4 shows the cumulative incidence of colorectal cancer in first-degree relatives of patients, by age at diagnosis of the case. "CRC" mean colorectal cancer. For example, the brother of an individual who was diagnosed with colorectal cancer at age 50 would have a 5% risk of colorectal cancer by age 70.

Figure C-5 shows the cumulative incidence of colorectal cancer in siblings of patients with adenomas, according to the patients' ages at the time of diagnosis and whether a parent had had colorectal cancer. For example, the brother of a patient with adenomas at age 50 would have a 9% risk for colorectal cancer by age 60, if his parent had colorectal cancer. The risk falls to 2.5% by age 60 if his sibling had an adenoma at age 50 but there was no family history of colorectal cancer. In comparison, the risk of colorectal cancer in the general population (spouse controls) is about 1% by age 60.

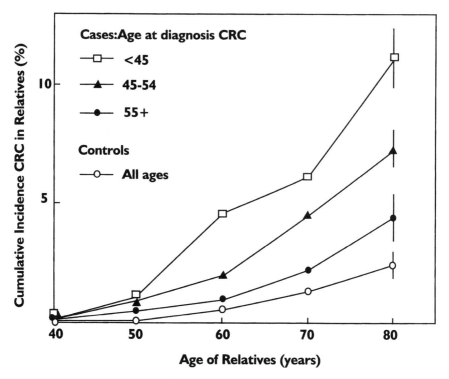

FIGURE C-4

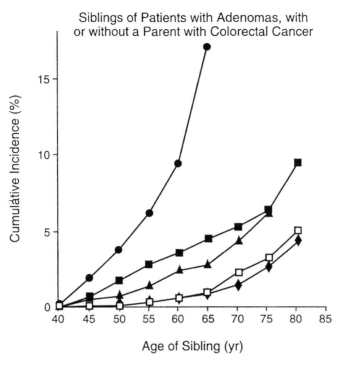

FIGURE C-5 Age of patient at diagnosis (yr) and parental history of colorectal cancer. ● <60, parent with colorectal cancer. ■ ≥60, parent with colorectal cancer. ▲ <60, no parent with colorectal cancer. ◆ ≥60, no parent with colorectal cancer. □ Spouse.

Index

About the Author

Kenneth Offit, M.D., M.P.H. is Chief of the Clinical Genetics Service in the Department of Human Genetics at Memorial Sloan-Kettering Cancer Center. He graduated from Princeton University and received an M.D. from Harvard Medical School and an M.P.H. from the Harvard School of Public Health. Dr. Offit is an Associate Professor of Medicine at the Cornell University Medical College and an Associate Member of the Memorial Sloan-Kettering Cancer Center. He has been active in research on the genetics of cancers of the breast and colon, as well as non-Hodgkin's lymphoma. His group identified the most common mutation predisposing to breast and ovarian cancer in Ashkenazi Jewish individuals. Dr. Offit is a member of the Cancer Genetics Working Group of the National Cancer Institute. He chaired the Subcommittee on Genetic Testing for Cancer Susceptibility of the American Society of Clinical Oncology.